D1359231

A MANUAL OF
LABORATORY DIAGNOSTIC TESTS

J. B. LIPPINCOTT COMPANY
PHILADELPHIA • TORONTO

A MANUAL OF
LABORATORY
DIAGNOSTIC
TESTS

☐
☐
☐
☐

FRANCES TALASKA FISCHBACH, R.N., B.S.N., M.S.N.

Assistant Professor in Health Restoration
University of Wisconsin–Milwaukee
School of Nursing
Milwaukee, Wisconsin

9 11 12 10 8

Library of Congress Cataloging in Publication Data

Fischbach, Frances Talaska.
  A manual of laboratory diagnostic tests.
  Bibliography:
  Includes index.
  1. Diagnosis, Laboratory—Handbooks, manuals, etc.
2. Diagnosis—Handbooks, manuals, etc. 3. Nursing.
I. Title.
RB37.F54   616.07′5   80-10163
ISBN 0-397-54242-9

The authors and publisher have exerted every effort to ensure that drug selection and dosage set forth in this text are in accord with current recommendations and practice at the time of publication. However, in view of ongoing research, changes in government regulations, and the constant flow of information relating to drug therapy and drug reactions, the reader is urged to check the package insert for each drug for any change in indications and dosage and for added warnings and precautions. This is particularly important when the recommended agent is a new or infrequently employed drug.

TO JACK AND FRANCES J.

PREFACE

A MANUAL OF LABORATORY DIAGNOSTIC TESTS is intended to be a quick reference for practitioners and a teaching-learning tool for students in a variety of health care areas: nursing, physical therapy, inhalation therapy, x-ray technology, medical technology, and others. The need for a book of this type became evident to me while working with nursing students, practicing nurses, and educators who were looking for a reliable, up-to-date resource in one volume.

My purpose in writing this book is twofold: First, I want to present current information on commonly ordered laboratory diagnostic tests; second, I hope to organize the data in a form that is orderly and easy to use and understand. There is an enormous quantity of information a health care practitioner could know about diagnostic tests. However, this book was written with the belief that the only valuable knowledge is knowledge that can be used. In our society, health care practice relies heavily on diagnostic testing. Health care professionals today are therefore expected to be thoroughly familiar with diagnostic tests and to be able to prepare patients for this testing.

A major feature of this book is its consistent format, with its resulting easy retrievability of information. Each chapter opens with an introduction that offers general information on the types of tests included and provides a background for the more specific details included with each individual test.

Every test description includes the same vital data organized into clearly identifiable sections: Normal Values, Background, Test Explanation, Procedure, Clinical Implications, Interfering Factors, Patient Preparation, and Patient Aftercare. Many tests also have a special feature, Clinical Alert, which highlights areas of concern that must be considered to assure patient safety and well being.

With the exception of the background description and the test explanation, tests are presented in outline form. This presentation enables readers to retrieve needed information quickly and easily; it also offers a quick comparison of related data in other tests. The background and explanation segments were written in a full-sentence format because the material lent itself more readily to this approach.

Each test includes carefully checked "Normal Values." The reader must bear in mind, however, that these values will vary from laboratory to laboratory, depending upon methods used. The section headed "Procedure" offers a list of the specific steps to be taken either in collecting the test specimen or in performing the test—whichever is more pertinent to the practitioner at the time. "Clinical Implications" includes the disorders or disease entities that cause either increases or decreases from the normal range. "Interfering Factors" offers a brief listing of any drug, food, condition, or activity that might alter the values, thereby giving false negative or false positive results. Any findings must be evaluated in relation to these factors, or the factor themselves must be avoided if possible.

Effort was made to provide information that can and should be used in the education of patients. "Patient Preparation" and "Patient Aftercare," in particular, suggest ways to make the patient more comfortable before and after a procedure and to acquaint the patient with adequate information about a given test. Each practitioner will decide how much or how little of this information will be given to the patient, depending upon the assessment of the patient's ability to understand, his or her desire for information, and his or her educational level. The practitioner will make this decision in collaboration with the patient and other health professionals involved in care.

The material for this book has been gathered and adapted from many sources. The organization of the material makes this book different from others available. Answers to four questions can be found in the discussion of each test: Why is the test ordered? What are the implications of an abnormal test result? How may the patient be prepared for the test? Is there any special information needed to administer the test?

The patient care plan cannot be implemented without the scientific knowledge about diagnostic tests and the facts that must be given to patients. We know that one of the most important professional functions is patient education. One area of patient education that has been most neglected is that concerning diagnostic testing. Many patients are fearful about the test, the procedure, and the outcome. Often they do not have a clear understanding of the reasons a test was ordered or the implications of an abnormal outcome. Most people want to know, and all patients have a right to know how they will be involved in diagnostic protocols.

In the appendices are tables of normal values with the common causes of alterations in values and tables of drugs which interfere with laboratory testing. The tables of normal values were compiled from the body of the manuscript. The tables of drug-induced modifications were compiled from the body of the manuscript and the most current reference available on this topic. These tables should be helpful to the reader for general reference; the drug table, especially, serves to emphasize the common interfering factor of drug usage on diagnostic testing.

If this book supplies the reader with the facts she or he needs and wants to know about diagnostic testing, if it helps to implement a better care plan and to give clear and accurate information to patients receiving diagnostic tests, then I will have succeeded in writing the kind of book that I set out to create.

Frances Talaska Fischbach
August 1979

ACKNOWLEDGEMENTS

I want to give special recognition to my research assistant, Timothy Philipp, for his dedicated work.

The following persons are acknowledged for providing information, encouragement, and help in manuscript preparation: Jeanne Ewens, Jack Fischbach, Michael Fischbach, Mary Fischbach, Paul Fischbach, Margaret Fischbach, Frances Talaska, Mary Bates, Dorothy Berns, Terry Denueve, Cathy Dodd, Marshal Dunning, Jane Fabian, Stuart Farber, M.D., Mary Lou Fischbach, Dorothy Fischbach, Gary Geis, Rasma Gilis, Ruth Gremminger, Jean Greve, Helen Hintz, Clara Hussing, M.D., Sister Juliana Kelly, Opal Kelly, Gordon Lang, M.D., Klay Lau, Robert Lipo, M.D., Beverly Luell, Barbara Maas, Peggy Margelowski, Randall Pollard, M.D., Carol Porth, Jeanne Salmon, Susan Saltzenheim, Mary Pat Schmidt, Carol Schuck, Lisa Sommers, Jean Sterzinger, Mary Sydel, and Raymond Zastrow, M.D.

I appreciate the help given by the staff of the laboratories, x-ray, and special diagnostic departments in Milwaukee, Wisconsin, of County General, Lutheran, Columbia, St. Mary's, St. Joseph's, Family, and Columbia Hospitals. I also appreciate the use of their manuals for reference.

Many special thanks are owed to Theresa M. Linietsky and Diana Intenzo for their painstaking editing and support during the preparation of the manuscript.

CONTENTS

1 □□ BLOOD STUDIES

INTRODUCTION

Composition

The average person has about five liters of blood (5 to 6 quarts) which may be separated into three liters of plasma and two liters of cells; the plasma is a liquid derived from the intestines and organs of the body, and the cells compose the solids formed mainly by the bone marrow. The normal adult's blood volume is estimated at one thirteenth of his total body weight.

The blood can be thought of as a tissue serving many functions. Without plasma, cells cannot circulate, and without cells, the vascular fluid alone cannot maintain life.

The cells are classified as white cells (leukocytes), red cells (erythrocytes), and platelets (thrombocytes); white cells are further divided into granulocytes, agranulocytes, and their related subclassifications:

A. Erythrocytes (red blood cells)
B. Leukocytes (white blood cells)
    1. Granulocytes (granular leukocytes)
        (a) Neutrophils
        (b) Eosinophils
        (c) Basophils
    2. Agranulocytes (agranular leukocytes)
        (a) Lymphocytes
        (b) Monocytes
C. Thrombocytes or Platelets

The cells vary in size with the white cells being the largest, the red cells next, and the platelets the smallest. Red cells greatly predominate; for every 500 red cells there are approximately 30 platelets and only one white cell.

Blood Disorders

Disorders of the red blood cells (RBC) are grouped into *anemias,* severe reductions in circulating red cells due to production and destruction disorders, and *polycythemias,* abnormal increases in circulating red cells.

Disorders of the leukocytes are termed either as *leukocytosis* (an increased number of cells) or *leukopenia* (a decreased number of cells). Since there are numerous types of white blood cells (WBC), variations in the counts of the different types of cells may reflect a wide range of disorders, including infection, leukemia, agranulocytosis, or granulocytopenia. Decreased counts of platelets or thrombocytes result in *thrombocytopenia*, which can become manifest in hemorrhage.

The production of red cells, platelets, and white cells is referred to as *hematopoiesis*, and occurs mainly in bone marrow. Under normal conditions, only mature cells enter the bloodstream from the bone marrow. In pathologic states, a variety of immature cells can be found in the circulating blood.

Therefore, examination of the blood and bone marrow constitutes the major means of determining certain types of blood disorders. The procedures involved in obtaining the specimens are peripheral blood smear, venipuncture, and bone marrow aspiration.

COLLECTION PROCEDURES

Peripheral Blood Smear

Capillary blood is preferred for a peripheral blood smear.
1. Capillary blood is obtained from:
    (a) The tip of a finger or earlobe in adults
    (b) The great toe or heel in infants.
    (c) The tip of the finger in infants over one year old.
2. Puncture site is washed with disinfectant (70 per cent alcohol) dried with sterile gauze, and skin is punctured no deeper than 2 mm. with a sterile disposable lancet. If betadine is used, it must be allowed to dry thoroughly to be effective.
3. First drop of blood is wiped away with sterile gauze and subsequent drops are collected in a microtube and slides.

CLINICAL ALERT
1. Avoid squeezing the extremity to obtain blood, because doing this will alter the composition of the blood.

2. If difficulty is encountered in obtaining blood:
   (a) Warm the extremity (warming the extremity must be done for all blood gases).
   (b) Allow the extremity to remain in a hanging position for some time.
3. Hematomas can be prevented by:
   (a) Using a clean needle stick.
   (b) Releasing tourniquet before blood is aspirated.
   (c) Applying sufficient pressure over puncture site after completion of the procedure.
Prolonged use of a tourniquet causes stasis of blood, produces hemoconcentration, and causes other changes that make the blood unsuitable for blood gases, blood count, blood pH, and some clotting.

Venipuncture

Venipuncture is a procedure necessary for most tests that require anticoagulation and large quantities of blood. It is the puncturing of a vein with a needle attached to a syringe.
1. Venous blood is usually obtained from the antecubital vein, although veins in other sites may be chosen. There is no variation in blood values if specimens are obtained from various veins.
2. A tourniquet is placed and tightened on the upper arm to cause venous congestion and prevent venous return.
   (a) Blood pressure cuff that is inflated to a level between systolic and diastolic pressure can be used as a tourniquet.
3. Patient is asked to make a fist and to open and close his hand several times.
4. The puncture site is cleansed with 70 per cent alcohol and dried with sterile gauze. If betadine is used, it must be allowed to dry thoroughly.
5. The vein is cleanly punctured with a sterile, 20 gauge 2.5 cm. (1 inch) needle, attached to a syringe. The level of the needle is pointed up.
6. After the vein is entered (blood appears in the syringe or tube), the tourniquet is loosened. If a syringe without a vacuum is used, apply *gentle* suction to obtain specimen. Excessive suction can collapse the vein.

7. Remove needle and apply sterile gauze with pressure to stop bleeding. Cover puncture site with an adhesive bandage.

CLINICAL ALERT
1. If oozing from the puncture site is difficult to stop, elevate area and apply a pressure dressing. Stay with the patient until bleeding stops.
2. Never draw blood for any laboratory test from the same extremity that is being used for I.V. medications, I.V. fluids, or blood.
3. In patients with leukemia, agranulocytosis, and in others with lowered resistance, the finger stick and ear lobe puncture are more likely to cause infection than venipuncture. If a capillary sample is necessary in these patients, the alcohol should remain in contact with the skin for at least seven to ten minutes.

If a betadine swab is used, the skin is scrubbed, allowed to dry (this can take up to two minutes), and then wiped off with alcohol and dried with sterile gauze.

BONE MARROW SMEAR

Normal Values

Rust red color, thick fluidlike consistency with visible amounts of fatty material and pale gray-white marrow fragments. (Bone marrow is that organ located within cancellous bone and in cavities of long bones).

Explanation of Test

A smear is obtained by aspiration or biopsy to see if the bone marrow is performing its function of manufacturing normal red and white cells and platelets. The developmental stages of the most immature cells to those ready to be released into the circulating blood can be seen.

Indications for Test

A bone marrow smear is of particular help in diagnosing (a) aplastic anemia, (b) pernicious anemia, (c) leukemia, (d) pur-

TABLE 1–1. QUANTITATIVE MARROW REPORT*

Formed Cell Elements	Normal (mean %)	Range (%)
Undifferentiated cells	0.0	0.0–1.0
Reticulum cells	0.4	0.0–1.3
Myeloblasts	2.0	0.3–5.0
Promyelocytes	5.0	1.0–8.0
Myelocytes		
Neutrophilic	12.0	5.0–19.0
Eosinophilic	1.5	0.5–3.0
Basophilic	0.3	0.0–0.5
Metamyelocytes		
Neutrophilic	25.6	17.5–33.7
Eosinophilic	0.4	0.0–1.1
Basophilic	0.0	0.0–0.2
Segmented granulocytes		
Neutrophilic	20.0	11.6–30.0
Eosinophilic	2.0	0.5–4.0
Basophilic	0.2	0.0–3.7
Monocytes	2.0	1.6–4.3
Lymphocytes	10.0	3.0–20.7
Megakaryocytes	0.4	0.0–3.0
Plasma cells	0.9	0.1–1.7
Erythroid series		
Pronormoblasts	0.5	0.2–4.2
Basophilic normoblasts	1.6	0.25–4.8
Polychromatic normoblasts	10.4	3.5–20.5
Orthochromatic normoblasts	6.4	3.0–25
Promegaloblasts	0	0
Basophilic megaloblasts	0	0
Polychromatic megaloblasts	0	0
Orthochromatic megaloblasts	0	0
Myeloid: erythroid ratio (M:E) ratio of WBC to nucleated RBC	3.0–4.1	6.1–2.1
Conclusion		

*From Platt, William R.: COLOR ATLAS AND TEXTBOOK OF HEMATOL-OGY. Philadelphia, J. B. Lippincott Co., 1969.

pura, (e) agranulocytosis, and is even more helpful in determining hematopoiesis. However, a bone marrow smear does not always provide specific or even relevant information, and is not diagnostically sufficient in and of itself. The presence or the suspicion of a blood disorder is not always an indication of the need to study the bone marrow. The decision to employ this procedure is made for each patient on the basis of the history, physical examination, and examination of his peripheral blood.

Procedure

1. Patient is positioned on his back or side according to site selected. The posterior iliac crest is the preferred site in all patients over the age of 12 to 18 months. Other sites include the anterior iliac crest, sternum, spinous vertebral processes T10 through L4 ribs, and tibia in children.

   The sternum usually is not used in children because the cavity is too shallow, danger of mediastinal and cardiac perforation is too great, and observation of procedure is associated with apprehension and lack of cooperation.
2. The area is shaved, if necessary, cleansed, and draped as for any minor surgical procedure.
3. A local anesthetic of procaine or lidocaine is injected. The infiltration of the medication is accompanied by pain from needle insertion and a burning sensation.
4. A short, rigid, sharp-pointed needle with stylet is introduced through the periosteum into the marrow cavity. The stylet is removed from the needle and 0.2 to 0.5 ml. of marrow fluid is aspirated.

   When the bone marrow is entered, a feeling of pressure is experienced. Moderate discomfort, which only lasts a few seconds, *may* be felt when aspiration is done, especially if the iliac crest is the chosen site. There is no way to prevent or lessen this discomfort.
5. After the needle is removed, pressure is applied to the site until any bleeding ceases and a small sterile dressing is applied to puncture site. Slides are usually smeared at the bedside.
6. Total procedure time is no more than five minutes.
7. Label specimen container with patient's name, date, and room number, and take it immediately to the laboratory.

Clinical Implications

1. A specific and diagnostic bone marrow picture is associated with many diseases. The report indicates the presence, absence, and ratio of cells which are characteristic of the suspected disease. However, bone marrow interpretation is a complicated task and requires considerable training and

experience. Only a highly trained hematologist can be expected to evaluate a marrow specimen accurately.
2. Bone marrow examination may reveal:
   (a) Leukemia
   (b) Deficiency states including vitamin B_{12}, folic acid, iron, and pyridoxine
   (c) Toxic states producing marrow depression or destruction
   (d) Neoplastic diseases in which the marrow is invaded by tumor cells.
3. Agranulocytosis (a decrease in the production of certain types of white cells) occurs when the bone marrow activity is severely depressed, usually due to radiation therapy and drugs used in cancer therapy. This means that the patient can be in danger of death due to overwhelming infection.

Patient Preparation

1. Instruct the patient about the procedure and purpose of the test.
2. Reassure the patient that many people are extremely fearful about this test, especially if they have had it done previously.
4. Advise the patient that analgesics or sedatives may be ordered.
3. If iliac crest is the site used, prepare patients for pain by having them hold onto a pillow and bite into it if pain is experienced.

Patient Aftercare

1. Observe for bleeding at puncture site, signs of shock, and continued pain, which may indicate fracture.
2. Recommend bed rest for 30 minutes; then normal activities may be resumed.
3. Administer analgesics or sedatives if necessary. Slight soreness over puncture site area for three to four days after procedure is normal and is no cause for alarm.

CLINICAL ALERT

1. Bone marrow aspiration is usually contraindicated in patients with hemophilia and other bleeding dyscrasias. However, the importance of further information that could be obtained by this method should be weighed against the risks.
2. Complications include bleeding and sternal fractures. Osteomyelitis and death due to injury to heart or great vessels are rare, but do occur.
3. Pressure over the puncture site will control excessive bleeding which sometimes occurs in patients with thrombocytopenia and other bleeding disorders.

COMPLETE BLOOD COUNT (CBC)

Explanation of Test

The CBC is a basic screening test in all patients and is one of the most frequently ordered laboratory procedures. The significant findings in the CBC give valuable information about the patient's diagnosis, prognosis, response to treatment, and recovery.

The complete blood count (CBC) consists of:
  White Blood Count (WBC)
  Differential white cell count (Diff)
  Red Blood Count (RBC)
  Hematocrit (Hct)
  Hemoglobin (Hgb)
  Red Blood Cell Indices
    Mean Corpuscular Volume (MCV)
    Mean Corpuscular Hemoglobin (MCH)
    Mean Corpuscular Hemoglobin Concentration (MCHC)
  Stained red cell examination (film or peripheral blood smear)
  Platelet count often included in CBC
These tests will be described in detail in following pages.

WHITE BLOOD CELL COUNT (WBC) (LEUKOCYTE COUNT)

Normal Values

5000–10,000/cu.mm.

Leukocyte Function

The main function of leukocytes is to fight infection, defend the body by phagocytosis against invasion by foreign organisms, and to produce, or at least transport and distribute, antibodies in the immune response. Behaving as separate yet related systems, the various types of leukocytes serve different functions. These functions will be discussed in detail in subsequent test descriptions.

Types of Leukocytes

Leukocytes, or white blood cells, are divided into two main groups: granulocytes and agranulocytes. These are further classified as follows:

Granulocytes		Agranulocytes	
Neutrophils	60–70%	Lymphocytes	20–40%
Eosinophils	1–4%	Monocytes	2–6%
Basophils	0.5–1%		

The granulocytes receive their name from the granules which are present in the cytoplasm of neutrophils, basophils, and eosinophils. However, each of these cells also contains a multi-lobed nucleus which accounts for their also being called *polymorphonuclear leukocytes.* In laboratory terminology, they are often called "polys (PMN's)."

The agranulocytes, which consist of the lymphocytes and monocytes, do not contain granules and have spherical nuclei; thus, the term *mononuclear leukocytes* is applied to these cells.

Leukocyte Formation

Since granulocytes and monocytes are formed in the red bone marrow, all of these cells can be considered myelogenous. The lymphocytes are formed in the lymphatic tissue which includes the spleen, thymus, and tonsils. After formation they are transported in the blood to the different regions, organs, or tissues of the body where they are needed. Vitamins, folic acid, and amino acids are used by the body in the formation of the leukocytes.

The endocrine system is an important regulator of the number of leukocytes in the blood. Hormones affect production of the leukocytes in the blood-forming organs, their storage and release from the tissue, and their disintegration. A local inflammatory process exerts a definite chemical effect on the mobilization of the leukocytes.

The life span of leukocytes varies from 13 to 20 days, after which the cells are destroyed in the lymphatic system, many being excreted from the body in fecal matter.

Granulocyte Development

Granulocytes develop through the following progression:
1. Myeloblasts (immature cells normally found in bone marrow) increased numbers found in granulocytic leukemia
2. Promyelocytes (immature cells normally can be found in blood in granulocytic [myelocytic] leukemia)
3. Myelocytes (found in the bone marrow)
4. Metamyelocytes (cells found in granulocytic [myelocytic] leukemia or severe infection)
5. "Bands" (applies to neutrophils in early stages of maturity; increased numbers found in blood when leukocyte count is elevated)
6. "Polys" (mature cells sometimes referred to as "segs")

Staining Properties

Neutrophils, basophils, and eosinophils are distinguished from one another by the staining properties of the granules in their cytoplasm.
　Neutral staining reaction: Neutrophils
　Acid stain reaction: Eosinophils
　Basic stain reaction: Basophils

Agranulocyte Development

Agranulocytes develop through the following progression:

Lymphocytes
1. Lymphoblast (immature cell found in lymphocytic leukemia)
2. Prolymphocyte (immature cell found in lymphocytic leukemia)
3. Lymphocyte (mature cell)

Monocytes
1. Monoblasts
2. Promonocyte (immature cells seen in monocytic leukemia)
3. Monocyte (mature cell)

Explanation of Test

Measurement of the total number of circulating leukocytes is an important procedure in the diagnosis and prognosis of the disease process, because specific patterns of leukocyte response can be expected in different types of diseases. It is known that certain diseases are accompanied by a specific type of white blood cell increase or decrease that is proportional to the severity of the signs and symptoms of the disease.

Since leukocytes are affected by so many diseases, the leukocyte count serves as a useful guide to the severity of the disease process. The differential count (count of the numbers of different types of leukocytes; see page 17) will identify certain persons with increased susceptibility to infection.

Leukocytes and differential counts by themselves are of little value as aids to diagnosis unless the results are related to the *clinical condition of the patient;* only then is a correct and useful interpretation possible. Serial examinations have diagnostic and prognostic value. Disorders of the WBC are often associated with changes in the red blood and platelet counts. The stained red cell examination is done with the differential count. The same blood slide is examined to detect variations in structure, size, shape, color, and content of the red blood cells.

Procedure

1. A venous blood sample of seven ml. or a finger stick sample is obtained.
2. Record time specimen is obtained (*e.g.,* 7:00 A.M.)

Clinical Implications

A. *Leukocytosis* (an increase of white blood cells above 10,000 per cu. mm.)
   1. Leukocytosis of 20,000 is considered slight;
      up to 30,000 is moderate;
      up to 50,000 is high.
   2. Leukocytosis is usually due to an increase of only *one* type of white cell and is given the name of the type of cell which shows the main increase:
      (a) Neutrophilic leukocytosis or neutrophilia
      (b) Lymphocytic leukocytosis or lymphocytosis
      (c) Eosinophilic leukocytosis or eosinophilia
      (d) Monocytic leukocytosis or monocytosis
      (e) Basophilic leukocytosis or basophilia
      An increase in circulating leukocytes is rarely due to a proportional increase in leukocytes of all types. When it occurs it is usually due to hemoconcentration.
   3. In certain diseases (such as measles, pertussis and sepsis), the increase of leukocytes is so great that the blood picture suggests leukemia. *Leukocytosis of a temporary nature is distinguised from leukemia, in which the leukocytosis is permanent and progressive.* The absence of anemia helps to distinguish severe infections from leukemia.
   4. Leukocytosis occurs in acute infections in which the degree of increase of white cells depends upon:
      (a) The severity of the infection
      (b) The patient's resistance
      (c) Patient's age
      (d) Marrow efficiency and reserve
   5. Other causes of leukocytosis include:
      (a) Hemorrhage
      (b) Trauma or tissue injury as occurs in surgery
      (c) Malignant disease, especially of the GI tract, liver, bone, and metastasis
      (d) Toxins as uremia, coma, eclampsia
      (e) Drugs, especially ether, chloroform, quinine, adrenalin
      (f) Serum sickness
      (g) Circulatory disease
      (h) Tissue necrosis

(i) Leukemia (in acute leukemia there is an increase in the total WBC with a decrease in normal appearing cells.)

6. Occasionally leukocytosis is found when there is no evidence of clinical disease. Such a finding suggests the presence of occult disease.

7. Steroid therapy modifies the leukocyte response.
    (a) When ACTH is given to a healthy person, leukocytosis occurs.
    (b) When ACTH is given to a patient with severe infection, the infection can spread rapidly without producing the expected leukocytosis; thus what would normally be an important sign is obscured.

B. *Leukopenia* (a decrease of white blood cells below 4000) Occurs during and following:

1. Viral infections
2. Hypersplenism
3. Bone marrow depression due to:
    (a.) Drugs
        (1.) Antimetabolites
        (2.) Barbiturates
        (3.) Benzine
        (4.) Antibiotics
        (5.) Antihistamine
        (6.) Anticonvulsives
        (7.) Antithyroid drugs
        (8.) Arsenicals
        (9.) Cancer chemotherapy causes a decrease in leukocytes (leukocyte count is used as a link to disease).
    (b.) Heavy metals
    (c.) Radiation
    (d.) Agranulocytosis
    (e.) Acute leukemia
    (f.) Pernicious and aplastic anemia
    (g.) Multiple myeloma
    (h.) Alcoholism
    (i.) Diabetes

Note: Alcoholism and diabetes tend to decrease mobilization of leukocytes; this may contribute to increased susceptibility to pneumonia and other infections.

CLINICAL ALERT

Agranulocytosis (marked neutropenia and leukopenia) is extremely dangerous and is often fatal because the body is unprotected against invading agents. Without treatment, death usually occurs three to six days after agranulocytosis appears. Patients who exhibit this disorder must be protected from infection by means of reverse isolation techniques with strictest emphasis on hand washing technique.

Interfering Factors

1. Hourly rhythm: There is an early morning low level and late afternoon high peak.
2. Age: In newborns and infants the count is high (10,000–20,000) and gradually decreases in children until the adult values are reached at about age 21.
3. Food, exercise, emotions: Eating, moderate physical activity, emotional upheaval, and pain will cause a slight increase in values.
4. Phase of reproductive cycle: Menstruation, last month of pregnancy, and obstetrical labor will cause an increase in values.
5. Stress: Fever, convulsions, anesthesia, paroxysmal tachycardia, following severe electric shock, and prolonged cold baths will cause an increase in values.
7. Chronic leukemic: Count may be falsely low in chronic lymphatic leukemia due to increased fragility of the cells.
8. Drugs: There are many drugs which can cause increased or decreased numbers of leukocytes. See appendix for complete listing.

DIFFERENTIAL WHITE BLOOD CELL COUNT (DIFF) (DIFFERENTIAL LEUKOCYTE COUNT)

Normal Values	Relative Values	Absolute Values
Neutrophils	60–70% (56% average)	(No. per cu. mm.)
Eosinophils	1–4% (2.7% average)	3,000–7,000
Basophils	0.5–1% (0.3% average)	50–400
Lymphocytes	20–40% (34% average)	25–100
Monocytes	2–6%	1,000–4,000
		100–600

Explanation of Test

The total leukocyte count of the circulating white blood cells is differentiated according to the five types of leukocyte cells, each of which performs a specific function.

Cell	Cause
Neutrophils	Bacterial infections, inflammatory disorders, stress, certain drugs
Eosinophils	Allergic disorders and parasitic infestations
Basophils	Blood dyscrasias and myeloproliferative diseases
Lymphocytes	Viral infections (measles, rubella, chicken pox, bacterial infections, infectious diseases)
Monocytes	Severe infections when the infection is becoming controlled

The differential count is expressed as a percentage of the total number of white cells. The distribution of the number and type of cells and the degree of increase or decrease is diagnostically significant.

The differential count expressed in per cent is the *relative* number of each type of leukocyte in the blood. The absolute number of each type of leukocyte is obtained mathematically by multiplying the percentile value of one type of leukocyte by the total leukocyte count.

Formula

$$\begin{array}{ccccc} \text{Absolute value} & & \text{Relative value} & & \text{Total WBC count} \\ \text{WBC/cu. mm.} & = & (\%) & \times & \text{(cells/cu. mm.)} \end{array}$$

The differential count alone has a limited value; it must always be interpreted in relation to the total leukocyte count. The reason for this interpretation can be explained in the following way: If the percentage of one type of cell is increased, it can be inferred that cells of that type are relatively more numerous than normal, but it is not known if this reflects an absolute decrease in cells of another type or an actual absolute increase in the number of cells that are relatively increased. On the other hand, if the relative percentile values of the differential are known and if the total leukocyte count is known, it is possible to calculate absolute values that are not subject to misinterpretation.

SEGMENTED NEUTROPHILS (POLYMORPHONUCLEAR NEUTROPHILS, PMN, OR "SEGS" OR "POLYS")

Normal Values

50–60% of total white cell count
3000–7000 per cu. mm.
0–3% of the total count of stabs or band cells

Background

The neutrophils are the most numerous and most important type of white cells in the body's reaction to inflammation. They constitute a primary defense against microbial invasion through the process of phagocytosis. These cells can also cause some damage to body tissue by their release of enzymes and endogenous pyrogens.

In their immature stage of development they are referred to as "stab" or "band" cells. The term "band" stems from the appearance of the nucleus which has not assumed the lobed shape type of the mature cell.

Clinical Implications

A. *Neutrophilia* (neutrophilic leukocytosis, increased percentage of circulating neutrophils)
   1. Causes of neutrophilia
      (a) Systemic and localized infections
      (b) Tissue or cell damage
      (c) Metabolic or drug intoxication
   2. Conditions causing neutrophilia
      (a) Bacterial and parasitic infections
      (b) Metabolic disturbances such as diabetic and uremic coma, gout, and eclampsia
      (c) Blood disorders such as hemorrhage, granulocytic leukemia, myeloproliferative disorders

(d) Hemolysis

(e) Drugs such as digitalis, mercury, ACTH, sulfonamides, arsenicals, potassium chlorate, benzene, venoms

(f) Tissue breakdown as in burns, myocardial infarction, tumors, gangrene, pus formation, hemolytic transfusion reactions, after surgery, cancer of liver, G.I. tract, and bone marrow

(g) Allergies

B. *Comparison between Neutrophilia and Total WBC*

1. Increase in percentage of neutrophils represents severity of infection. Total WBC indicates the patient's power of resistance.

2. If leukocyte count and percentage of neutrophils increase proportionately, there is a moderate infection with good resisting power by the patient.

3. If the neutrophil count is increased to a notably greater extent than the total count, no matter how low the count, there is either a lost resistance or severe infection.

4. In general, the degree of neutrophilia is proportionate to the amount of tissue involved in the inflammation. The neutrophilic-promoting substances are probably derived from necrotic cells.

5. The more the body is able to localize the infection, the more localized is the process and the more pronounced is the neutrophilia.

C. *Stab or Band Cells*

1. Any stimulus that causes an increase in neutrophils also causes early and immature neutrophils to be released into the blood.

An increase in these cells is known as a "shift to the left" and is an indication of a regenerative response.

2. Conditions causing an increase in percentage of stabs or band cells:

(a) Infectious states

(b) Chemotherapeutic drugs

(c) Disorders of cell production characterized by rapid proliferation of leukocytes such as leukemia.

    3. There are instances when the presence of early and immature neutrophils is the only indication that infection is present.

        (a) In elderly persons or in instances when the infection is overwhelming, there can be an increase in immature neutrophils with little or no leukocytosis.

        (b) On the other hand, absence of severe infection indicates a poor prognosis.

    4. In pernicious anemia and chronic morphine addiction, only adult or mature hypersegmented neutrophils are associated with increased neutrophils.

        An increase in mature cells is known as a "shift to the right."

D. *Neutropenia* (a decreased percentage of neutrophils)

    1. Neutropenia most often is due to defects in production so that an adequate input of the cells to the blood cannot be achieved. The cells disappear rapidly from the circulation.

    2. Conditions causing neutropenia

        (a) Acute viral infections such as influenza, infectious hepatitis, measles, mumps, poliomyelitis

        (b) Blood diseases such as aplastic and pernicious anemia and agranulocytosis and acute lymphoblastic leukemia.

        (c) Toxic agents such as Addison's disease, thyrotoxicosis, and acromegaly.

        (d) Hormonal diseases such as Addison's disease, thyrotoxicosis, and acromegaly.

    3. Neutropenia, instead of an expected neutrophila, may occur in massive infections, especially in debilitated patients.

        A neutropenia of less than 500 increases a patient's susceptibility to bacterial infections dramatically. If this occurs, institute necessary measures to protect the patient.

Interfering Factors

1. Age

    (a) Children respond to infection with a greater degree of neutrophilic leukocytosis than adults.

(b) Some elderly patients respond weakly or not at all, even when the infection is severe.

2. Resistance
   (a) People of any age who are weak and debilitated may fail to respond with a significant neutrophilia.
   (b) When an infection becomes overwhelming, the patient's resistance is exhausted and as death approaches, the number of neutrophils decreases greatly.

3. Steroids
   Tissue resistance is weakened when ACTH is given to a person suffering from a severe infection, so that the expected neutrophilia does not occur.

4. Patients treated with myelosuppresive chemotherapy

5. Dependent upon marrow efficiency and reserve.

EOSINOPHILS

Normal Values

1–4% of total leukocyte count (relative value)
   or
50–250/cu. mm.

Background

Although their exact function is unknown, eosinophils are polymorphonuclear granulocytes that may play a role in the breakdown of protein material. It is known, however, that the eosinophil response is produced by allergies, foreign proteins, and protein breakdown products, and that they are inflammatory exudates. Moreover, there is experimental evidence suggesting that the eosinophil plays a specialized role in phagocytizing antigen-antibody complexes.

Explanation of Test

1. Used to diagnose allergic infections, and infestations with worms and other large parasites severity, and the response to treatment.

2. Also the basis for the Thorn Test, which is used to evaluate the adrenal response to ACTH (see page 23)

Procedure

1. Note the time the blood sample is obtained (*e.g.*, 3:00 P.M.).
2. If the count is done separately, a blood sample of seven ml. is obtained.

Clinical Implications

A. Eosinophilia—an increase of circulating eosinophils greater than 5 per cent or more than 500.
    1. Causes
        (a) As response to hyperimmune, allergic, and degenerative reactions.
        (b) There is a relative and absolute increase in eosinophils in association with antigen-antibody reactions.
            (1.) Allergies
            (2.) Parasitic disease such as trichinosis
            (3.) Addison's disease
            (4.) Lung and bone cancer
            (5.) Chronic skin infections such as psoriasis, pemphigus, and scabies
            (6.) Myelogenous leukemia
            (7.) Hodgkin's disease
            (8.) Polycythemia
            (9.) Subacute infections
            (10.) Familial eosinophilia (rare)
            (11.) Polyarteritis nodosa
            (12.) Many tumors

B. Eosinopenia—a decrease in the amount of circulating eosinophils
    1. Usually due to an increased adrenal steroid production that accompanies most conditions of bodily stress.
    2. Decrease associated with:
        (a) Infectious mononucleosis
        (b) Hypersplenism
        (c) Congestive heart failure
        (d) Cushing's syndrome
        (e) Aplastic and pernicious anemia
        (f) Use of certain drugs—ACTH, epinephrine, and thyroxin
        (g) Infections with neutrophilia

3. Eosinophils disappear early in pyogenic infections when there is a leukocytosis with a marked shift to the left (increase in immature white cells).

C. *Eosinophilic myelocytes*

In the differential count, all the eosinophils are placed in one group, except the eosinophilic myelocytes which are counted separately because they have a greater significance, being found only in leukemia or leukemoid blood pictures.

Interfering Factors

1. Hourly rhythm
   (a) The normal eosinophil count is lowest in the morning, then rises from noon until after midnight.
   (b) For this reason, serial eosinophil counts should be repeated at the same time in the afternoon each day.
2. Stress
   Stressful situations, such as in burns, postoperative states, lupus erythematosis, electroshock, eclampsia, and labor will cause a decreased count.
3. Steroid therapy
   (a) Eosinophilia can be masked by steroid use; infections can be fatal.
   (b) It is not clear why eosinophils disappear promptly from the blood following injection of ACTH.

THORN ACTH TEST

Background

Administration of ACTH produces in 4 hours a decrease of 50 per cent or more in the eosinophil count in persons with a normally functioning adrenal cortex.

Explanation of Test

1. Useful in diagnosing Addison's disease as a test of adrenal cortex reserve before surgical procedures; and as a test to

distinguish functional hypopituitarism from organic disease of the adrenal cortex.

Procedure

1. No food, after 8 P.M.; only water allowed
2. A venous blood sample is drawn in the morning and an eosinophil count is done.
3. ACTH (25 mg.) is injected intramuscularly to stimulate the adrenal cortex. (Note the time: 8 A.M.)
4. Four hours later a second venous sample is obtained and eosinophil count is again obtained.

Clinical Implications

If adrenal cortex insufficiency is present, as in Addison's disease, the second eosinophil count will be decreased less than 20 per cent.

BASOPHILS

Normal Values

0.5–1.0% of the total leukocyte count
or
25–100/cu. mm.

Background

Basophils comprise a small percentage of the total leukocyte count—about 0.5 per cent. Their function is not clearly understood, although they are considered to be phagocytic and to contain heparin, histamines, and serotonin.

Explanation of Test

Basophil counts are used to study allergic reactions. There is a positive correlation between high basophil counts and high concentrations of blood histamines.

Clinical Implications

A. *Increased Count* (Basophilia)
1. Associated most commonly with granulocytic and basophilic leukemia and myeloid metaphasia.
2. Associated less commonly with:
   (a) Chronic inflammation
   (b) Polycythemia vera
   (c) Chronic hemolytic anemia
   (d) Following splenectomy
   (e) The healing phase of inflammation
   (f) Following radiation

B. *Decreased Count*
   Associated with:
   1. Acute allergic reactions
   2. Hyperthyroidism
   3. Stress reactions such as myocardial infarction and bleeding peptic ulcer
   4. Hypersensitivity reactions such as urticaria and anaphylactic shock
   5. Following prolonged steroid therapy

C. *Mast Cells*
   1. Also called tissue basophils, because like basophils they store and produce heparin, histamine, and serotonin.
   2. Normally never found in the peripheral blood and rarely seen in healthy bone marrow.
   3. Numbers of tissue mast cells are associated with:

(a.) Rheumatoid arthritis	(f.) Macroglobulinemia
(b.) Urticaria	(g.) Mast cell leukemia
(c.) Anaphylactic shock	(h.) Lymphoma invading
(d.) Hypoadrenalism	bone marrow
(e.) Lymphoma	(i.) Urticaria pigmentosa

MONOCYTES
(MONOMORPHONUCLEAR MONOCYTES)

Normal Values

2–6 of total leukocyte count relative value
or
100–600/cu. mm.

Background

These agranulocytes, the monomorphonuclear monocytes, are the body's second line of defense against infection and are the largest cells of normal blood. Through phagocytosis, these cells ingest microbes and very small cells. Histiocytes, which are large macrophagic phagocytes, are classified as monocytes in a differential leukocyte count. Histiocytes and monocytes are thought to be capable of reversible transformation from one to the other.

Phagocytic cells of varying size and mobility remove injured and dead cells, microorganisms, and insoluble particles from the circulatory blood. Monocytes escaping from the upper and lower respiratory tracts and the gastrointestinal and genitourinary organs perform a scavenger function, clearing the body of debris.

Monocytes are known to circulate in certain conditions in which their macrophagic properties act specifically—tuberculosis, leprosy, lipoid storage, disease and subacute bacterial endocarditis (infectious leukocytosis).

Procedure

A blood sample of seven ml. is obtained.

Clinical Implications

A. *Monocytosis* (increase in the number of monocytes)
1. By itself the monocyte count is not as diagnostically significant as other types of leukocytosis.
2. Conditions causing increase in monocytes:
    (a) Viral infections (infectious mononucleosis, chickenpox, mumps)
    (b) Bacterial and parasitic infections (subacute endocarditis, tuberculosis, Weil's disease, thyphoid fever, malaria, brucellosis, amebic dysentery, ulcerative colitis, regional enteritis.)
    (c) Collagen diseases
    (d) Hemotalogic disorders—myelocytic leukemia, lymphomas, and multiple myeloma

3. Phagocytic monocytes (macrophages) may be found in small numbers in the blood in many conditions:
   (a) Severe infections
   (b) Lupus erythematosus
   (c) Hemolytic anemias
   (d) Agranulocytosis
   (e) Thrombocytopenic purpura
   (Phagocytic cells are normally found in the bone marrow, not the blood. Examples of phagocytic cells: (1.) Farata cell—seen frequently in subacute bacterial endocarditis and (2.) Tart cell)

B. *Decreased Monocyte Count* (not usually identified with specific diseases)

RED BLOOD CELL COUNT (RBC)
(ERYTHROCYTE COUNT)

Normal Values

Men: 4.2–5.4 million/cu. mm. (average 4.8)
Women: 3.6–5.0 million/cu. mm. (average 4.3)
Values vary according to individual laboratory standards

Background

A. *Erythrocyte Function*
The main function of the red blood cell or erythrocyte is to carry oxygen from the lungs to the body tissue and to transfer carbon dioxide from the tissues to the lungs. This process is achieved by means of the *hemoglobin* in the red cells which combines easily with oxygen and carbon dioxide. The combination of hemoglobin and oxygen gives arterial blood a bright red appearance. Since venous blood has a low oxygen content it appears dark red.

To enable the maximum amount of hemoglobin to be utilized, the red cell is shaped like a biconcave disk which affords more surface area for the hemoglobin to combine with oxygen. The cell is also able to change its shape when necessary to allow for passage through the smaller capillaries.

B. *Erythrocyte Formation* (Erythropoiesis)

Red blood cells are formed in the red bone marrow and progress through the following stages of development:

Hemocytoblast (precursor of all blood cells)

Prorubricyte or basophil erythroblast (synthesis of hemoglobin begins)

Rubricyte (nucleus begins to shrink; more hemoglobin synthesizes)

Normoblast (nucleus starts to disintegrate and to be absorbed; more hemoglobin is synthesized)

Reticulocyte (as nucleus continues to be absorbed, remaining strands of the endoplasmic reticulum can still be noted)

Erythrocyte (mature red cell without nucleus or reticulum)

Normally the mature erythrocyte, without nucleus, is the major cell released into the circulation. Frequently, when the hematopoietic (blood-forming) system is faced with a heavy demand for red blood cell replacement (due to hemorrhage or disease), immature blood cells are released into the blood system. Such cells can be recognized by their structural components and their particular stage of development.

The mature erythrocyte, once released into the circulation, has a life span of about 120 days. When worn out, it is removed from the circulation by phagocytes in the spleen, liver, and red bone marrow (reticuloendothelial system).

Millions of red blood cells are destroyed daily, while millions are formed to replace them. It is estimated that about two million erythrocytes are produced per second. For the red blood count (RBC) to remain constant, about 1/120 of the total erythrocyte mass (approximately 35 trillion) must be replaced daily. To maintain health, the number of erythrocytes and the amount of hemoglobin they contain must remain fairly constant.

If the number of red cells in the blood is reduced, the bone marrow can increase its rate of production. The trigger of this increased production is the lack of oxygen in the body system which stimulates the production of erythropoietin, a hormone that in turn stimulates the production of red blood cells.

Explanation of Test

The RBC determines the total number of red blood cells or erythrocytes found in a cubic millimeter of blood. It is an important measurement in the determination of anemia or polycythemia.

Procedure

Automated electronic devices are generally used to determine the number of red blood cells.

Clinical Implications

A. *Decreased Values*
1. Anemias
Due to:
(a) Decreased red blood cell production
(b) Increased red blood cell destruction
(c) Blood loss
(d) Dietary insufficiency of iron and certain vitamins, especially B_6, B_{12}, and folic acid, which are essential in the production of erythrocytes.
2. Diseases of bone marrow function
(a) Hodgkin's disease
(b) Multiple myeloma
(c) Leukemia
3. Hemolytic and pernicious anemia
4. Lupus erythematosus
5. Addison's disease
6. Rheumatic fever
7. Subacute endocarditis
B. *Increased values*
1. Polycythemia vera
2. Secondary polycythemia
(seen in erythropoietin-secreting tumors, in renal disorders such as hypernephroma and renal cysts, and in cancer of the liver.)
3. Severe diarrhea

4. Dehydration
5. Acute poisoning
6. Pulmonary fibrosis
7. During and immediately following hemorrhage

Interfering Factors

Physiological Variation
1. Posture—When blood sample is obtained from a healthy person in a recumbent position, the count is lower than normal. (If the patient is anemic, the count will be even lower.)
2. Exercise—Extreme exercise and excitement produce higher counts than those obtained under basal conditions. Counts obtained under these conditions are of doubtful clinical value.
3. Dehydration—Hemoconcentration in dehydrated adults due to severe burns, untreated intestinal obstruction, and severe, persistent vomiting may obscure significant anemia.
4. Age—The normal RBC of a newborn is higher than that of an adult with a rapid drop to the lowest point in life at 2 to 4 months. The normal adult level is reached at age 14, maintained until old age, when there is a gradual drop.
5. Altitude—The higher the altitude, the greater the increase in RBC. Decreased oxygen content of the air stimulates the RBC to rise (erythrocytosis).
6. Pregnancy—There is a normal decrease in RBC when the body fluid increases in pregnancy with the normal number of erythrocytes becoming more diluted.
7. There are many drugs which may cause *reduced* RBC's. See appendix for complete listing.
8. Drugs which may cause *increased* RBC's include:
   (a.) Gentamicin
   (b.) Methyldopa

ANEMIAS

Background

Anemia, in general terms, is a decrease in the number of circulating erythrocytes, a decrease in hemoglobin concentration, or both hemoglobin being more important. Anemia may be suspected if there is a red blood count of less than 4.2 million/cu. mm. in males, and less than 3.6 million/cu. mm. in females. The hemoglobin might be less than 12 gm. in males, and less than 10.6 gm. in females. A combination of these deficiencies would also suggest anemia. The causes of anemia as well as its classification vary, depending on a variety of factors.

Causes of Anemia

1. Deficiencies in:
    (a) Dietary iron and absorption of iron
    (b) Vitamin B_{12}
    (c) Folic acid
2. Increased demand for iron during
    (a) Pregnancy
    (b) Growth periods
    (c) Blood regeneration
3. Disorders of the erythrocytes
4. Bone marrow damage or hyperactive spleen
5. Bleeding (iron loss)
    (a) From gastrointestinal tract (due to cancer)
    (b) From trauma

Etiologic Classification of Anemias*

A. *Anemias Due to Excessive Blood Loss*
    1. Acute posthemorrhagic anemia (normocytic, normochromic)
    2. Chronic posthemorrhagic anemia (normocytic, normochromic)
B. *Anemias Due to Deficient Red Cell Production*
    1. Deficiency of factors related to erythropoiesis
        (a) Iron-deficiency (iron-deficiency anemia)
        (b) Vitamin B_{12} and folic acid deficiencies
            (1.) Pernicious anemia
            (2.) Megaloblastic anemia (megaloblasts are large primitive erythrocytes)
    2. Anemias of bone marrow failure
        (a) Hypoplastic and aplastic anemias
        (b) Sideroblastic anemias

*Adapted from Berkow, Robert (ed.): *The Merck Manual of Diagnosis and Therapy.* 13th Ed., Rahway, N.J. Merck Sharp & Dohme Research Laboratory, 1977, pp. 258–259.

C. *Anemias Due to Excessive Red Cell Destruction* (Hemolytic Anemias)
  1. Hemolysis principally attributed to intrinsic erythrocyte defects
     (a) G 6PD
     (b) Hereditary spherocytosis (congenital spherocytic anemias)
  2. Hemolysis principally attributed to extra-erythrocyte factors
     (a) Trauma
     (b) Chemical agents or drugs (toxic hemolytic anemias)
     (c) Infections
     (d) Systemic disease
     (e) Autoimmune reactions
     (f) Paroxysmal hemoglobinopathies
D. *Anemias Due to Both Decreased Production and Increased Destruction of Red Cells*
  1. Defective hemoglobin synthesis
     (a) Hemoglobinopathies (sickle cell anemia and related disorders)
     (b) Thalassemias
  2. Anemias associated with chronic diseases (infection, cancer, rheumatoid arthritis)
  3. Anemia of renal disease
  4. Anemia of liver disease
  5. Anemia of myxedema
  6. Anemia due to bone marrow invasion (myelophthistic anemias)

HEMATOCRIT (HCT); PACKED CELL VOLUME (PCV)

Normal Values

  Men: 40–54/100 ml. (varies widely)
  Women: 37–47/100 ml.
Microhematocrit (done on small amount of blood, usually drawn from finger prick)

Men: 45–47
Women: 42–44
Infants: 44–62

Explanation of Test

The purpose of this test is to determine the relative volume of plasma, the total red blood cell mass (ratio of plasma to cells in the blood), and to roughly measure the concentration of erythrocytes. The word hematocrit means "to separate blood," which underscores the mechanism of the test, since the plasma and blood cells are separated by centrifusion.

The tube used in this test is the Wintrope tube, which is filled to a set mark with venous blood to which an anticoagulant has been added. The tube is then centrifuged to separate the cellular elements from the plasma. The height of the packed cells in the tube indicates the hematocrit. The measure is recorded in terms of the volume of cells found in 100 ml. of blood.

Procedure

A capillary blood stick is done, usually on the finger.

Clinical Implications

1. Increased Values
   Found in:
   - (a) Erythrocytosis
   - (b) Polycythemia
   - (c) Severe dehydration
   - (d) Shock, when the hemoconcentration rises considerably
2. Decreased values
   Found in:
   - (a) Anemia—an hematocrit of 30 or less means the patient is moderately to severely anemic.
   - (b) Leukemia
   - (c) Hyperthyroidism
   - (d) Cirrhosis
   - (e) Acute massive blood loss

(f) In hemolytic reaction due to:
  (1) Transfusion of incompatible blood
  (2) Reaction to chemicals or drugs
  (3) Reaction to infectious agent
  (4) Reaction to physical agent—severe burn and prosthetic heart valves

3. The hematocrit is unreliable immediately after even a moderate loss of blood and immediately after transfusions.

4. Hematocrit may be normal following acute hemorrhage. During the recovery phase, the hct and RBC will drop remarkably.

5. Usually the hematocrit parallels the RBC when the cells are of a normal size. As the number of normal sized erythrocytes increases so does the hematocrit.
  (a) However, for the patient with microcytic or macrocytic anemia, this relationship does not hold true.
  (b) If a patient has an iron deficiency anemia with small red cells, the hematocrit decreases because the microcytic cells pack to a smaller volume. *The RBC, however, may be normal.*

Interfering Factors

1. Normally, the value slightly decreased in the physiologic hydremia of pregnancy.

2. The normal value for infants is higher because the newborn has many macrocytic red cells.

3. There is a tendency toward lower values in men and women after age 50, corresponding to lower values for erythrocyte counts in this age group.

HEMOGLOBIN (Hgb)

Normal Values

Women: 12–15 gm./100 ml.
Men: 14–16.5 gm./100 ml.

Newborn: (both genders) 14–20 gm./100 ml.
Varies widely according to the standard used.

Background

Hemoglobin, the main component of erythrocytes, serves as the vehicle for the transportation of O_2 and CO_2. It is composed of (1) amino acids that form a single protein called globin, and (2) a compound called "heme," which contains iron atoms and the red pigment porphyrin. Each erythrocyte contains about 200 to 300 million molecules of hemoglobin.

The iron pigment is that portion of the hemoglobin which combines readily with oxygen and gives blood its characteristic red color. When hemoglobin carries its full complement of oxygen, the blood (arterial) is scarlet red; when it loses its oxygen, the blood (venous) turns dark red.

Each gram of hemoglobin can carry 1.34 ml. of oxygen. The oxygen-combining capacity of the blood is directly proportional to the hemoglobin concentration rather than to the red blood cell count (RBC) since some red cells contain more hemoglobin than others. This is why hemoglobin determinations are more important in the evaluation of anemia than the erythrocyte count (RBC).

The complex arrangement of the amino acids in the globin portion of the hemoglobin accounts for numerous types of hemoglobin which have been identified by hemoglobin electrophoresis. The normal forms of hemoglobin are referred to as A_1, A_2, and F (fetal hemoglobin). The most serious abnormal form is hemoglobin S which is associated with sickle cell anemia.

The heme portion of hemoglobin provides another method of classifying hemoglobin, which is based on the type of compound the heme forms. Examples include oxyhemoglobin, carboxyhemoglobin and methemoglobin (see page 58).

While oxygen transport is the main function of hemoglobin, it also serves as one of the primary buffer substances in the extracellular fluid and helps maintain acid-base balance by the process called chloride shift. Chloride moves or shifts in and out of the red blood cells according to the level of oxygen in the blood plasma. For each chloride ion which enters the red blood cell, a bicarbonate ion is released. Thus a hemoglobin measurement is important in determining acid-base balance.

Explanation of Test

The hemoglobin determination test is used to:
1. Screen for disease associated with anemia
2. Determine the severity of anemias
3. Follow the response to treatment for anemias
4. Aid in determining acid-base balance

Procedure

A venous blood sample of two ml. is obtained.

Clinical Implications

A. As an indication of anemia:
    1. It is difficult to say explicitly what hemoglobin level represents the presence of anemia per se, because of the variable adaptability and efficiency of the body in response to blood hemoglobin concentrations.
    2. An arbitrary level of 12 gm. is acceptable.
        (a) This level must be evaluated along with the erythrocyte count
        (b) If the erythrocytes are normal in size (normocytic) and contain normal amounts of hemoglobin (normochromic), the erythrocyte count and the hemoglobin concentrations give compatible information.
    3. The total amount of circulating hemoglobin is of greater physiologic importance than the number of erythrocytes because the symptoms of anemia are caused by an insufficient amount of circulating hemoglobin.
B. *Decreased Levels*
    Found in:
    1. Anemia states (especially iron-deficiency anemia)
    2. Hyperthyroidism

3. Cirrhosis of the liver
4. Severe hemorrhage
5. Hemolytic reactions due to:
   (a) Tranfusions of incompatible blood
   (b) Reactions to chemicals and drugs
   (c) Reactions to infectious agents
   (d) Reactions to physical agents (severe burns and artificial heart valves)
   (e) Accompanying a variety of systemic diseases:
      (1) Hodgkin's disease
      (2) Leukemia
      (3) Lymphoma
      (4) Systemic lupus erythematosus
      (5) Carcinomatosis
      (6) Sarcoidosis
      (7) Renal cortical necrosis
C. *Increased Levels*
   Found in:
   1. Hemoconcentration of the blood (any condition such as polycythemia and severe burns in which the number of circulating erythrocytes rises above normal)
   2. Chronic obstructive pulmonary disease
   3. Congestive heart failure
D. *Unreliable Levels*
   After transfusions, hemorrhages, burns
   (Hgb and Hct are both high during and immediately after hemorrhage)

Interfering Factors

1. People living at high altitudes will have increased values.
2. Excessive fluid intake will cause a decreased value.
3. Normally the value is higher in infants before active erythropoiesis begins.
4. Hemoglobin levels are normally decreased in pregnancy.
5. Drugs which may cause *increased* levels of hemoglobin include:
   (a) Gentamicin
   (b) Methyldopa
6. There are many drugs which may cause *decreased* levels of

hemoglobin. See appendix for a complete listing of the drugs.

RED BLOOD CELL INDICES; COLOR INDEX (C.I.)

Background

Red blood cell indices include the mean corpuscular volume, (MCV), the mean corpuscular hemoglobin (MCH), and the mean corpuscular hemoglobin concentration (MCHC), which are calculated from the RBC count, Hgb, and Hct. In most laboratories these percentages will be recorded on all hemoglobins and hematocrits (H & H). These tests are determined on the same blood sample used for hemoglobin, hematocrit, and RBC count.

Explanation of Test

The purpose of determining blood indices is to corroborate and correlate the fundamental results obtained in the routine complete blood count—the hematocrit, the red blood cell count, and the hemoglobin concentration. In this way, the types of anemia may be objectively classified, and the red blood cell variations may be specifically studied.

Results from the MCV, MCH, and MCHC require an accuracy of at least ± five per cent in red blood cell count, hemoglobin, and hematocrit determinations because it is essential to use accurate data to calculate these values. In addition, it is useful to compare the appearance of the red blood cell on the stained film with the calculated values and then compare the calculated values with each other. For example, very low values for MCH are inconsistent with macrocytosis.

On the basis of the red blood cell indices, the erythrocytes can be characterized as normal in every respect, or as abnormal in volume or hemoglobin contents. In deficient states the anemias can be classified by cell size as *macrocytic, normocytic, simple microcytic,* or by cell size and color as *microcytic hypochromic* (Table 1–2).

TABLE 1–2. MORPHOLOGIC CLASSIFICATION OF ANEMIAS

Type of Anemia	Blood Constants	
	MCV (μ)	MCHC (gm./100 ml.)
Microcytic hypochromic	60–87	20–30
Macrocytic normochromic	103–160	32–36
Normocytic normochromic	87–103	32–36
Microcytic normochromic	60–87	32–36

(From Bauer, John D., et al.: BRAY'S CLINICAL LABORATORY METHODS, 8th ed., St. Louis, The C. V. Mosby Company, 1974, p. 201.)

MEAN CORPUSCULAR VOLUME (MCV)

Normal Values

87–103 cu. μ
89±7 Basal adult values
(Higher values in infants and newborns)

Explanation of Test

This description of individual cell size is the best index for classifying anemias and is based on the visual or electronic counting of erythrocytes. It is an index that expresses the volume occupied by a single red cell and is a measure in cubic microns of the mean volume.

Normal values are modified by erythropoietin and iron supply.

Procedure

A venous sample of seven ml. is collected.

Clinical Implications

A. *Decreased Values*
   Found in:
   1. Iron-deficiency anemia
   2. Pernicious anemia
   3. Thalassemia

    4. Anemia of chronic blood loss

    5. Chlorasis

B. *Increased Values*

    Found in:

    1. Liver diseases

    2. Alcoholism

    3. Sprue

    4. Anti-metabolite therapy

    5. Deficiency of folate or vitamin B_{12}

    Microcytic anemia is characterized by a decrease in MCV (75 or less).

    Macrocytic anemia is characterized by an increase in MCV (115 or greater).

C. *Unreliable Values*

    1. It is possible to have a wide variation of cells (macrocytes and microcytes) in the blood smear and still have a normal MCV.

        (a) This may occur when there is a large number of reticulocytes in the blood (Reticulocytes usually have a larger volume than mature red cells).

        (b) Thus, MCV must be elevated in relation to the blood smear.

    2. In sickle cell anemia and other anemias characterized by abnormal erythrocyte shape, the MCV is of doubtful value because the hematocrit is not reliable in these diseases.

MEAN CORPUSCULAR HEMOGLOBIN CONCENTRATION (MCHC)

Normal Values

32–36 gm./100 ml. (of whole blood)

27–31 pg. (picograms of hemoglobin per red blood cells)

33 ± 3 Coulter counter 33 ± 2

Explanation of Test

This test is a measure of the concentration or proportion of hemoglobin in an average (mean) cell. For a given MCHC, the smaller the cell, the higher the concentration. The percentage represents grams of hemoglobin per 100 ml. of whole blood.

This test is most valuable in evaluating therapy for anemia because the two most accurate hematological determinations (hemoglobin and hematocrit, not RBC) are used in the test.

Procedure

A venous blood sample of seven ml. or a capillary blood sample is obtained.

Clinical Implications

A. *Decreased Values*
1. A decreased MCHC signifies that a unit volume of packed RBC's contains less hemoglobin than normal, or that hemoglobin has been replaced by erythrocytic stomal material as in:
   (a) Iron-deficiency
   (b) Macrocytic anemias
   (c) Pyridoxine responsive anemia
   (d) Thalassemia
2. Hypochromic anemia is characterized by a MCHC of 30 or less.

B. *Increased Values*
1. An increased MCHC usually indicates spherocytosis.
2. MCHC is *not* increased in pernicious anemia.

C. *Full Saturation*
Occurs at about 38 per cent (greater values are rarely observed).

MEAN CELL HEMOGLOBIN (MCH)

Normal Values

27–32 picograms (pg.) (Normally higher in newborns and infants)

Explanation of Test

This is a measure of the amount of weight of hemoglobin in a single red blood cell, regardless of size. This index is of value in diagnosing severely anemic patients, but it is not as useful as MCHC because the red cell count is not always accurate.

The MCH is expressed as micrograms or picograms of hemoglobin per red blood cell.

Procedure

A venous blood sample of seven ml. or a capillary blood sample is obtained.

Clinical Implications

1. An *increase* of the MCH is associated with macrocytic anemia.
2. A *decrease* of the MCH is associated with iron-deficiency anemia.

STAINED RED CELL EXAMINATION (FILM) (STAINED ERYTHROCYTE EXAMINATION)

Normal Values

Size
   Normocytic (normal size)
   Microcytic (smaller size)
   Macrocytic (larger size)
Color
   Normochromic (normal)
   Hypochromic (less color)
Shape
   Target cells (leptocytes) (thin and less hemoglobin)
   Spherocytes (small and round)
   Sickle cells (crescent or sickled)
   Schistocytes (fragmented, spiral or triangular)
Structure
   Normoblasts (immature cell with dissolving nucleus)
   Metarubricyte (nucleated erythrocyte)
   Megaloblast (large cell with nucleus)

Explanation of Test

The stained film examination furnishes the best means of studying the blood to determine variations and abnormalities in erythrocyte size, shape, structure, hemoglobin content, and staining properties. It is useful in diagnosing blood disorders such as anemia, thalassemia, and leukemia. This examination also serves as a guide to therapy and as an indicator of harmful effects of chemotherapy and radiation.

Procedure

A blood sample of seven ml. is collected.

Clinical Implications

A. *Variations in Staining, Color, and Red Cell Inclusion*
   Normally, the erythrocytes have a tendency to absorb acid stains. The depth of staining furnishes a rough guide to the amount of hemoglobin in the erythrocyte.
   1. *Normochromic cells* are those erythrocytes that are normal in hemoglobin content and color (central area is pale and stains pinkish orange).
   2. *Hypochromic Cells*
      (a) When the amount of hemoglobin is diminished, the central area which is normally pale and stains a pinkish-orange color, becomes larger and paler and stains a lighter color.
      (b) Hypochromic cells usually appear in most of the anemias and are an indication that the bone marrow is regenerating to meet the demand for circulatory cells in the blood.
   3. *Basophilic Stippling* (the inclusion variation that occurs most frequently)
      (a) This term refers to the bodies included or enclosed in the cell, such as granules, crystals, and pigments.
      (b) Basophilic stippling will appear in the stained film examination of every patient in which there are symptoms of *lead poisoning.*

(c) Except in lead poisoning, basophilic stippling indicates a serious blood disorder, usually related to excessive regeneration of erythrocytes or some impairment of hemoglobin synthesis. It is present in severe pernicious anemia, leukemia, and less commonly in other forms of anemia.

4. *Polychromatophilia*
   (a) Cells having a number of RBC's that do not take an acid stain, and instead stain with a basic stain to shades of blue.
   (b) Cells which stain in this manner are most numerous in acute blood loss anemia and hemolytic anemias.

5. *Malarial Stippling*
   (a) The term applied to the fine granular appearance of erythrocytes that harbor the parasites of tertiary malaria
   (b) The very fine granules, Schüffner's dots, which stain purplish red

6. *Other Inclusion Variations*
   (a) *Howell-Jolly bodies* (appear after removal of the spleen)
   (b) *Cabot rings* (indicate severe anemia)

B. *Variations in Size and Shape*
   1. *Normocytes* are cells that are normal in size and shape (biconcave disc).
   2. *Poikilocytosis* is the presence of erythrocytes showing abnormal variations and irregularities in shape.
      (a) The cause of abnormally shaped RBC's is defective cell formation, usually due to the presence of abnormal hemoglobins.
      (b) Erythrocytes that vary from the normal shape are present in most types of anemia, including severe anemia, and are numerous and most bizarre.
         Irregularities in shape are especially conspicuous in leukemia and pernicious anemia.
      (c) The abnormally shaped cells most commonly seen are:

(1.) *Target cells*
- (a.) These are erythrocytes that are thinner than normal with a small amount of hemoglobin in the center *(leptocytes)*.
- (b.) These cells are numerous in chronic anemias, liver disease, hemoglobin C disease, and thalassemia, also called hereditary leptocytosis.

(2.) *Spherocytes*
- (a.) These are erythrocytes that are a little smaller than normal and are round, rather than biconcave in shape.
- (b.) Their presence is associated with:
  1. Thalassemia major
  2. Hemoglobin C disease
  3. Congenital hemolytic anemia

(3.) *Sickle cells*
- (a.) These are erythrocytes that assume a crescent or sickle shape due to the presence of the abnormal hemoglobin, (Hgb S).
- (b.) They occur in the hemolytic anemias.

(4.) *Schistocytes*
- (a.) These are fragmented erythrocytes with extremely bizarre shapes (triangular or spiral).
- (b) They occur in the hemolytic anemias.

C. *Variations in Size*

Normal values: 7 to 8 microns

Anisocytosis

1. Term used to identify abnormal variations in size of erythrocytes.
2. Is due to abnormal cell development caused by
   - (a) Congenital structural defects
   - (b) Lack in folic acid

(c) Lack of vitamin B_{12} and iron

3. *Microcytes*
    (a) Abnormally small erythrocytes (6 microns)
    (b) Microcytosis is associated with:
        (1.) Iron-deficiency anemia
        (2.) Spherocytic anemia
        (3.) Thalassemia major

4. *Macrocytes*
    (a) Are abnormally large erythrocytes (9 microns)
    (b) Macrocytosis is associated with pernicious anemia and folic acid deficiency anemia. In pernicious anemia, anisocytosis is extremely pronounced with megalocytes present.
    (c) Cells of larger than normal size are normally seen in newborns.

CLINICAL ALERT
Marked abnormalities in size and shape of red blood cells without a known cause is an indication for more complete blood studies.

D. *Variations in Structure*
    Normal mature red blood cells are unique in that they do not have a nucleus. Normal immature cells are called *normoblasts*.
    1. *Nucleated red blood cells*
        (a) These are the variations in structure that are counted and reported as NRBC per 100 WBC.
        (b) *Metarubricyte* is another term for a nucleated erythrocyte.
        (c) The presence of NRBC's is an indication of a severe anemia and indicates that the body is making an excessive demand on the blood-forming organs to regenerate erythrocytes.
    2. *Megaloblasts*
        (a) These are distinct cells with a nucleus, not merely larger normoblasts.
        (b) These cells are not found in normal bone marrow.

(c) They are larger than normal cells, containing an increased amount of hemoglobin with a typical nucleus.

(d) The presence of megaloblasts indicates a change in the type of blood formation, as in pernicious anemia. Megalocytes are rarely found in any other condition.

OTHER ERYTHROCYTE TESTS

ERYTHROCYTE FRAGILITY (OSMOTIC FRAGILITY AND AUTOHEMOLYSIS)

Osmotic Fragility

Normal Values. Fragility: Hemolysis begins at 0.45–0.39% saline solution

Hemolysis ends at 0.33–0.30% saline solution

Background. Although destruction of red blood cells (hemolysis) occurs at a normal rate, a dramatic increase in the rate of destruction can result in anemia. It is important to know if the increased destruction is due to unusual fragility of the erythrocytes which makes them susceptible to easy damage, thereby shortening their life span.

Explanation of Test. Osmotic fragility is determined by exposing red cells to a hypotonic sodium chloride solution which causes water to enter the cell more rapidly than it leaves. As a result, the cell swells and at some point ruptures, causing the hemoglobin to disperse (hemolysis).

In the fragility test the red cells are exposed to a hypotonic solution of varying strength, ranging from 0.7 to 0.3 per cent. In each solution the cells will swell to some extent. The point at which hemolysis begins is noted along with the point at which it is completed. If the cells burst in relatively high salt concentrations, they are identified as having increased fragility. Those that burst in lower salt concentrations have decreased fragility.

Clinical Implications

A. Increased Fragility (>0.5 per cent) occurs in:
1. Hereditary spherocytosis
2. Hemolytic jaundice
3. Autoimmune anemia (ABO and RH) incompatibility
4. Chemical poisons
5. Burns

B. Decreased Fragility (< 0.3 per cent) occurs in:
1. Obstructive jaundice
2. Thalassemia
3. Sickle cell anemia
4. Iron-deficiency anemia
5. Polycythemia vera
6. Liver disease
7. Following splenectomy
8. 46-C disease

Decreased fragility indicates that red cells are excessively flat. Occurs in iron-deficiency anemia, thalassemia, and sickle cell disease.

Autohemolysis

Normal Values
0.4–4.5
0–0.7 glucose added
0–15 ATP added

Background. Autohemolysis is determined by measuring the amount of spontaneous hemolysis that will occur in blood over a 24 to 48 hour period under special laboratory conditions. Normal blood undergoes very little spontaneous hemolysis in the laboratory.

Explanation of Test. In the test, ATP (adenosine triphosphate) and glucose are added to blood which is incubated for 24 to 48 hours. The results are helpful in differentiating between hereditary spherocytosis and congenital nonspherocytic hemolytic anemia.

1. In hereditary spherocytosis there is a marked diminishing of hemolysis.
2. In congenital nonspherocytic hemolytic anemias, the hemolysis diminishes to a much less degree.

HEINZ-EHRLICH BODY STAIN (BEUTLER'S METHOD)

Normal Values

Negative in healthy individuals.

Explanation of Test

These tests are ordered to detect the presence of Heinz-Ehrlich bodies in the red blood cells. Heinz bodies are granules which contain precipitated denatured hemoglobin. Their presence is usually associated with hemolytic anemias and indicates some injury to the erythrocyte due to some type of oxidative activity that interferes with the normal functioning of hemoglobin, such as occurs in patients with glucose-6-phosphate dehydrogenase deficiency (G6PD).

G6PD is an enzyme that accounts for a small portion of glucose metabolized by erythrocytes. When red cells are exposed to an oxidative substance, greater amounts of glucose must be metabolized. A deficiency of G6PD will hamper the red cells' ability to metabolize the necessary additional glucose, and will result in hemolysis of the erythrocyte and formation of Heinz bodies.

Clinical Implications

1. G6PD deficiency is indicated if more than 40 per cent of the cells have 5 or more Heinz bodies. Affected individuals are often of Dutch, German, or French ancestry.
2. Heinz bodies are also found in splenectomized patients who

had unstable hemoglobin syndromes or thalassemia prior to surgery.
3. Heinz bodies are associated with acute hemolytic crisis and may be associated with methemoglobinemia.
4. Drugs related to hemolytic anemias.
   (a) 50 to 75 per cent of the erythrocytes may contain Heinz bodies in hemolytic anemias caused by drug poisoning.
   (b) These drugs have an oxidating activity that interferes with the normal functioning of hemoglobin in some individuals.
   (c) Drugs that cause this effect include:
       (1.) Drugs used in treatment of malaria
       (2.) Sulfonamides
       (3.) Antipyretics and analgesics
       (4.) Nitrofurans such as Furadantin and Furacin
       (5.) Phenolhydrazine
       (6.) Tolbutamide
       (7.) Large doses of vitamin K

ERYTHROCYTE SEDIMENTATION RATE (ESR)

Normal Values

Method		
Westegren	Men	0–15 mm./hr.
	Women	0–20 mm./hr.
	Children	0–10 mm./hr.
Cutler	Men	0–8 mm./hr.
	Women	0–10 mm./hr.
	Children	4–13 mm./hr.
Landon Adams	Men	0–6 mm./hr.
	Women	0–9 mm./hr.
	Children	0–20 age 4–11—12 mm./hr.
		age 12–15—7.5 mm./hr.

Wintrobe	Men	9.0 mm./hr.
	Women	0–15.0 mm./hr.
	Children	0–13.0 mm./hr.
Smith	Adults	0–10 mm./hr.

Explanation of Test

Erythrocyte sedimentation rate (ESR), is the rate at which erythrocytes settle out of unclotted blood in one hour. This test is based on the fact that inflammatory and necrotic processes cause an alteration in blood proteins, resulting in an aggregation of red cells, which make them heavier and more likely to fall rapidly when placed in a special vertical test tube. The faster the sedimentation rate or settling of cells, the higher the ESR (as indicated in the listing above, the range of normal values will differ depending on the method or type of tube used).

Sedimentation is due the surface changes of the erythrocytes which cause them to clump or aggregate together in a column-like manner (rouleau formation). These changes are related to alterations in the plasma, particularly in the physical state of the plasma proteins.

This test is useful in diagnosing occult disease, in differential diagnosis, and in following individual cases It is most often used as a gauge for determining the progress of an inflammatory disease, rheumatic fever, rheumatoid arthritis, respiratory infections, and acute myocardial infarction. It is a nonspecific test (not considered diagnostic for any particular disorder).

In many diseases the ESR rate is normal; in a variety of disease states the rate is rapid, and in some cases it is proportional to the severity of the disease. An abnormal rate indicates a pathologic state rather than a functional disturbance.

Procedure

A venous blood sample of seven ml. is obtained.

Clinical Implications

A. *Increased Values* found in:
1. All of the collagen diseases
2. Infections
3. Inflammatory diseases
4. Carcinoma
5. Acute heavy metallic poisoning
6. Cell or tissue destruction
7. Toxemia
8. Syphilis
9. Nephritis
10. Pneumonia
11. Severe anemia
12. Rheumatoid arthritis

B. *Decreased Values*
   Found in:
1. Polycythemia vera
2. Sickle cell anemia
3. Congestive heart failure
4. Hypofibrinogemia due to any cause

C. *Varied Values*
1. In acute disease, the change in rate may lag behind the temperature elevation and leukocytosis for six to 24 hours, reaching a peak after several days.
2. In convalescence the increased rate tends to persist longer than the temperature or the leukocytosis.
3. *In unruptured acute appendicitis*, even when suppurative or gangrenous, the rate is normal, but if abscess or peritonitis develops, the rate increases rapidly.
4. Musculoskeletal Conditions
   (a) In rheumatic, gonorrheal, and acute gouty arthritis, the rate is significantly increased.
   (b) In osteoarthritis the rate is slightly increased.
   (c) In neuritis, myositis, and lumbago, the rate is within normal range.
5. Cardiovascular Conditions
   (a) In myocardial infarction the ESR is increased.
   (b) In angina pectoris the rate is not increased.

6. Malignant Diseases
   (a) In multiple myeloma, lymphoma, and metastatic cancer, the rate is very high
   (b) However, there is little correlation between the degree of elevation of the ESR and the prognosis in any one case.

Interfering Factors

1. The blood sample should not be allowed to stand because the rate will increase.
2. In refrigerated blood the sedimentation rate is greatly increased. Refrigerated blood should be allowed to return to room temperature before the test is performed.
3. Factors leading to increased rate:
   (a) The presence of fibrinogen, globulins, and cholesterol
   (b) Pregnancy after 12 weeks until about the fourth week postpartum
   (c) Young children
   (d) Menstruation
   (e) Certain drugs (see below)
4. Factors leading to reduced rates
   (a) High blood sugar
   (b) High albumin level
   (c) High phospholipids
   (d) In newborn (because of decreased fibrinogen level of the blood)
   (e) Certain drugs (see below)
5. Drugs
   (a) Those that increase levels:
      (1.) Dextran
      (2.) Methyldopa
      (3.) Methysergide
      (4.) Oral Contraceptives
      (5.) Penicillamine
      (6.) Procainamide
      (7.) Theophylline
      (8.) Trifluperidol
      (9.) Vitamin A

(b) Those that decrease levels
    (1.) Ethambutol
    (2.) Quinine
    (3.) Salicylates
    (4.) Drugs that cause a high blood glucose level (cortisone and ACTH)

TESTS FOR HEMOGLOBIN DISORDERS

Hemoglobin Electrophoresis

There are many different types of hemoglobin which result from variations in the amino acid structure of the globin portion of the hemoglobin. The most common form of normal hemoglobin found in the adult is hemoglobin A_1. Two other normal hemoglobins found in only trace amounts in the adult are A_2 and F (fetal hemoglobin).

Of the various types of abnormal hemoglobin (hemoglobinopathies), the best known are hemoglobin S, which is responsible for sickle cell anemia, and hemoglobin C, which may result in a mild hemolytic anemia.

Normal and abnormal hemoglobins can be detected via the process of electrophoresis which matches hemolyzed red cell material against standard bands for the various hemoglobins known.

Interfering Factors.   The results may be questionable if a blood transfusion has been given in the preceding four months.

FETAL HEMOGLOBIN (HEMOGLOBIN F) (ALKALI RESISTANT HEMOGLOBIN)

Normal Values

Adults: 0–2%
Newborns: 60–90%
Before age 2: 0–4%

Explanation of Test

Fetal hemoglobin, also called hemoglobin F, is a normal hemoglobin which is manufactured in the red blood cells of the fetus and infant and composes 50 to 90 per cent of the hemoglobin in the newborn. The remaining portion of the hemoglobin in the newborn is made up of hemoglobin A_1 and A_2, the adult types.

In laboratory testing, hemoglobin F is the only hemoglobin known to be alkali–resistant. Adult hemoglobin does not resist alkali denaturation when analyzed in the laboratory.

Under normal conditions, the manufacture of fetal hemoglobin is replaced by the manufacture of adult hemoglobin during the first year of life. But if hemoglobin F persists and composes more than five per cent of the hemoglobin after six months of age, an abnormality should be expected, especially thalassemia. Therefore, determination of hemoglobin F is useful in the diagnosis of thalassemia, an inherited abnormality in the manufacture of hemoglobin, characterized by microcytic, hypochromic anemia.

Procedure

A venous blood sample of seven ml. is obtained.

Clinical Implications

Increased Values—occur in:
1. Thalassemia
2. Hereditary familial fetal hemoglobinemia
3. Spherocytic anemia
4. Sickle cell anemia
5. Hemoglobin H disease
6. As a compensatory mechanism in anemia
7. As a result of leakage of fetal blood into the maternal bloodstream during pregnancy.

In *thalassemia minor,* continued production of fetal hemoglobin may occur on a minor scale with values of five to ten per cent. In *thalassemia major,* the values may reach 40 to 90 per cent. This continued production of hemoglobin F leads to a severe anemia. In thalassemia minor, the patient usually lives; in thalassemia major, death usually occurs.

Interfering Factors

If analysis of specimen is delayed for more than two to three hours, the specimen may falsely appear to have higher quantities of hemoglobin F.

HEMOGLOBIN S (SICKLE CELL TEST)

Normal Values

Normal Adult: 0

Background

Sickle cell anemia is caused by an abnormal form of hemoglobin, known as hemoglobin S. The molecular structure of this form of hemoglobin causes it to become increasingly insoluble when unoxygenated (about 50 times more than normal hemoglobin). The hemoglobin thus becomes more viscous and tends to precipitate or bond in such a way as to cause the red cells to sickle in shape. The abnormally shaped cells are unable to pass freely through the capillary system, resulting in increased viscosity of the blood and sluggish circulation. Frequently the blood supply to certain organs is cut off by the backup of cells in the capillary system.

Sickle cell disorder is genetically transmitted via a recessive gene. A person with one recessive gene is said to have sickle cell trait, but will not suffer the ill effects of the disease itself. When two such genes are present, sickle cell anemia results.

Explanation of Test

This blood measurement is routinely done as a screening test for sickle cell disorder (anemia/trait), or to confirm these disorders. The purpose of the test is to detect the presence of hemoglobin S, an inherited, recessive gene. An examination is made of the erythrocytes for the sickle-shaped forms characteristic of sickle cell anemia or trait. This is done in the laboratory by removing oxygen from the erythrocyte. In erythrocytes with normal hemoglobin the shape is retained, but erythrocytes containing hemoglobin S will assume a sickle-shape. However, the distinction between sickle cell trait and sickle cell disease is done by electrophoresis which identifies a hemoglobin pattern.

Clinical Implications

A. *Positive Test*
1. Means that great numbers of erythrocytes have assumed the typical sickle-cell (crescent) shape.
2. Positive tests are 99% accurate
B. *Sickle Cell Trait*
1. Definite confirmation of sickle cell trait by hemoglobin electrophoresis reveals the following A/S heterozygous pattern:
   Hgb S   20–40%
   Hgb A$_1$ 60–80%
   Hgb F   small amount
2. This means that this patient has inherited a normal hgb A gene from one parent and an hgb S gene from the other.
3. This patient does not have any clinical manifestations of the disease, but some of the children of this patient may inherit the disease if this person marries a mate with the same recessive gene pattern.
4. The diagnosis of sickle cell trait does not affect longevity and is not accompanied by signs and symptoms of sickle cell anemia.
C. *Sickle Cell Anemia*
1. Definite confirmation of sickle cell anemia by hemoglobin electrophoresis reveals the following S/S. homozygous pattern:
   Hgb S 80–100%
   Hgb F makes up the rest
   Hgb A 0%

2. This means that an abnormal S gene has been inherited from both parents.
3. Such a patient has all the clinical manifestations of the disease.

Interfering Factors

1. False negatives—occur in:
   (a) Infants before three months
   (b) Polycythemia
   (c) Protein abnormalities
2. False positives—occur:
   Up to four months after transfusions with RBC's having sickle cell trait.

CLINICAL ALERT
1. A positive diagnosis of this disorder has genetic implications.
2. A person with sickle cell disease should avoid situations in which hypoxia may occur:
   (a) Traveling to high altitude regions
   (b) Traveling in an unpressurized aircraft
   (c) Performing very strenuous exercise
3. On account of general anesthetics and the state of shock creating hypoxia, surgical or maternity patients with sickle cell disease need very close observation to avoid hypoxia.

METHEMOGLOBIN (Hgb M); SULFHEMOGLOBIN; CARBOXYHEMOGLOBIN

Background.   While abnormalities in the globin portion of the hemoglobin are responsible for hemoglobinopathies, such as sickle cell anemia, the ability of the heme portion of hemoglobin to combine with elements other than oxygen can lead to such complexes as methemoglobin, sulfhemoglobin, and carboxyhemoglobin.

Methemoglobin

Normal Values
2% of total hemoglobin
0.5% gm./dl.

Explanation of Test. This test is used to diagnose hereditary or acquired methemoglobinemia (Hgb M), with the suspected patient having symptoms of anoxia or cyanosis without evidence of cardiovascular or pulmonary disease.

Methemoglobin is formed when the iron in the heme portion of deoxygenated hemoglobin is oxidized to a ferric form rather than to a ferrous form. In the ferric form, oxygen and iron cannot combine. The formation of methemoglobin is a normal process and is kept within bounds by the reduction of methemoglobin to hemoglobin.

When a high concentration of methemoglobin is produced in the erythrocytes, it reduces the capacity of the red blood cells to combine with oxygen. Thus, anoxia and cyanosis result. When these symptoms appear without evidence of cardiovascular or pulmonary disease, the erythrocytes are examined in an effort to diagnose methemoglobinemia which may be either hereditary or acquired.

Clinical Implications
A. *Hereditary Methemoglobinemia*
  1. The Hgb M content may be as high as 40 per cent of the total hemoglobin structure.
  2. Associated with polycythemia (but not with hemolytic anemia)
  3. Possible family history
  4. Treatment includes intravenous methylene blue and oral ascorbic acid.
B. *Acquired Methemoglobinemia*
  1. Associated with:
     (a) Black water fever
     (b) Paroxysmal hemoglobinuria
     (c) Clostridia infection
     (d) Ingestion of colored wax crayons or chalk
     (e) Exposure to excessive radiation

2. Most common cause is toxic effect of drugs or chemicals
   (a) Aniline dyes and derivatives
   (b) Sulfonamides
   (c) Nitrates and nitrites
   (d) Acetanilid
   (e) Phenacetin
   (f) Chlorates
   (g) Benzocaine
   (h) Lidocaine

Exposure to these agents is not always obvious:
   (a) May result from eating Polish sausage and spinach which are rich in nitrite and nitrate
   (b) Nitrate may also be absorbed from silver nitrate used to treat extensive burns.
   (c) Excessive intake of Bromo-Seltzer is a common cause of methemoglobinemia. (The patient appears cyanotic, but otherwise feels well.)

CLINICAL ALERT
Because of fetal hemoglobin being more easily converted to methemoglobin than adult hemoglobin, infants are more susceptible than adults to methemoglobinemia caused by drinking well water containing nitrites, and bismuth preparations for diarrhea that may be reduced to nitrites by bowel action.

Sulfhemoglobin

Background. Sulfhemoglobin is an abnormal hemoglobin pigment produced by the combination of inorganic sulfides with hemoglobin.

Clinical Implications

1. Once sulfhemoglobin is formed, it remains stable and is irreversible, disappearing with the red blood cells after completion of the 120 day life span of the erythrocyte.
2. Sulfhemoglobin is observed in patients who take oxidant drugs such as phenacetin (excessive intake of Bromo-Seltzer).

Carboxyhemoglobin

Normal Values
0–2.3% of total hemoglobin
In smokers: 2.1–4.2% of total hemoglobin

Background. Carboxyhemoglobin is formed when hemoglobin is exposed to carbon monoxide. The affinity of hemoglobin for carbon monoxide is 218 times greater than for oxygen.

Clinical Implications
1. Since carboxyhemoglobin is not capable of transporting oxygen, hypoxia results.
2. Death may result from anoxia and irreversible tissue changes.
3. Carboxyhemoglobin produces a cherry-red or violet color of the blood and skin.

PAROXYSMAL NOCTURNAL HEMOGLOBINURIA (PNH) (SCREENING ACID SERUM TEST, PRESUMPTIVE ACID SERUM TEST, AND HAM TEST-ACIDIFIED SERUM LYSIS TEST)

Normal Values

Negative

Background

PNH is a rather uncommon disease that is characterized by the intermittent appearance of hemoglobin in the urine which is more marked during and after sleep, and may be related to increased susceptibility of the red cells to an acid pH. It is associated with pancytopenia that occurs in anemia, leukopenia, and thrombocytopenia. The actual cause of the disease is unknown. It is known that the red cells appear to be sensitive to the increase of carbon dioxide that occurs during sleep, and which lowers the pH of the plasma. The plasma is darker in the morning than during the rest of the day because of hemolysis.

Explanation of Test

These tests are carried out to make a definitive diagnosis of paroxysmal nocturnal hemoglobinuria (PNH). The basis of this test is that the cells peculiar to PNH have membrane defects which make them extra sensitive to complement in the plasma. Under certain conditions in the laboratory, osmotic lysis of the cells is demonstrated by activating the serum complement by slightly acidifying the serum (Ham's test) or by means of an osmotic solution of sucrose. Cells from patients with PNH will undergo marked hemolysis after 15 minutes in the laboratory test.

Procedure

A venous blood sample of 20 ml. is obtained.

Clinical Implications

1. These tests are almost never positive in any other disease than PNH, and are seldom negative in patients with PNH.
2. The tests are performed on patients who have hemoglobinuria, or those with bone marrow aplasia, (hypoplasia) or undiagnosed hemolytic anemias.

Interfering Factors

False positive results may be obtained when blood contains large numbers of spherocytes.

TESTS OF OTHER BLOOD COMPONENTS

RETICULOCYTE COUNT

Normal Values

Adults: 0.5–1.5% of total erythrocytes or about 60,000 reticulocytes/cu. mm.

Children: 0.5–4.0% of total erythrocytes
Infants: 2–5% of total erythrocytes
Reticulocyte index = one

Background

A *reticulocyte* is a young non-nucleated cell of the erythrocyte series formed in the bone marrow. As an immature red cell it contains reticular material (from the dissolving nucleus) which will stain a gray-blue when tested in the laboratory. Reticulum is present in newly released blood cells and lasts about four days before the cell reaches its full mature state. Normally a small number of these cells are found in the circulating blood (about 0.5 to 1.5 per cent of the total red blood count), see the normal value. The number of reticulocytes per 1,000 erythrocytes yields the reticulocyte count.

In order for the reticulocyte count to be meaningful, it must be viewed in relation to the total number of erythrocytes.
1. An increase in the reticulocyte count indicates that red cell production (erythropoiesis) has been accelerated and that mature red cells are being prematurely destroyed.
2. A decrease in number indicates that red cell production by the bone marrow has been reduced.

Explanation of Test

A reticulocyte count is used:
1. To differentiate anemias due to bone marrow failure from those due to hemorrhage or hemolysis (red cell destruction)
2. To check the effectiveness of treatment in pernicious anemia and the recovery of bone marrow function in aplastic anemia
3. To determine the effects of radioactive substances on exposed workers

Procedure

A blood sample of seven ml. is obtained.

Clinical Implications

An increased count (reticulocytosis) means that hyperactive erythrocyte production is occurring as the bone marrow replaces cells lost or destroyed. Identifying reticulocytosis may lead to the recognition of an otherwise occult disease such as hidden chronic hemorrhage or unrecognized hemolysis (sickle cell anemia and thalassemia).

A. *Increased Levels*

Found in:

1. Hemolytic anemias
2. Sickle cell disease
3. Metastatic carcinoma
4. Leukemia
5. Three to four days following hemorrhage
6. Hereditary spherocytosis
7. After splenectomy
8. Following treatment of anemias (therapeutic diagnostic test):
    (a) Increase may be used as an index of the effectiveness of treatment.
    (b) After adequate doses of iron in iron-deficiency anemia, the rise in reticulocytes may exceed 20 per cent.
    (c) There is a proportional increase when pernicious anemia is treated by transfusion.

B. *Decreased Levels*

A decreased reticulocyte count means that bone marrow is not producing enough erythrocytes.

Found in:

1. Iron-deficiency anemia
2. Aplastic anemia (A persistent deficiency of reticulocytes suggests a poor prognosis)
3. Untreated pernicious anemia
4. Chronic infection
5. Radiation therapy

Interfering Factors

The reticulocyte count is normally increased in pregnancy and infants.

HISTIOCYTE SMEAR

Normal Values

None, not normally found in circulating *blood.*

Explanation of Test

A blood smear is examined to identify and count the number of histiocytes present. Histiocytes or reticulum cells are not blood cells but tissue cells derived from reticuloendothelial tissue. Histiocytes are not normally found in the blood but are known to circulate in the blood in certain conditions in which their macrophagic properties act specifically, as in tuberculosis, leprosy, subacute endocarditis and lipid storage diseases. Histiocytes may be classified as monocytes in a differential leukocyte count.

Procedure

1. Usually four blood smears are taken from a puncture site.
2. The earlobe is rubbed for one to two minutes, wiped with alcohol, and pricked with a needle.
3. Obtaining a venous blood sample is the other procedure method.

Clinical Implications

1. Histiocytes are found in:
    (a) Subacute bacterial endocarditis
    (b) Typhoid fever
    (c) Hemolytic anemia
    (d) Hodgkin's disease
    (e) Reticulum cell sarcoma
    (f) Severe diarrhea in children
    (g) Tuberculosis
    (h) Leprosy
    (i) Fat storage disease

(j) Lymphoma
(k) Some parasitic diseases
(l) Histiocytic leukemia

LYMPHOCYTES (MONOMORPHONUCLEAR LYMPHOCYTES)

Normal Values

20–40% of total leukocyte count (relative value) or 1000–4000/cu. mm.

Explanation of Test

These agranulocytes are small motile cells that migrate to areas of inflammation both in the early and late stages of the inflammation process. They may possibly convert to tissue macrophages and plasma cells. These cells are the source of serum globulin and possibly of immune bodies; therefore they play an important role in immunologic reactions. It is believed that lymphocytes do not form antibodies per se, but they may contribute to formation by being responsible for the storage of immunologic memory. This means that a second contact with an antigen elicits an accelerated and increased response. They are found in the blood in infectious leukocytosis at the recovery stage of disease.

Procedure

A venous blood sample of seven ml. is obtained.

Clinical Implications

A. *Lymphocytosis*—an increase in the amount of circulating lymphocytes
   1. Above 9,000/cu. mm. in infants and young children

Above 7,000/cu. mm. in older children

Above 4,000/cu. mm. in adults

2. Conditions causing lymphocytosis:
   (a) Most viral upper respiratory infections
   (b) Other viral diseases such as mumps, pertussis, infectious mononucleosis, infectious hepatitis, viral pneumonia and measles
   (c) Bacterial infections such as tuberculosis, brucellosis, syphilis and healing infections
   (d) Hormonal disorders such as hypothyroidism and hypoadrenalism
   (e) Lymphocytic leukemia, lymphocytic lymphosarcoma, leukosarcoma
   (f) Diarrhea

B. *Lymphopenia* (a decrease in the amount of circulating lymphocytes)

Occurs in:
   (a) Hodgkin's disease
   (b) Lupus erythematosus
   (c) After administration of ACTH and cortisone
   (d) After burns or trauma
   (e) Chronic uremia
   (f) Cushing's syndrome
   (g) Early acute radiation syndrome

CLINICAL ALERT

A decreased lymphocyte count greater than 500 means that a patient is dangerously susceptible to infection, especially viral infections. *Institute measures to protect patient from infection.*

Morphologic Forms of Lymphocytes

A. *Virocytes* (also called stress lymphocytes or Downy type cells)

1. Are small atypical cells that appear in viral diseases such as mononucleosis, viral hepatitis, viral pneumonia, and viral upper respiratory tract infections.

2. May also be found in numerous nonviral conditions:

(a) Fungoid and protoxoid infections

(b) Autoimmune states

(c) Allergic reactions

(d) After transfusions and tissue grafts

3. When seen in stress response, are called stress lymphocytes

4. May be found in apparently healthy children

5. Up to ten per cent of all lymphocytes can be considered normal.

Note: Any amount of atypical lymphocytes are reported.

B. *Transformed Lymphocytes*

1. Examples

(a) Lymphocytoid cells which may be seen in macroglobulinemia

(b) Turk cells and Reider cells which are seen in acute lymphatic leukemia

(c) Vacuolated lymphocytes which are seen in lipidosis

2. Culturing of lymphocytes in laboratory

(a) Stimulates small lymphocytes to transform into large atypical cells which produce immunoglobulins.

(b) Transformation response is impaired in culturing of lymphocytes from patients with:

(1) Hodgkin's disease

(2) Lymphatic leukemia

(3) Lymphocytosis

(4) Agammaglobulinemia

(c) Transformation response increased in sarcoidosis

3. Other uses of transformation test are to determine histiocompatibility of recipient and donor for tissue grafts.

(a) Lymphocytes from donor not related to recipient stimulates the production of up to 3 per cent of transformed lymphocytes in recipient.

(b) Lymphocytes from siblings react less strongly.

(c) No reaction occurs on cultures from fraternal twins.

ROSETTE TEST FOR T AND B LYMPHOCYTES

Normal Values

B-cells 10–30% of total lymphocytes
T-cells 70–90% of total lymphocytes

Explanation of Test

Lymphocytes can be divided into two categories, T and B cells, according to their primary function within the immunity system. The test is done to evaluate the immune system by identifying specific cells involved in the immune response.

T and B cells can be identified with an electromicroscope according to certain distinguishing surface marks (rosettes): T cells are smooth; B cells have projections.

The majority of circulating lymphocytes are T cells having a life span of months to years. B cells comprise ten to 30 per cent of the lymphocytes and have a life span measured in days.

The purpose of the test is based on the fact that temporary or permanent faulty functioning of the immune system results in the invasion of the body by bacteria, viruses, and cancer cells.
B Lymphocytes
1. Are considered "bursa or bone marrow dependent", although exact site of B cell production has not been identified
2. Are responsible for humoral immunity (in which antibodies are present in the serum)
3. Begin producing antibodies in the primary antibody production within 48 to 72 hours after initial contact with antigen
T Lymphocytes
1. Are thymus dependent and are known to be produced by the thymus
2. Are responsible for cellular immunity
3. Function to:
    (a) Interact with antigen
    (b) Destroy tumor cells
4. Cause rejection of transplants

Cellular Immunity
1. Response appears in:
    (a) Rejection of transplanted organs
    (b) Contact allergies
    (c) Tuberculosis
    (d) Autoimmune diseases
    (e) Immunity to viruses, protozoa, and fungi
    (f) Fight against cancer
2. Stimulation of the cellular immune response (immuno-therapy) is useful in cancer treatment when combined with other therapies, primarily in the prevention of subsequent metastasis.
3. Depression or weakening of the cellular immune response is important in the prevention of rejection of transplanted organs, especially in kidney recipients who have been presensitized by a prior graft, multiple blood transfusions, or multiple pregnancies.

Procedure

A venous blood sample of ten ml. is obtained.

Clinical Implications

A. *T cells*
    1. Increased in Grave's disease
    2. Decreased in:
        (a) DeGeorge syndrome (genetic absence of both thymus and parathyroid glands)
        (b) Hodgkin's disease
        (c) Chronic lymphocytic leukemia
        (d) Long-term immunosuppressive drug therapy
B. *B cells*
    1. Increased in active erythematosus
    2. Decreased in:
        (a) X-linked agammaglobulinemia
        (b) Myeloma
        (c) Chronic lymphocytic leukemia

SUDAN BLACK B STAIN (SBB) FOR PHOSPHOLIPIDS

Normal Values

Lymphocytes will not stain with this method. Granulocytic cells will stain with this method. Normal blood is used as a control.

Explanation of Test

This technique is used in the diagnosis of leukemia. The Sudan B Stain is useful in differentiating acute granulocytic leukemia from acute lymphocytic leukemia. Lymphocytes and lympho-blasts (immature lymphocytes) do not stain with SBB and are said to be sudanophobic. Cells of the granulocytic and monocyte series contain granules that take the stain and are said to be sudanophilic.

Sudan Black B also stains a wide variety of lipids including neutral fats, phospholipids, and steroids.

Procedure

A bone marrow aspirate must be taken.

Clinical Implications

1. Positive staining of primitive cells indicates myelogenous origin of cells.
2. The test is SBB positive in acute granulocytic leukemia.
3. The test is SBB negative in acute lymphocytic leukemia.

PERIODIC ACID SCHIFF STAIN (PAS)

Normal Values

Granulocytes stain PAS positive
Agranulocytes stain PAS negative

Explanation of Test

This staining technique is used to identify reactions to amyloid, a glycoprotein, and to classify immature cells of the blood and bone marrow.

The PAS reaction for glycogen is one of the histiological methods that are helpful in the diagnosis of amyloid diseases such as acute lymphocytic leukemia and erythroleukemia. Amyloidosis is a disease process of unknown cause, characterized by waxy deposits in the liver, kidney, spleen, heart, skin, and alimentary tract. This staining technique is also useful in differentiating erythemic myelosis from sideroblastic anemia.

Methods used other than PAS are Metachromatic Methyl and Crystal Violet, thioflavine T, and Congo red.

Procedure

A bone marrow aspirate must be taken.

Clinical Implications

1. The test is positive in:
   (a) Acute lymphocytic leukemia
   (b) Erythroleukemia
   (c) Severe iron-deficiency anemia
   (d) Thalassemia
   (e) Amyloidosis
   (f) Strongly positive lymphocytes in the circulatory blood suggest malignant lymphoma
2. Blast cells that stain Schiff positive are:
   (a) Erythroblasts of erythroleukemia
   (b) Thalassemia sideroblastic anemia
   (c) Mucin
   (d) Hyaline
   (e) Basement membranes
   (f) Fungus
   (g) Amyloid
   (h) Glycogen
   (i) Gaucher cells
   (j) Megakaryocytes

Interfering Factors

Results of test reflect the adeptness and skill of the laboratory technician.

LEUKOCYTE ALKALINE PHOSPHATASE STAIN (LAP); ALKALINE PHOSPHATASE STAIN

Normal Values

30–130 Each laboratory establishes its own range.

Explanation of Test

This test is usually ordered to differentiate granulocytic leukemia from leukemoid reactions. The enzyme, alkaline phosphatase, is present in leukocytes; enzyme activity is represented by granulation in the cytoplasm of neutrophilic granulocytes. High concentrations of this enzyme will be found in normal white blood cells and low to negative concentrations in leukemic leukocytes.

Procedure

A venous blood sample of seven ml. is obtained.

Interfering Factors

Value is normally increased in pregnancy.

Clinical Implications

1. In chronic granulocytic anemia, the range is from 0 to 13, meaning that none or little alkaline phosphatase activity is demonstrable.
2. Values below normal may be found in:
    (a) Acute and chronic granulocytic leukemia,
    (b) Paroxysmal nocturnal hemoglobinuria,

    (c) Aplastic anemia,

    (d) Infectious mononucleosis,

    (e) Hereditary hypophosphatasia,

    (f) Many infections

3. Values above normal may be found in:

    (a) Neutrophilic leukemoid reactions,

    (b) Polycythemia vera,

    (c) Thrombocytopenia infection,

    (d) Myelofibrosis.

4. A leukemoid reaction is a blood picture that looks like leukemia, but is not.

BUFFY COAT SMEAR

Normal Values

Atypical Mononuclear cells	The buffy coat of the
Megakaryocytes	blood of healthy
Metamyelocytes and Myelocytes	people contains
Normal white cell components	these cells.

Explanation of Test

This diagnostic smear of the leukocytes is most commonly done on leukemic and cancer patients with metastatic relapse to the bone marrow. The purpose of this test is to search for either cells or tumor cells.

Procedure

A venous blood sample of five ml. is obtained.

Clinical Implications

1. Abnormal cells such as tumor cells and LE cells are an indication of:

(a) Leukemia
(b) Cancer metastatic to the bone
(c) Lupus erythematosus

TESTS OF COAGULATION AND HEMOSTASIS

Introduction

A wide variety of laboratory tests are available to determine the nature and extent of coagulation disorders. These tests are generally related to the physiologic response of the body to bleeding disorders and to injury of blood vessels.

Mechanism of Hemostasis. Several mechanisms arrest bleeding: (1) The skin, subcutaneous tissue, and muscle comprise the body's first line of defense. They may be considered the *extravascular resistance* to bleeding. (2) Blood vessel walls contract to reduce the quantity of blood flowing through them. This response is the *vascular resistance* to bleeding. (3) Platelets adhere to each other and to the damaged endothelium, and initiate clotting factors. (4) The clotting factors of the blood react via a cascading mechanism to generate thrombin and to deposit fibrin. Platelet response plus the clotting factor reactions comprise the *intravascular resistance* to bleeding.

Laboratory diagnostic tests are usually effective in determining the cause of a hemorrhagic disorder. However, judged by the result of laboratory tests, patients can still appear to be normal and yet have a history of bleeding.

Bleeding does not necessarily indicate a hemorrhagic disorder due to defective hemostasis, nor does the absence of current bleeding rule out an existing hemorrhagic disorder. It is important to remember that the most common cause of hemorrhaging of any sort is thrombocytopenia, the deficiency of platelets. Liver disease, uremia, thrombocytopenia, and DIC disease, as well as the administration of Coumadin (warfarin sodium) and heparin, account for most of the hemorrhagic disorders seen in routine medical practice. It is relatively infrequent to see hemophilias.

Disseminated intravascular coagulation (DIC) disease is an acquired hemorrhagic disease in which there is continuous generation of thrombin that causes bleeding. The causative factors of DIC include:

1. Incompatible blood transfusion
2. Paroxysmal nocturnal hemoglobinuria
3. Malaria
4. Cold hemoglobinuria
5. Sickle cell disease
6. Injection of hypotonic solutions
7. Abruptio placenta
8. Retained dead fetus
9. Amniotic fluid imbalance
10. Trauma and crushing injuries
11. Cancer
12. Rocky Mountain spotted fever
13. Hageman factor contact by collagen

Note: The treatment for DIC is heparin, which may seem paradoxical. The reason heparin is given is that this drug blocks thrombin formation, thus causing bleeding to stop.

Laboratory Investigation.   Generally, a set routine of coagulation studies is followed. Enough blood is collected at one time to provide the specimens needed for the various tests.

1. Usually at least 20 ml. of blood is obtained using the two-syringe technique.
    (a.) Five cc. of blood is obtained in the first syringe and this specimen is discarded
    (b.) 15 to 20 cc. of blood is obtained in the second syringe and this specimen is examined
2. Coagulation studies, also called "coagulation profile," or "coagulogram" are indicated:
    (a.) In screening of preoperative patients
    (b.) With coagulation disorder symptoms, such as:
        (1.) Easy bruising
        (2.) Prolonged bleeding
        (3.) Heavy nosebleeds
        (4.) Excessive menstrual flow
        (5.) Family history of abnormal heavy bleeding

This sequence of tests is recommended in the investigation of a hemorrhagic disorder.

1. Tests for vascular function and platelet function
   (a.) Bleeding time
   (b.) Capillary fragility test or Rumple-Leede test
2. Tests for overall clotting ability
   (a.) Clotting time
   (b.) Activated partial thromboplastin time
3. Tests of stage III
   (a.) Fibrinogen level
   (b.) Thrombin time
   (c.) Fibrinolysis tests
4. Tests of stage II
   (a.) Prothrombin time
   (b.) Prothrombin consumption
5. Tests of stage I
   (a.) Activated partial thromboplastin time
   (b.) Prothrombin consumption
   (c.) Platelet function time tests
6. Tests of platelet function
   (a.) Platelet count
   (b.) Bleeding time
   (c.) Platelet aggregation studies
7. Tests of stage IV
   (a.) Euglobulin lysis
   (b.) Clot lysis test
   (c.) Partial thromboplastin time
8. Tests for circulating anticoagulants

Four primary screening tests are performed in the initial laboratory investigation of suspected coagulation disorders:

1. Platelet count, size, and shape
2. Bleeding time provides information about the ability of platelets to perform their normal function and the ability of the capillaries to constrict their walls.
3. Partial thromboplastin time determines the ability of the blood to clot
4. Prothrombin time measures the activity of clotting factors
   Other commonly ordered tests include:
1. Clot retraction

2. Fibrinogen level
3. Definitive coagulation studies (e.g., factor assays)

When a hemostatic defect has been identified as due to a problem in coagulation, and the problem has been suspected of being in the fibrinolytic system, specific tests provide the most reliable and precise method of establishing an accurate diagnosis. These tests will be performed only in certain laboratories. They are the following:

1. Euglobulin clot lysis—identifies increased plasminogen activator activity (plasmin is *not* usually present in the blood plasma).
2. Dilute whole blood clot lysis test—detects physiologic amounts of fibrinolytic activity
3. Whole blood clot lysis test—identifies severe pathologic fibrinolysis.

CLINICAL ALERT
All patients who are known to have hemorrhagic or bleeding tendencies, or who are being examined through coagulation studies, should be observed closely, and a careful drug history and family history of bleeding should be obtained.

Assessment of Patient
1. Examine skin for bruising on extremities and other parts of the body that patient cannot easily see.
2. Record the appearance of petechiae that may occur after a blood pressure reading or application of tourniquet for venipuncture. These may be the first indication of a bleeding tendency.
3. Note bleeding from the nose or gums.
4. Estimate quantity of blood appearing in vomitus or expectoration, urine, stools, and increased menstrual flow.
5. Record bleeding from injection sites.
6. Intracranial bleeding may develop. Watch for symptoms associated with cerebrovascular disease and increased intracranial pressure.

7. Determine whether the patient has a history of taking coumarin drugs and aspirin in any form.
8. Procedure alert. When a blood sample is obtained for Pro Time, PTT, and TT, sodium citrate (anticoagulant) is added to the syringe or vacucontainer.

BLEEDING TIME (DUKE AND IVY METHODS)

Normal Values

3–10 minutes in most laboratories
  Duke Method < 8 minutes (usually 1–6 minutes)
  Ivy Method 2–9.5 minutes

Explanation of Test

This is one of the four primary screening tests for coagulation disorders. A small stab wound is made in either the earlobe or forearm; the time to stop bleeding is recorded, and a measurement is made of the rate at which a platelet clot is formed. The duration of bleeding from a punctured capillary depends upon the quantity and quality of platelets, and the ability of the blood vessel wall to constrict.

The bleeding time test is of significant value in detecting vascular abnormalities, and of moderate value in detecting platelet abnormalities or deficiencies. Its principal use today is in the diagnosis of von Willebrand's disease, an inherited defective molecule of factor VIII, and a type of pseudohemophilia. It has been established that aspirin may cause bleeding in some normal persons, but the bleeding time has not proved to be consistently valuable in identifying such persons. While the bleeding time is classically recognized as prolonged in thrombocytopenia, the test is an indirect method of identifying the condition. A stained red cell examination and platelet count are more effective than bleeding time in confirming the diagnosis of thrombocytopenia.

Procedure

Two procedures are followed: (1) the Duke method and (2) the Ivy method.

DUKE METHOD

1. In the modified Duke method, the area used for puncture is just above the rounded, fatty portion of the earlobe, which is highly vascular.
   - (a.) The ear is quickly pierced with a hemolet ("ear sticker") to make a wound three mm. deep.
   - (b.) A stopwatch is started. Pressure should not be exerted on the ear to initiate bleeding.
   - (c.) The blood should be allowed to fall freely on 4" × 4" gauze sponges or filter paper.
   - (d.) The wound is blotted every 30 seconds until all bleeding has stopped.

IVY METHOD

2. In the Ivy method, the area three finger-widths below the antecubital space is cleansed with alcohol and allowed to dry.
   - (a.) A blood pressure cuff is placed on the arm above the elbow and inflated to 40 mm. of mercury.
   - (b.) A cleansed area of the forearm without superficial veins is selected. The skin is stretched laterally and tautly between the thumb and forefinger.
   - (c.) The skin is punctured with a sterile disposable device to a uniform depth of 5 mm. and width of 1 mm.
   - (d.) Start a stopwatch. The edge of a 4" × 4" filter paper used to collect the blood through capillary action by gently touching the drop every 30 seconds. The blood pressure gauge is removed when bleeding stops spontaneously and a sterile dressing is applied.
3. The results of both procedures are reported in this way:
   - (a.) The end point is reached when blood no longer drops from the ear or forearm puncture

Clinical Implications

1. Bleeding time is prolonged in:
   - (a.) Thrombocytopenia
   - (b.) Platelet dysfunction syndromes

    (c.) Vascular defects

    (d.) Severe liver disease

    (e.) Leukemia

    (f.) Aplastic anemia

    (g.) DIC disease

2. Bleeding time can be either normal or prolonged in von Willebrand's disease. It will definitely be prolonged if aspirin is administered prior to testing.

3. A single prolonged bleeding time does not prove the existence of hemorrhagic disease because a larger vessel may have been punctured. The puncture should be done twice (on the opposite ear or opposite arm) and the average of the bleeding times taken.

Interfering Factors

1. The normal range may vary when the puncture is not of standard depth and width.

2. Touching the incision during the test will break off any fibrin particles and prolong the bleeding time.

3. Heavy alcohol consumption (as in alcoholics) may cause bleeding time to be increased.

4. Prolonged bleeding time will result from the ingestion of ten gm. of aspirin (acetylsalicylic acid) up to five days before the test.

5. Other drugs that may cause the bleeding time to be increased include:

    (a.) Dextran

    (b.) Streptokinase-streptodornase (used as fibrinolytic agent)

    (c.) Mithramycin

    (d.) Pantothenyl alcohol

Patient Preparation

1. Explain the purpose and procedure of the test to patient.

2. Warn patient to take no aspirin for at least five days before the test.

3. Advise outpatients not to drink alcoholic beverages before coming for test.

CLINICAL ALERT

If the puncture site is still bleeding beyond 15 minutes, the test should be discontinued by applying pressure to area. Report to physician.

TOURNIQUET TEST; RUMPEL-LEEDE POSITIVE PRESSURE TEST; CAPILLARY FRAGILITY TEST; NEGATIVE PRESSURE TEST

Normal Values

Occasional petechiae or none
  Positive pressure test—Occasional (5–10) petechiae or none
  Negative pressure test—1–2 petechiae

Explanation of Test

This test is done to demonstrate a Stage I defect of capillary fragility that is due to an abnormality in the capillary walls or thrombocytopenia. Positive or negative pressure is applied to various areas of the body via a blood pressure cuff or a suction cup. The degree of increased capillary fragility is reflected in the number of petechiae (nonraised, round red spots) appearing in a given area of observation.

The forearm, wrists, hands, and fingers are examined for petechiae. The distribution of petechiae is usually irregular and no effort is made to count the number in a given area. The test is graded 1+ to 4+, depending on whether there are few or many spots.

Procedure

1. In the positive pressure touniquet test, a blood pressure cuff is applied to the upper arm and inflated to 70 to 90 mm. of mercury or to midway between the patient's systolic and diastolic pressure. The inflated cuff is removed after five

minutes. The arm, wrist, and hand are then inspected for petechiae.
2. In the negative pressure test, a lubricated suction cup of two cm. diameter is applied to the skin of the upper arm. Pressure is applied to the skin for one minute. The suction cup is released and five minutes later the skin is inspected for petechiae. This is not commonly done, but a description is included here because it is referred to in the literature about bleeding disorders.

Clinical Implications

1. Increased petechiae formation occurs most commonly in thrombocytopenia and less commonly in (a) thrombasthenia, (b) vascular purpura, (c) senile purpura, and (d) scurvy.
2. The number and size of petechiae are roughly proportional to the bleeding tendency and possibly to the degree of thrombocytopenia. However, the test can be positive because of capillary fragility in the presence of a normal platelet count.
3. Results will be normal in coagulation disorders and vascular disorders.
4. Positive 1+ is a few petechiae over anterior forearm.
   2+ is many petechiae over anterior forearm.
   3+ is multiple petechiae over the whole arm and top of hand.
   4+ confluent petechiae in all areas of arm and top of hand.

Interfering Factors

1. Menstruation: Capillary fragility is normally increased before menstruation.
2. Infectious disease: Capillary fragility is increased in measles and influenza.
3. Age: Women over 40 with decreasing estrogen levels may have a positive test which is not indicative of a coagulation disorder.
4. Readministration: Repetition of the test on same arm within one week of the first test may lead to error.

5. Variation: Results may vary because of differences in texture, thickness, and temperature of the skin.

Patient Preparation

Explain purpose and procedure of the test.

> **CLINICAL ALERT**
> Do not repeat this test on the same arm for at least one week because the results will be unreliable. Use the opposite arm for a repeat test.

COAGULATION TIME (CT); WHOLE BLOOD CLOTTING TIME; LEE-WHITE CLOTTING TIME

Normal Values

5–10 minutes.

Explanation of Test

This is one of the oldest tests in use and is a relatively insensitive test for coagulation. The basis for this test is that whole blood will form a solid clot when exposed to a foreign surface such as a glass test tube. Clotting time is the time required for the solid clot to form.

Whole blood clotting time is in popular use, but it is the least effective test and of least value in the diagnosis of actual or potential hemostatic failure. It has been replaced in many laboratories by the partial thromboplastin time (PTT) test. One of the reasons the test has been replaced is that mild hemophiliacs may have a normal coagulation time. The primary use of this test is in monitoring and regulating patients on heparin therapy. A normal CT does not rule out a clotting defect.

Procedure

1. A venous sample of three ml. is obtained in a plastic syringe.
2. The clinician should remain at patient's side and immediately transfer the blood to glass test tubes.

3. Using a stopwatch, the clinician should start timing the test when the blood comes in contact with the glass.
4. One method of performing the test is to put one ml. of blood into each of two dry test tubes. Tube number one is tilted every 30 seconds until a solid clot forms which allows for complete inversion of the test tube without flow of blood. Then Tube number 2 is tilted. The reported value is the length of time it takes for the last tube to clot.

Clinical Implications

1. Severe deficiencies of any of the coagulation factors must be present before the coagulation time will be prolonged. Fibrinogen, for example, needs to be decreased to 50 mg. per cent or less before the coagulation time is affected; the normal range of fibrinogen is 200 to 400 mg./100 ml.
2. When prothrombin is diminished to a level of 30 per cent of normal, there will be a small change in coagulation time, giving a result in the range of 12 minutes. This, of course, does not give very great sensitivity since the upper limit of normal is ten minutes.
3. Prolonged coagulation time will be noted in afibrinogenemia and marked hyperheparinemia.

Interfering Factors

1. Quality of venipuncture: The venipuncture must be carefully done because either tissue thromboplastin obtained as a contaminant when the venipuncture is done, or hemolyzed red blood cells suctioned when the blood is drawn, can cause a marked shortening of the coagulation time. The time required for a severe hemophiliac's blood to clot can be shortened from one hour to a normal value when a poor venipuncture is done.
2. Type of test tube: The coagulation time will be lengthened to 20 to 40 minutes if plastic or silicone coated test tubes are used.
3. Drugs which may cause the coagulation time to be *increased* include:
   (a.) Mithramycin
   (b.) Tetracyclines

(c.) Anticoagulants

(d.) Azathioprine

(e.) Carbenicillin

4. Drugs which may cause the coagulation time to be *decreased* include:

   (a.) Corticosteroids

   (b.) Epinephrine

Heparin Therapy: Protocols and blood coagulation tests

1. Heparin combines in the blood with an alpha globulin (heparin cofactor) for a potent antithrombin.

2. The intravenous injection of heparin will give an immediate anticoagulant effect, so it is used when rapid effects are desired.

3. Because of heparin not remaining in the blood very long, the clotting time is measured before each injection.

4. The coagulation time is ordinarily maintained at two to two and one half times the normal limit.

5. To evaluate the effect of heparin, the blood is tested for coagulation time:

   (a.) Before therapy is started for baseline

   (b.) One hour before next dose is administered

   (c.) Dependent upon the status of patient during heparin therapy (signs of bleeding)

6. Protamine sulfate is the antidote for heparin overdose and hemorrhage.

THROMBIN TIME; THROMBIN CLOTTING TIME

Normal Values

15 seconds—However, there are so many modifications of this test that "normals" vary widely. Check your laboratory values.

Explanation of Test

Stage III defects of fibrinogen abnormalities can be detected by this method. It is a valuable test for detecting hypofib-

In the circulating blood there appears to be a balance between the factors acting to stimulate the formation of thrombin and the forces acting to delay its formation. This balance maintains blood in its fluid state. When the blood vessels are injured or when blood is removed from a vessel, the balance is upset and coagulation occurs. A number of coagulation factors have been identified that are involved in four progressive stages of clotting. The Roman Numerals assigned to the coagulation factors identify their order of discovery, rather than their involvement in the stages of clot formation.

Stage	Components of Stages	Clotting Factors
Stage I **Phase I** Platelet activity. Platelets serve as a source of thromboplastin. **Phase II** Thromboplastin (Factor III, an enzyme thought to be liberated by damaged cells, is formed by six different factors plus calcium.)	90% of all coagulation disorders are due to defects in Phase I. Platelet counts <1000,000/cu. mm. indicate moderate interference with Phase I activity. Calcium Factor V Factor VIII Factor IX Factor X are involved in this forma- Factor XI tion of tissue thromboplastin Factor XII (intrinsic prothrombin activa- tion).	INTERNATIONAL NOMENCLATURE Factor I = Fibrinogen Factor II = Prothrombin (Vitamin K functions in the production of prothrombin) Factor III = Tissue thromboplastin Factor IV = Calcium ions Factor V = Platelet phospholipids & calcium ions Factor VI = This factor is no longer considered to be a distinct part of coagulation Factor VII = A coenzyme (stable factor) Factor VIII = Antihemophilic globulin Factor IX = Christmas factor (Hemophelia) Factor X = Stuart-Prower factor. Factor X must be activated to convert prothrombin to thrombin Factor XI = Plasma thromboplastin antecedent (PTA) Factor XII = Hageman factor Factor XIII = Fibrin stabilizing factor (FSF)
Stage II Prothrombin, Factor II, is converted to thrombin in the presence of *calcium*.	Factor II Factor X are involved in this conversion Factor VII of fibrinogen to fibrin.	
Stage III Thrombin interacts with fibrinogen, (Factor I) to form the framework of the clot. **Stage IV** Fibrinolytic system (antagonistic system to the clotting mechanism; check and balance system is activated)	At the end of Stage III, Factor XIII functions in the stabilization of the clot.	

[87]

*Note: The 13 clotting factors of the blood are proteins. They are present in the blood plasma in an inactive form.

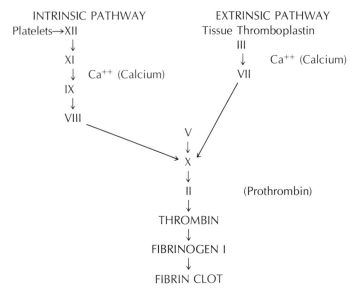

Fig. 1–1. *Mechanism of fibrin clot formation. (Diagram developed by author, with M. Schmidt.)*

rinogenemia and may also be used for control of heparin therapy. The test measures the time needed for plasma to clot in the laboratory when thrombin is added. Normally, a clot is formed instantly; if not, a fibrinogen deficiency is present.

Procedure

If the test is used to monitor heparin therapy, blood is drawn one hour before administration of anticoagulant. A seven ml. venous blood sample is obtained and an anti-coagulant, sodium citrate, is added to the syringe.

Clinical Implications

1. No clot will form if afibrinogenemia is present.
2. A small visible clot will form in hypofibrinogenemia, but the thrombin clotting time is prolonged.
3. The time is also prolonged during:

(a) Anticoagulant therapy when heparin is present in the blood
(b) In the dysproteinemias such as multiple myeloma

PARTIAL THROMBOPLASTIN TIME (PTT); ACTIVATED PARTIAL THROMBOPLASTIN (APTT)

Normal Values

PTT: 30–45 seconds
APTT: 16–25 seconds
The basis of this test is fibrin clot formation.

Explanation of Test

The PTT, which is a one stage clotting test, is an important and sensitive screening test for coagulation disorders and is of most value in detecting deficiencies of Stage II clotting mechanism. Specifically, it is used to detect deficiencies of the components of the intrinsic thromboplastin system. This method will detect not only those abnormalities that are identified by the whole blood clotting time, and some that might be missed by the whole blood clotting time, but will also reveal abnormalities characterized by defects in the second stage of the coagulation mechanism. The PTT is sometimes preferred over the coagulation time test for monitoring heparin therapy.

Note: PTT and APTT test for the same functions. Deficiency of Factor VII is not measured in this test system.

The APTT is a modified PTT which is used frequently to monitor heparin therapy because it is a more sensitive test than PTT and takes less time to perform.

The APTT is also used to detect circulating anticoagulants. Both classic hemophilia A and hemophilia B can be complicated by the presence of circulating anticoagulants. These circulating anticoagulants are antibodies, most of which are induced in hemophiliacs by the transfusion of plasma from normal persons. The prolonged PTT of hemophiliacs can be corrected by transfusions, but if the anticoagulants (inhibitors of clotting) develop, the PTT again becomes prolonged. The APTT will determine whether or not the cause of the prolonged PTT time is due to the development of anticoagulants.

Procedure

A venous sample of seven ml. is obtained, using sodium citrate added as an anticoagulant in the syringe.

Clinical Implications

A. PTT
   1. The PTT is prolonged in all coagulation defects of Stage II.
   2. The PTT is usually prolonged in von Willebrand's disease and is accompanied by a consistently diminished factor VIII level.
   3. The PTT and prothrombin time will detect approximately 95 per cent of coagulation abnormalities. When a PTT is performed in conjuction with a prothrombin time (PT), a further clarification of coagulation defects is possible. For example, a normal PT and an abnormal PTT means that the defect lies within the first stage of the clotting mechanism.

B. APTT
   1. Causes of prolonged APTT are:
       (a.) Hemophilia
       (b.) Vitamin K deficiency
       (c.) Liver disease
       (d.) Presence of circulating anticoagulants
       (e.) DIC disease
   2. Shortened APTT occurs in:
       (a.) Extensive cancer, except when the liver is involved
       (b.) Immediately after acute hemorrhage

4. Anticoagulants which develop in the treated hemophiliac are detected by prolonged APTT. Anticoagulants also can be detected:
   (a.) Following repeated blood transfusions
   (b.) Drug sensitivity in lupus erythematosus
   (c.) Tuberculosis
   (d.) Chronic glomerulonephritis

PROTHROMBIN TIME (PRO TIME PT)

Normal Values

11–16 seconds or 100%; each laboratory will set its own normals.

Explanation of Test

Prothrombin is a protein produced by the liver and is used in the clotting of blood. Production of prothrombin depends on an adequate intake and absorption of Vitamin K. During the clotting process, prothrombin is converted to thrombin. The prothrombin content of the blood will be reduced in patients with liver disease.

Prothrombin time is one of the four most important screening tests used in diagnostic coagulation studies. It indirectly measures the ability of the blood to clot, and directly measures a defect in Stage II of the clotting mechanism. The clotting abiliy of five plasma coagulation factors (prothrombin, fibrinogen, Factor V, Factor VII, and Factor X) is measured; this ability is referred to as the "prothrombin time." This test is commonly ordered in conjunction with the management of coumadin anticoagulant therapy.

Procedure

1. A venous sample of seven ml. is obtained prior to administering.

2. In the laboratory, a calcuim-binding anticoagulant (sodium citrate) is added to the sample.

Oral Anticoagulant Therapy—Oral anticoagulant drugs, such as coumadin and dicumarol (4-hydroxy-coumarin), commonly are used to treat blood clots. However, heparin is used first in treatment because it is rapid acting and also partially lyses the clot.

1. These drugs act in the liver to delay coagulation by interfering with the action of Vitamin K dependent factors (II, VII and X). Coumadin is an indirect anticoagulant; heparin is a direct anticoagulant.
2. Drug therapy delays coagulation, and causes the pro time to increase.
3. The usual procedure is to run a prothrombin time test every day; after the pro time is determined, the dosage of the anticoagulant is adjusted and administered.
4. Coumadin requires 16 to 48 hours to cause a measurable change in the pro time.

Drug Therapy and Pro Time Protocols

1. Cardiac patients usually are maintained at a pro time of 16 to 24 seconds or two to two and one-half times normal.
2. In the treatment of blood clots the pro time is maintained within the range of 28 to 40 seconds. If the pro time drops below 28 seconds, the treatment may be ineffective and old clots may expand or new clots may form. If the pro time rises above 40 seconds, hemorrhage may occur.

Clinical Implications

1. Conditions accompanied by an increased pro time include:
    (a.) Prothrombin deficiency
    (b.) Vitamin K deficiency
    (c.) Hemorrhagic disease of the newborn
    (d.) Liver disease (e.g., alcoholic hepatitis)
    (e.) Anticoagulant therapy
    (f.) Biliary obstruction
    (g.) Salicylate intoxication
    (h.) Hypervitaminosis A
    (i.) DIC disease

Interfering Factors

1. Diet: Excessive amounts of fatty foods will increase the body's absorption of Vitamin K.
2. Alcohol: Prothrombin time is increased due to liver disease.
3. Diarrhea and vomiting: These conditions will increase pro time.
4. Quality of venipuncture: It is important that a clean and careful venipuncture is done, otherwise the pro time can be shortened.
5. There are many drugs known to cause increases or decreases in prothrombin time. See appendix for a complete listing.

Patient Preparation

1. Explain the purpose and frequency of the test. Patients on long term anticoagulant therapy must understand the need for regular monitoring through frequent blood testing. *Do not refer to anticoagulants as "blood thinners."* One exploration might be: "Your blood will be tested periodically to determine the pro time, which is an indication of how quickly the blood clots." The dose of the anticoagulant will be increased, decreased, maintained, or discontinued on the basis of this test.
2. Caution the patient to avoid self-medication. Explain that many drugs, including medicines available without a prescription, can either increase or decrease the effect of the anticoagulants and alter the results of the test.
3. Instruct patient never to start or stop taking any drug without the doctor's permission, for this will affect the pro time.

CLINICAL ALERT

1. If prothrombin time is excessively prolonged (>40 seconds) Vitamin K is administered intramuscularly. Ordinarily intramuscular injections are contraindicated during anticoagulant therapy because large painful hematomas may form at the injection site. As values get into danger zones, assess carefully for bleeding, including: (a) craniotomy checks; (b) lung auscultation, especially of the upper lobes; (c) occult blood of the urine using Hemastix (a cellulose strip, impregnated with a peroxide and orthotolidine).

2. Patients who are being monitored by pro time for long-term anticoagulant therapy should not take any drugs unless absolutely necessary.

3. When unexpected changes in anticoagulant doses are required to maintain a stable pro time, or when there is a consistent change in pro time, a drug interaction should be suspected.

4. *Blood for pro time should be drawn for a base line and prior to administration of anticoagulants.*

5. Protamine sulfate is the antidote for heparin.

PLATELET COUNT

Normal Values

150,000–350,000/cu. mm.

Phase platelets—the normal value, also as above, can be slightly higher than, or the same as, the standard method. This is the preferred method.

Background

Platelets (or thrombocytes) are the smallest of the formed elements in the blood. These cells are non-nucleated, round or oval, flattened disk-shaped structures. Platelet activity is necessary for blood clotting.

A *deficiency of platelets leads to prolonged bleeding time or impaired clot retention.*

Functions of Platelets

1. Coagulation/clotting of blood
2. Vascular integrity and vasoconstriction
3. Adhesion and aggregation activity in the formation of a platelet plug that occludes (plugs) breaks in small vessels.

4. Ability to take up, store, transport, and release vasoactive serotonin, platelet factor III.
5. Clot retraction action

Platelet Formation

Platelet (thrombocyte) development takes place primarily in the bone marrow and possibly in the lungs. Thrombocytes are fragments of megakaryocytes, the largest of all bone marrow cells. The life span of a platelet is approximately 7.5 days. Normally, two thirds of all the body platelets are in the circulating blood and one third are in the spleen.

Explanation of Test

This test is indicated when the platelet count is below normal on a peripheral blood smear. This measurement is helpful in evaluating bleeding disorders that occur in liver disease, thrombocytopenia, uremia, and with anticoagulant therapy. The test is also used in following the course of diseases and disorders associated with bone marrow failure, as in leukemia, aplastic anemia, and the use of toxic drugs.

Other tests to study platelet function:
1. *Platelet count*—measures number of platelets.
2. *Clot retraction*—is a rough measurement of platelet function.
3. *Bleeding time*—measures number of platelets, adhesiveness, and platelet factor III content or release.
4. *Prothrombin consumption* test—detects a significant decrease of platelet factor III.
5. Special platelet function tests—such as platelet aggregation.

Procedure

A venous blood sample of seven ml. is obtained and an anticoagulant (EDTA) is added to the syringe.

Clinical Implications

1. Abnormally *increased* numbers of platelets (thrombocythemia/thrombocytosis) occur in:

(a.) Cancer
(b.) Chronic myelogenous and granulocytic leukemia
(c.) Polycythemia vera
(d.) Splenectomy
(e.) Trauma
(f.) Asphyxiation
(g.) Rheumatoid arthritis
(h.) Iron-deficiency and posthemorrhagic anemia
(i.) Acute infections
(j.) Heart disease
(k.) Cirrhosis
(l.) Chronic pancreatitis
(m.) Tuberculosis

In 50 per cent of those patients who exhibit an unexpected increase in platelets, a malignancy will be found. This malignancy is usually disseminated, advanced, or inoperable.

2. Abnormally decreased numbers of platelets (thrombocytopenia) occur in:
(a.) Idiopathic thrombocytopenic purpura
(b.) Pernicious, aplastic, and hemolytic anemias
(c.) After massive blood transfusion
(d.) Pneumonia
(e.) Allergic conditions
(f.) Exposure to DDT and other chemicals
(g.) During cancer chemotherapy
(h.) Infection
(i.) Lesions involving the bone marrow
(j.) Toxic effects of many drugs. Note: The dose of any drug does not have to be high to have a toxic effect. The development of toxic thrombocytopenia depends on the ability of the body to metabolize and secrete the toxic substance.

Drugs Known to Cause Toxic Thrombocytopenia (decrease in number of platelets):

1. Antineoplastic agents
2. Arsenobenzene
3. Arsphenamine
4. Benzene
5. Bismuth
6. Busulfan
7. Carbamazepine
8. Chloramphenicol

9. Chloroquine
10. Chlorothiazide
11. Chlorpropamide
12. Colchicine
13. DDT
14. Diazoxide
15. Diethylstilbestrol
16. Diphenylhydantoin
17. Gold
18. Heparin
19. Isoniazid
20. Mepazine
21. Mephenytoin
22. Meprobamate
23. Methotrexate
24. Oxyphenbutazone
25. Penicillins
26. Phenindione
27. Phenylbutazone
28. Potassium Perchlorate
29. Prednisone
30. Pyrazinamide
31. Ristocetin
32. Salicylamites
33. Stilbestrol
34. Streptomycin
35. Sulfamethoxazole
36. Sulfamethoxypyridazine
37. Sulfisoxazole
38. Sulfonal Ureas (Oral hypoglycemic agent)
39. Thioridazine
40. Thiourea
41. Tolbutamide

See appendix for listing of other drugs which may cause a decrease in the numbers of platelets.

3. A *decrease* in platelets of <20,000 cu. mm. may be associated with a tendency to:
   (a.) Spontaneous bleeding
   (b.) Prolonged bleeding time
   (c.) Petechiae
   (d.) Ecchymosis
   (e.) DIC disease
   (f.) Poor clot retraction

Note: The precise number of platelets necessary for hemostasis is not firmly established. Generally, platelet counts of greater than 50,000 cu. mm. are not associated with spontaneous bleeding. Those occasional patients with platelet counts in the 50,000 to 100,000 range will bleed excessively during surgical procedures.

Interfering Factors

1. Normally decreased first day of an infant's life
2. Normally increased at high altitudes
3. Normally increased after strenuous exercise and excitement

4. Normally increased in winter
5. Normally decreased before menstruation
Note: These physiologic variations in the number of platelets in the blood indicate the balance between their production and their utilization loss or destruction.

CLINICAL ALERT
Observe patients with serious platelet deficits for signs and symptoms of G.I. bleeding, hemolysis, hematuria, petechiae vaginal bleeding, epistasis, and bleeding from gums. When hemorrhage is apparent, use emergency measures to control bleeding and notify attending physician.

CLOT RETRACTION

Normal Values

After one hour the blood clot appreciably shrinks or retracts from the sides of the test tube and becomes more firm. The clot maintains its molded shape when it is removed from the container in which it has formed. Clot retraction is nearly complete in 4 hours and definitely completed in 24 hours. If clot retraction is normal and complete, approximately half the total volume is clot and the other half is serum.

Explanation of Test

This test is a rough measurement and is used to confirm a platelet problem such as thrombocytopenia.

In this test, blood is allowed to clot in a test tube without an anticoagulant. This test is based on the fact that whole blood that clots normally will retract or recede from the sides of its container resulting in the separation of transparent serum and the contracted blood clot. Since platelets play a major part in the mechanism of clot retraction, this reaction is impaired when platelets are decreased or function abnormally. This reaction is also influenced by the fibrinogen content of the plasma, the ratio of the plasma volume to red cell mass, and the activity of a retraction-promoting principle in the serum. Results are determined at 1 hour and at 24 hours.

Procedure

1. About five ml. of venous blood is collected in a tube without anticoagulant.
2. Clot begins separating from tube walls in 30 minutes to 1 hour; clot usually separated completely in 12 to 24 hours.
3. For 72 hours the retracted clot does not change appreciably.

Clinical Implications

1. There is a distinct parallel between the quality of the clot and the number of platelets.
   A defective clot is soft and soggy, is readily torn, and, after removal from its container, flattens out as a shapeless mass from which serum continues to ooze.
2. Poor or decreased clot retraction occurs in:
   (a.) Thrombocytopenia
   (b.) von Willebrand's disease when platelets are deficient in quality
   (c.) Disorders due to increase in red cell mass
3. Clot retraction appears to be increased in severe anemia and hypofibrinogenemia as a result of small clot formation occurring from an increase in plasma volume.

Interfering Factors

1. If the hematocrit is high because of polycythemia or hemo-contraction, clot retraction will be decreased.
2. In increased fibrinolysis the clot will lyse in 10 to 30 minutes, and it will appear that no retraction has taken place.

PROTHROMBIN CONSUMPTION TEST (PCT); SERUM PROTHROMBIN TIME

Normal Values

15 seconds or more, measured one hour after coagulation
>80 per cent consumed in one hour

Explanation of Test

In this test, a measurement is made of the prothrombin remaining in the serum after the coagulation of whole blood. After a clot has formed, 25 per cent or less of prothrombin should remain in the serum. A patient with a defect in Stage I will not convert as much prothrombin to thrombin in coagulation; thus, a great deal of prothrombin may be left in the serum.

The PCT is used to diagnose a defect in the clotting mechanism. This measurement, also called Serum Prothrombin Time, is one of the most accurate tests used to detect Stage I deficiencies. The outstanding advantage of PCT is its sensitivity to a clinically significant decrease of platelet factor III.

Procedure

A venous blood sample of seven ml. is obtained. No anticoagulant is added to the syringe.

Clinical Implications

1. The more prolonged the PCT, the better the coagulation mechanism is functioning.
2. A shortened PCT indicates a deficiency of platelets and factors which are necessary for production of thromboplastin and may indicate the presence of anticoagulants. Shortened PCT is probably due to a deficiency of any one of the factors required in Stages I and II of coagulation (a pro time is done in conjunction with PCT for Stage II).
3. Because normal platelet function is necessary for the generation of plasma thromboplastin, there is no point in doing a PCT when thrombocytopenia is present.
4. A shortened PCT may be associated with the following:
   - (a.) Circulating anticoagulants
   - (b.) Hemophilias
   - (c.) Hypoprothrombinemia
   - (d.) Thrombocytopenia
   - (e.) Thrombocytopathies
   - (f.) DIC disease

Interfering Factors

Hemolysis of red cells due to excessive suction in drawing the blood, or in rough handling of the blood, can give results over 35 seconds.

REFERENCES

Austen, D. E. G., and Rhymes, I. L.: A LABORATORY MANUAL OF BLOOD COAGULATION. Oxford, Blackwell Scientific Publications, 1975.

Bauer, John D., Ackerman, Philip G., and Toro, Gelson: CLINICAL LABORATORY METHODS. 8th Ed., St. Louis, The C. V. Mosby Company, 1974.

Berkow, Robert (ed.): THE MERCK MANUAL OF DIAGNOSIS AND THERAPY. 13th Ed., Rahway, N.J., Merck Sharpe & Dohme Research Laboratories, 1977.

Collins, R. Douglas: ILLUSTRATED MANUAL OF LABORATORY DIAGNOSIS. 2nd Ed., Philadelphia, J. B. Lippincott Company, 1975.

Davidson, I., and Henry, J. B. (eds.): TODD-SANFORD CLINICAL DIAGNOSIS BY LABORATORY METHODS. 15th Ed., Philadelphia, W. B. Saunders Company, 1974.

Desforges, Jane F., and Merritt, John A.: DIAGNOSTIC PROCEDURES IN HEMATOLOGY. Chicago, Year Book Medical Publishers, Inc., 1971.

Frankel, S., and Reitman, S.: CLINICAL LABORATORY METHODS AND DIAGNOSIS, A TEXTBOOK ON LABORATORY PROCEDURES AND THEIR INTERPRETATION. St. Louis, The C. V. Mosby Company, 1974.

French, Ruth M.: GUIDE TO DIAGNOSTIC PROCEDURES. 4th Ed., New York, McGraw-Hill Book Company, 1975.

Garb, Solomon: LABORATORY TEST IN COMMON USE. 6th Ed., New York, Springer Publishing Company, 1976.

Linman, James W.: HEMATOLOGY: PHYSIOLOGIC, PATHOPHYSIOLOGIC AND CLINICAL PRINCIPLES. New York, Macmillan Publishing Company, 1975.

Meyer, John S., et al.: REVIEW OF LABORATORY MEDICINE. 2nd Ed., St. Louis, C. V. Mosby Company, 1975.

Pamahac, Patricia: LABORATORY METHODS IN CLINICAL SEROLOGY. Milwaukee County General Hospital, 1976. (Unpublished)

Platt, William R.: COLOR ATLAS AND TEXTBOOK OF HEMA-
    TOLOGY. Philadelphia, J. B. Lippincott Company, 1979.
Poller, L. (ed.): RESEARCH ADVANCES IN BLOOD COAGULA-
    TION. No. 2. Edinburgh, Churchill Livingstone, 1977.
Semrad, Alice M. (ed.): COMPREHENSIVE REVIEW FOR MEDI-
    CAL TECHNOLOGISTS. St. Louis, C. V. Mosby Company,
    1975.
Tilkian, S. M., Conover, M. H., and Tilkian, A. G.: CLINICAL IM-
    PLICATIONS OF LABORATORY TESTS. 2nd Ed., St. Louis,
    C. V. Mosby Company, 1979.
Wallach, Jacques: INTERPRETATION OF DIAGNOSTIC TESTS
    —A HANDBOOK SYNOPSIS OF LABORATORY MEDI-
    CINE. 3rd Ed., Boston, Little, Brown and Company, 1978.
Weed, Robert I. (ed.): HEMATOLOGY FOR INTERNISTS. 7th Ed.,
    Boston, Little, Brown and Company, 1971.
Zuck, Thomas F. (ed.): HUMAN HEMOSTASIS—1975. Washington,
    D.C., American Association of Blood Banks, 1975.

2 □□ URINALYSIS

INTRODUCTION

Overview of Urine Formation

Urine, a very complex fluid, is composed of 95 per cent water and five per cent solids. It is the end product of the metabolism carried out by billions of cells, resulting in an average urinary output of one to one and one half liters (approximately 1.5 qts.) per day (less in summer; more in winter).

The formation of urine takes place in the kidneys, the two small fist-sized organs located outside the peritoneal cavity on each side of the spine at about the level of the last thoracic and upper two lumbar vertebrae. The kidneys, along with the skin and respiratory system, are the chief excretory organs of the body. Each kidney is a highly discriminating organ which maintains the internal environment by selectively excreting or retaining various substances according to specific body needs. The importance of urine formation and excretion as a regulating function is profoundly emphasized in situations in which kidney function is suddenly lost. Under these circumstances, death occurs within a few days.

The main functional unit of the kidney is the nephron. There are about one million nephrons per kidney, each composed of two main parts: a glomerulus, which is essentially a filtering system, and a tubule through which the filtered liquid passes. Each glomerulus consists of a capillary network surrounded by a membrane called Bowman's capsule, which continues on to form the beginning of the renal tubule. The afferent arteriole carries blood from the renal artery into the glomerulus, where it divides to form a capillary network. These capillaries reunite to form the efferent arteriole through which blood leaves the glomerulus. The blood vessels then follow the course of the tubule, forming a surrounding capillary network.

There is a tremendous blood flow through the kidneys. It is believed that 25 per cent of the blood from the left heart passes through the kidneys. One liter of urine can be thought of as the end result of more than 1000 liters of blood passing through the kidneys. The blood enters the glomerulus of each nephron by passing through the afferent arteriole into the glomerular capillaries.

Urine formation begins in the glomerular capillaries, with dissolved substances passing into the proximal tubule as a result of the force of blood pressure in the large afferent arteriole and the pressure in Bowman's capsule. As the filtrate passes along the tubule, more solutes are added by excretion from the capillary blood and secretions from the tubular epithelial cells. Solutes and water pass back into the blood by tubular reabsorption. Urine concentration and dilution take place in the renal medulla. The kidney has the remarkable ability to produce dilute or concentrated urine according to the needs of the individual and to regulate sodium excretion. Blood chemistry, blood pressure, fluid balance, nutrient intake, and state of health are key elements in metabolism. They are also key elements in establishing the character of urine.

Urine contains thousands of dissolved substances, although the three principal constituents are water, urea, and sodium chloride. More solids are excreted from the body in the urine than by any other method. Its composition depends greatly on the quality and the quantity of the excreted waste material. Some constituents of the blood such as glucose have a renal threshold; that is, a certain elevated level must be reached in the blood before this constituent will be excreted in the urine. Almost all substances found in the urine are also found in the blood, although in different concentrations. Urea, for example, is present in the blood, but at a much lower concentration than in the excreted urine.

URINE TESTING

Urinalysis is an essential procedure for hospital admissions and physical examinations. It is one of the most useful indicators of health and disease, and it is especially helpful in the detection of renal or metabolic disorders. It is an aid in diagnosing and following the course of treatment in diseases of the kidney and urinary system, and in detecting disorders in other parts of the body such as metabolic or endocrinic abnormalities in which the kidneys function normally.

Laboratory Testing

In the laboratory, urinalysis is carried out by an instrument which is designed to test and record the levels of specific substances in urine, (glucose, protein, ketones, bilirubin, occult blood, pH), as well as its specific gravity. Fifty specimens may be loaded for testing at one time. Analysis results are automatically printed so that the data obtained can be fed directly into a computer.

Dipsticks

While laboratory facilities allow for a wide range of urine tests, modern tablets, tapes, and dipstick tests are available for urinalysis. These devices are useful because they do not require a laboratory and can be read directly by patients as well as by clinicians, physicians, and technologists.

Dipsticks, similar in appearance to blotter paper, are actually miniature laboratories. These chemically impregnated reagent (reactive) strips allow for quick determination of the following properties of urine: pH, protein, glucose, ketones, bilirubin, hemoglobin (blood), nitrite, urobilinogen. The tip of the dipstick is impregnated with chemicals which react with specific substances in the urine to produce colored end products. In some tests, the depth of color produced is related to the concentration of the substance in the urine. Color standards are provided against which the color can be compared. The reaction rates of the impregnated chemicals are standard for each dipstick, and color changes must be matched at the correct time after each stick is dipped into the urine specimen. These matching methods are included in the instructions which accompany each type of dipstick. When more than one reaction is arranged on a single stick, (e.g., pH, protein, glucose), the chemical reagents for each test are separated by a water permeable barrier made of plastic.

In addition to dipsticks there are other reagent strips, chemical tablets and treated slides for special determinations such as bacteria, PKU, mucopolysaccharide, salicylate, and cystinuria.

Procedure

1. Use fresh urine.
2. Dip reagent strip in urine, remove, and compare each reagent area with the corresponding color chart on the bottle label at the number of seconds specified on bottle (*i.e.*, 30 seconds).

Interfering Factors

1. If dipsticks are kept too long in the urine or urine stream, the chemicals impregnated in the cellulose may be overly dissolved resulting in an inaccurate reading.

2. When not in use, the container for the tablets, tapes, or dipsticks should be tightly closed to keep the reagents dry. If the dipsticks, tapes, or tablets absorb moisture from the air before they are used, they will not give correct results.

3. Certain drugs give false positive reactions. (See individual tests).

TYPES OF URINE SPECIMENS

During the course of 24 hours, the composition of urine continuously changes. For this reason, various types of urine specimens are collected for urinalysis:

Single, random specimen
Timed, short-term specimen
Timed, long-term specimen (12 or 24 hours)

SINGLE, RANDOM SPECIMEN

Most testing is done on a random specimen of urine freshly voided by the patient. Since the composition of urine changes over the course of the day, the time of day when the specimen is collected may influence the findings. The first voided morning specimen is particularly valuable, for it is usually concentrated and more likely to reveal abnormalities and formed substances. Since the chemical testing involved in urinalysis measures the concentration of substances, the results will vary whether or not the urine is dilute. Significant abnormalities will be missed in dilute urine which is collected during the day. Morning specimens are also relatively free of dietary influences since they are collected after a period of fasting.

Procedure

1. Patient is instructed to void directly into a clean, dry container or into a clean, dry bedpan and then transfer the specimen directly into an appropriate container.

2. Specimens from infants and young children can be collected in a disposable collection apparatus consisting of a plastic bag with an adhesive backing around the opening

to fasten it to the child so that voiding is done directly into the bag.

3. All specimens should be covered and sent immediately to the laboratory.
4. If a urine specimen is likely to be contaminated with vaginal discharge or menstrual blood, then a clean specimen must be obtained using the same procedure for bacteriologic examination (page 354).

Interfering Factors

1. Glycosuria appears more often after meals.
2. Proteinuria may occur following activity or upon assuming an upright position.
3. Hemoglobin may appear in the urine following exertion.
4. In urinary infections the number of bacteria in the urine varies during the day.
5. Feces, vaginal secretion, and menstrual fluid can contaminate specimen.
6. If specimen is kept unrefrigerated for more than one hour before analysis, changes in the constitution of the urine may occur:
   (a) Bacteria in the urine "split" the urea, converting it to ammonia and producing an alkaline urine.
   (b) Casts decompose in urine after several hours.
   (c) Red blood cells are lysed by hypotonic urine.
   (d) Marked changes in pH may affect cellular components.

CLINICAL ALERT
1. If specimen is kept for more than one hour before analysis, it should be refrigerated to avoid changes in the urine.
2. If specimen is contaminated by feces or vaginal discharge, a clean voided specimen must be obtained.

TIMED, LONG-TERM SPECIMEN (24 HOURS)

Explanation of Test

Some diseases or conditions require that a 24-hour urine specimen be collected in order to truly and accurately evaluate kidney function. Substances excreted by the kidney are not excreted at the same rate or in the same amounts during various periods of the day and night. Therefore, a random urine specimen would not give an accurate picture of the processes taking place. For measurement of total urine protein, creatinine, electrolytes, etc., more accurate information is obtained from urine collected over a 24-hour period. This involves collecting the specimen in a suitable receptacle and either adding a preservative to it or keeping it refrigerated.

Procedure

1. At the beginning of the collection of a 24-hour timed urine specimen (or any timed specimen), the patient is asked to void, the specimen is *discarded,* and the time noted.
2. The time the test begins is placed on the label along with the time the collection should end.
3. All urine passed over the next 24 hours is collected in a large container (usually made of polyethylene), labeled with the patient's name and marked for the particular test ordered. It is not necessary to measure urine unless explicitly stated for individual tests.
4. To conclude the collection, the patient must void 24 hours after the first voiding. Urine from this last voiding must be added to the specimen in the container.

    NOTE: Since the patient may not always be able to void on command, a last specimen should be obtained as close as possible to the stated end of time for the next test and the exact time marked on the bottle.
5. Storage:
    (a) In the hospital, nonrefrigerated tests may be kept in a soiled utility room or in the patient's bathroom.
    (b) If refrigeration is necessary, the urine specimen must be refrigerated immediately after the patient has voided.

Clinical Implications

1. Responsibility for the collection of urine specimen should be assigned to a specific person.

2. All persons instructing a patient about 24-hour urine collections should make certain that the patient understands that he must void and empty his bladder at the time the 24-hour collection is to start and that this specimen is to be discarded.
3. Do not predate and pretime the laboratory slips, for it is rare for patients to urinate on the hour.
4. It cannot be stressed enough that the marking of exact time is crucial and that it is not important whether this is 15 or 30 minutes more or less than 24 hours, provided the information is accurate.
5. The patient should be reminded to try to urinate near the end of the collection period.
6. Whenever a preservative has to be used (such as the hydrochloric acid preservative used for 24-hour urine collection of VMA), the patient should be warned to take precautions against spilling any liquid from the container.
7. Patients who are using bedpans should be instructed to void before having a bowel movement. Otherwise they may forget and urinate into the pan while having a bowel movement, thus spoiling the urine collection.

Interfering Factors

1. Failure of the patient or attending personnel to comprehend the procedure is the most common source of error.
2. Toilet paper in collection container may decrease the actual amount of urine saved or possibly contaminate the specimen in some way.
3. Feces in collection container also may contaminate the specimen. For this reason, patients who are using bedpans should be instructed to void before having a bowel movement.

Patient Preparation

Most 24-hour urine specimens are started in the morning.
1. Empty bladder completely on awakening in the morning and discard this urine specimen. Record the time the discarded specimen was voided (7:08 A.M.), and begin the test (7:08 A.M.).

2. Save all urine passed during the rest of the day and night. Also save the first specimen of urine passed the next morning.
3. The bedpan, urinal, or the collection bottle itself, can be used for each voiding.
4. It is most important that ALL urine be saved and placed in the container. Ideally, the container should be stored in the refrigerator.
5. Test results are calculated on the basis of a 24-hour output and unless all urine is saved, results will not be accurate. (This is particularly important, for this test is expensive, complicated, and necessary for the evaluation and treatment of the patient's condition.)
6. The urine voided the next morning (as close to 7:00 A.M. as possible) is added to the collection container, and the 24-hour test is terminated. Write down the time of this last voiding.

ROUTINE URINALYSIS AND RELATED TESTS

Normal Values

General Characteristics and Measurements	Chemical Determinations	Microscopic Examination of Sediment
Color—yellow—amber— indicates a high specific gravity and small output of urine. Turbidity—clear Specific gravity—1.015–1.025 with a normal fluid intake pH—4.6–8—average person has a pH of about 6. (acid)	Glucose—negative Ketones—negative Blood—negative Protein—negative Bile-Bilirubin— negative	Casts negative—occasional hyaline casts Red Blood Cells negative Crystals negative White Blood Cells negative

Explanation of Test

Urinalysis is the means of determining the various properties of urine: color, odor, turbidity, specific gravity, pH, glucose, ketones, blood, protein, and bile as well as any abnormal constituents revealed by microscopic examination of the sediment.

A 10 ml. urine specimen is usually sufficient for conducting these tests.

SPECIFIC GRAVITY

Normal Values

1.003–1.035 (usually between 1.010 and 1.025)
1.025–1.030 + (concentrated urine)
1.001–1.010 (dilute urine)

Explanation of Test

Specific gravity is a means by which the kidney's ability to concentrate urine is measured. The test is conducted by comparing the weight of urine against the weight of distilled water, which has a specific gravity of 1.000. Since urine is a solution of minerals, salts, and compounds dissolved in water, the specific gravity is obviously greater than 1.000. The relative difference between the specific gravity and the specific gravity of urine reflects the degree of concentration of the urine specimen.

The range of urine specific gravity depends upon the state of hydration and varies with urine volume and the load of solids to be excreted. When fluid intake is restricted or increased, under standardized conditions, specific gravity measures the concentrating and diluting abilities of the kidney. Loss of these capacities is an indication of renal dysfunction.

Procedure

1. Urinometer

   Specific gravity is most frequently determined with a urinometer. This is a weighted instrument that contains a scale calibrated in specific gravity readings. The instrument is floated in a cylinder containing the urine specimen. The concentration of the urine will affect the degree to which the urinometer will float. The depth to which it sinks in the urine indicates the specific gravity.

2. Specimen collection
  (a) For regular urinalysis testing a random specimen is used.
  (b) When evaluation of specific gravity is ordered separately from the urinalysis, the patient should fast for 12 hours prior to the time the specimen is collected.

Clinical Implications

A. *Normal*
  Specific gravity varies inversely with urine excretion (decrease in volume; increase in specific gravity).
    Examples of conditions in which this relationship is affected:
    (a) Diabetes: increased volume; increased specific gravity
    (b) Hypertension: normal volume; decreased specific gravity
    (c) Early chronic renal disease: increased volume; decreased specific gravity
B. *Low Specific Gravity* (1.001–1.003)
    1. Diabetes insipidus
      (a) Low specific gravity and large urine volume
      (b) Due to absence of antidiuretic hormone (ADH)
          ADH triggers kidney absorption of water; without it kidneys produce excessive amounts of urine (sometimes 15–20 liters a day).
    2. Glomerulonephritis and pyelonephritis
      (a) Tubular damage affects kidney's ability to concentrate urine.
      (b) Decreased volume, low specific gravity
    3. Severe renal damage
        Fixed low specific gravity (1.010) which varies little from specimen to specimen.
C. *Increased Specific Gravity*
    1. Diabetes mellitus or nephrosis
        Abnormally large amounts of glucose and protein increase the specific gravity up to 1.050.
    2. Occurs in instances of excessive water loss (fever, vomiting, diarrhea).

Interfering Factors

1. Specific gravity is highest in the first morning specimen.
2. Specific gravity is elevated whenever there is an excessive loss of water. This may occur in:
   (a) Sweating
   (b) Fever
   (c) Vomiting
   (d) Diarrhea
3. Drugs causing false positive elevation
   (a) Dextran
   (b) Radiopaque contrast media used in x–rays of urinary tract.

CONCENTRATION

Normal Values

Methods of Concentration Testing:

Fishberg test—1:024 or higher on one specimen and up to 300 ml. of urine.

Vohhard—1.025 or higher-osmolality showed rise above 800 in osmolality, on at least one specimen in the afternoon.

Mosenthal—1.020 There must be at least a seven point difference between the lowest and highest specific gravity.

Explanation of Test

This test is carried out in patients with suspected renal disease and measures the kidneys' ability to concentrate urine after liquids have been withheld from the diet for a number of hours. The goal of the test is to see if the kidneys can produce urine with a specific gravity greater than 1.010.

In health, specific gravity normally ranges from 1.003 to 1.035 or higher. When fluids are restricted in accordance with this test, the urine produced is more concentrated and has a specific gravity higher than 1.020 to 1.025. Kidney dysfunction can result in *isosthenuria* (urine specific gravity remains consistently at 1.010) or *hyposthenuria* (urine specific gravity is less than 1.008). Whenever a more precise measurement is indicated, osmolality of urine can be determined. Osmolality is a measure of the number of particles in a given weight.

Procedure

A. *Pretest Preparation*
   1. All diuretics should be stopped 48 to 72 hours prior to the test and during the test.
   2. An adequate protein diet and normal hydration should be taken for three days before the test.
   3. No medications should be given.
B. *Test Procedure*
   1. The test begins at 6:00 P.M., after which time no fluids are permitted until the test is completed ("Dry" foods are permitted).
   2. At 10:00 P.M., the patient voids, *discards* the specimen, and may retire.
   3. The next morning, urine specimens are collected at 6:00 A.M., 7:00 A.M., and 8:00 A.M. Keep specimens separate. (Normally, kidneys concentrate urine at twice the rate during the night than during waking hours). If patient voids during the night, save this urine and send to laboratory in a separate labeled container.
   4. The volume of each urine specimen and the total volume of all three specimens are measured and recorded.
   5. The specific gravity or osmolality (see p. 193) of each specimen is measured.

Clinical Implications

1. A specific gravity of less than 1.020 on all specimens indicates renal disease. With severe involvement the specific gravity is persistently 1.010 or less.
   (a) Total loss of urinary concentrating ability with fixed specific gravity near 1:010 or osmolality between 300

and 400 mosm per mg. is not seen until very late in the course of renal disease.

(b) Abnormal concentration levels generally reflect progressive inability of kidneys to increase the osmotic pressure of urine above that of the glomerular filtrate in chronic renal failure.

2. A normal finding does not necessarily rule out active kidney disease.
3. A specific gravity of 1.020 occurs in:
    (a) Potassium deficiency
    (b) Hypercalcemia due to sarcoidosis
    (c) Bone disease (multiple myeloma; vitamin D intoxication or sensitivity)
    (d) Hyperparathyroidism
    (e) Renal parenchymal disease, such as pyelonephritis, which damages the tubules
    (f) Acute renal disease
2. The urine may be abnormally concentrated for a day or so after injection of dyes used in intravenous pyelograms (IVP).
3. Edema, sweats, diarrhea, and fever interfere with the water tests.
4. Concentration tests are meaningless in patients taking diuretics.
5. Patients who have been markedly overhydrated for several days prior to testing may have impaired concentration if dehydration is then imposed.

Interfering Factors

1. The test is unreliable when patient is pregnant, is on low salt or protein diets, or suffers from severe water or electrolyte imbalance, chronic liver disease, edema from renal disease, or heart failure. In these conditions the tubules may be unable to concentrate urine.

Patient Preparation

1. Explain the purpose and procedure of the test to the patient.
2. Instruct the patient to completely empty his bladder at each voiding.

CLINICAL ALERT
1. The fluid deprivation required in this test may be contraindicated in some patients with heart disease or early renal failure.
2. Accidental or deliberate fluid intake during the night will interfere with the results. Reschedule test if this occurs.

COLOR

Normal Values

Yellow is the normal color of urine. The specific gravity ranges from 1.011 to 1.019 and the urine output is one to one and a half liters per day.

Straw colored urine is normal and indicates a low specific gravity, usually under 1.010. (The exception is a patient with a 4+ sugar; urine is very light, looks like water, but the specific gravity is high.)

Amber colored urine is normal and indicates a low specific gravity and a small output of urine. Specific gravity is above 1.020 and output less than one liter per day.

Explanation of Test

Urine specimens may vary in color from pale yellow to dark amber. The intensity of the normal amber color may be directly related to the concentration or specific gravity of the urine. The color of normal urine is primarily due to urochrome (pigments which are present in the diet or formed from the metabolism of bile). Due to the presence of abnormal pigments, the color of urine changes in many disease states.

Procedure

Observe color of urine specimen.

Clinical Implications

1. A nearly *colorless* urine may be due to:
   - (a) Large fluid intake
   - (b) Reduction in perspiration
   - (c) Chronic interstitial nephritis
   - (d) Untreated diabetes mellitus
   - (e) Diabetes insipidus
   - (f) Alcohol ingestion
   - (g) Diuretic therapy
   - (h) Nervousness
2. An *orange-colored* urine may be due to:
   - (a) Concentrated urine
   - (b) Restricted fluid intake
   - (c) Excess sweating
   - (d) Fever
   - (e) Small quantities of bile pigment
3. A *brownish-yellow or greenish-yellow* color may indicate bilirubin in the urine.
   - (a) However, not all dark urines contain bilirubin.
   - (b) Stale urine containing bilirubin may be green due to an oxidation of the bilirubin to biliverdin.
   - (c) Bilirubin crystals in the sediment may cause the urine to have an opalescent appearance.
   - (d) *Yellow foam* may be due to biliverdin bile pigment.
   - (e) *Green foam* may be due to biliverdin bile pigment.
4. A *red or reddish dark brown* color may indicate hemoglobinuria and be due to blood, porphyrins, hemoglobin, myoglobin.
5. A *port wine* color may be due to porphyrins or a mixture of methemoglobin and oxyhemoglobin.
6. *Dark brown* urine may be due to porphyrias, melanin.
   - (a) May indicate a melanotic tumor.
   - (b) Dark urine is sometimes associated with Addison's disease.
7. *Brown-black* urine may be due to a great deal of hemoglobin, lysol poisoning, or melanin.
8. *Black* urine results from alkaptonuria, a disease of tyrosine metabolism, which causes the urine to turn black on standing.
9. *Smoky* color may be due to red blood cells.

Interfering Factors

1. The color of normal urine darkens on standing. This is due to the oxidation of urobilinogen to urobilin.
2. Some foods cause the urine to change color.
   (a) Beets will turn the urine *red.*
   (b) Rhubarb can cause color to be *brown.*
3. Many drugs cause the urine to change color.
   (a) Cascara and senna laxatives in acid urine will turn the urine *reddish-brown;* in alkaline urine it will turn the urine *red.*
   (b) *Orange* may be due to phenazopyridine (Pyridium), amidopyrine.
   (c) *Orange to orange-red* may be due to Pyridium, ethoxazene.
   (d) *Orange to purple-red* may be due to chlorzoxazone.
   (e) *Orange-yellow* in alkaline urine may be due to salicylazosulfapyridine, anisindione, or phenindione.
   (f) *Rust-yellow to brownish* may be due to sulfonamides, nitrofurantoins.
   (g) *Pink to red or red-brown* may be due to Dilantin (diphenylhydantoin), Doxidan (Dioctyl Calcium Sulfosuccinate), Ex-lax (phenolphthalein) and Phenothiazine (thiodiphenylamine).
   (h) *Magenta* may be due to Ex-lax.
   (i) *Red* may be due to amidopyrine, Pyridium, Neotropin, prontosil, aniline dyes, PSP and BSP dyes in alkaline urine, phenolphthalein and Pyridium in acid urine, or Desferal (deferoxamine)
   (j) *Purple-red* may be due to Ex-lax in alkaline urine.
   (k) *Dark-brown* may be due to phenolic drugs, phenylhydrazine.
   (l) *Brown-black* may be due to Jecotofer, cascara.
   (m) *Bright yellow* may be due to riboflavin or Pyridium in alkaline urine.
   (n) *Blue or green* may be due to methyline blue and amitriptyline.
   (o) Urine that *darkens* on standing may be due to anti-Parkinsonian agents such as Levodopa or Sinemet.
   (p) *Dark-colored* urine may be due to iron salts.
   (q) *Pink* to *brown* may be due to phenothiazine tranquilizer.
   (r) *Pale blue* may be due to Pyrenium (triamterene).

ODOR

The characteristic odor of normal, freshly voided urine is due to the presence of volatile acids.

Normal Values

Fresh urine from most healthy persons has an aromatic odor.

Clinical Implications

1. The sweet smell of acetone can be recognized in diabetic ketosis.
2. Heavily infected urine has a particularly unpleasant odor.
3. An inherited disorder of amino acid metabolism is characterized by the passage of urine in infants that smells like maple syrup. This condition is maple sugar urine disease.

Interfering Factors

1. Some foods such as asparagus, produce characteristic odors.
2. After urine stands for a long time, ammonia with its characteristic pungent odor, is formed by bacterial activity and the decomposition of urea in the specimen.

pH

Normal Values

Average range: 4.6 to 8
Average pH is about 6 (acid)
(The pH of normal urine can vary widely.)

Background

The symbol "pH" expresses the exact strength of the urine as a dilute acid or a base solution and measures the free hydrogen ion (H^+) concentration in the urine. (The lower the pH, the greater the acidity). pH, therefore, is an indication of the renal tubules' ability to maintain normal hydrogen ion concentration in the plasma and extra-cellular fluid. The kidneys maintain normal acid-base balance primarily through the reabsorption of sodium and the tubular secretion of hydrogen and ammonium in exchange. Secretion of an acid or alkaline urine by the kidneys is one of the most important mechanisms of the body for maintaining a constant body pH.

Urine becomes increasingly acidic as the amount of sodium and excess acid retained by the body increases. Alkaline urine, usually containing bicarbonate-carbonic acid buffer, is normally excreted when there is an excess of base or alkali in the body.

Ingestion of different foods and soda bicarbonate also affects the urinary pH. The usual diet, rich in animal protein, produces an acid urine (pH less than 7).

Control of pH

Control of urinary pH is important in the management of several diseases including bacteriuria and renal calculi, and in drug therapy in which streptomycin or Mandelamine (methenamine mandelate) is administered.

A. *Renal Calculi*

   Renal stone formation is partially dependent on the pH of urine. Patients being treated for renal calculi are frequently given diets or medication to change the pH of the urine so kidney stones will not form.

   1. Calcium phosphate, calcium carbonate, and magnesium phosphate stones develop in alkaline urine. In such instances the urine must be kept acid.

   2. Uric acid, cystine and calcium oxalate stones precipitate in acid urines. In the treatment of these urinary calculi, the urine should be kept alkaline.

B. *Drug Treatment*

   1. Streptomycin, neomycin, and kanamycin are effective in genitourinary tract infections provided the urine is *alkaline.*

2. During sulfa therapy, an *alkaline* urine should help prevent formation of sulfonamide crystals.
3. Urine should also be kept persistently *alkaline* in control of salicylate intoxication (excretion is enhanced) and during blood transfusions.

C. *Clinical Conditions*
1. The urine should be kept *acid* in the treatment of urinary tract infections and persistent bacteriuria and in the management of those urinary calculi which develop in alkaline urine.

D. *Diet*
1. A diet, with an emphasis on citrus fruits and most vegetables, particularly legumes, will help keep the urine alkaline.
2. A diet high in meat and cranberry juice will keep the urine acid.

Explanation of Test

Urine pH is an important screening test for diagnosing renal disease, respiratory disease, and certain metabolic disorders. It is also used to monitor specific programs of medication or diet when it is desirable to maintain the urine as acid or alkaline. Keeping the urine at a consistently high or low pH requires frequent testing of the urinary pH.

A. *Laboratory Measurement*
Measurement of urine pH is done in the laboratory by electronic techniques utilizing a pH meter.

B. *Dipstick Measurement*
1. Multiple reagent strips treated with chemicals provide a spectrum of color changes from orange to green-blue in the pH range of 5 to 9.
2. The dipstick is dipped into a urine specimen and the color change is compared to a standardized color chart on the bottle.

Clinical Implications

A. *If urine pH is to be useful, it is necessary to use the pH information in conjunction with other information.* For example, in renal tubular necrosis, the kidney is not able to excrete a urine that is strongly acid. Therefore, if a urine pH of 5 (quite acid) is measured, renal tubular acidosis is eliminated as a possibility.

B. *Acid Urine* (pH less than 7)
   1. Found in acidosis, uncontrolled diabetes, pulmonary emphysema, diarrhea, starvation, dehydration
   2. Rarely excreted in severe alkalosis
   3. Found in respiratory diseases where CO_2 retention occurs and acidosis develops

C. *Alkaline Urine* (pH more than 7)
   1. Found in urinary tract infections, pyloric obstruction, salicylate intoxications, renal tubular acidosis, and chronic renal failure
   2. Rarely excreted during severe acidosis
   3. Found in respiratory diseases involving hyperventilation and loss of CO_2 with alkalosis

Interfering Factors

1. On standing, the pH of urine specimens will become alkaline because CO_2 will diffuse into the air.
2. Alkaline urine specimens tend to cause hemolysis of red cells and the disappearance of casts.
3. High protein diets will cause excessively acid urine (pH less than 6).
4. Ammonium chloride and mandelic acid may produce acid urines.
5. Alkaline urine after meals is a normal response to the secretions of HCl acid in gastric juices.
6. Sodium bicarbonate, potassium citrate, and acetozolamide may produce alkaline urines.

CLINICAL ALERT
1. An accurate measurement of urinary pH can only be done on a fresh voided specimen. If the urine must be kept for any length of time before analysis, it should be refrigerated.
2. Alkaline urine occurs from vegetarian diets, citrus fruits, milk, and other dairy products.
3. Highly concentrated urine such as that formed in hot, dry environments is strongly acidic and may be irritating.

4. During sleep, decreased pulmonary ventilation causes respiratory acidosis, and urine becomes highly acid.
5. Chlorothiazide diuretic administration will cause an acid urine to be excreted.
6. Bacteria in urinary tract infection or bacterial contamination of the specimen will result in an alkaline urine. Bacteria in the urine will convert urea to ammonia.

TURBIDITY

Normal Values

Fresh urine is clear.

Explanation of Test

The appearance of cloudy urine provides a warning of possible abnormality such as the presence of pus, red blood cells, or bacteria. However, excretion of cloudy urine may not be abnormal since the change in urine pH may cause precipitation within the bladder of normal urinary constituents. Alkaline urine may appear cloudy because of the presence of phosphates, and cloudy acid urine because of urates.

Procedure

Observe the appearance of a fresh urine sample.

Clinical Implications

1. Pathologic urines are often turbid or cloudy, but so are many normal urines.
   Cloudy urine may result from precipitation of crystals due to rapid cooling of the urine.
2. Occasionally, urine turbidity may result from urinary tract infections.
3. Abnormal urines may be cloudy due to the presence of red blood cells, white blood cells, or bacteria.

Interfering Factors

1. After ingestion of food, urates or phosphates may produce cloudiness in normal urine.
2. Vaginal contamination from female patients is a common cause of turbidity.
3. "Greasy" cloudiness may be caused by large amounts of fat.
4. Many normal urines will develop a haze or turbidity after refrigeration or standing at room temperature.

BLOOD OR HEMOGLOBIN (HEME)

Normal Values

Negative

Explanation of Test

Blood in the urine is usually occult blood which has been hemolyzed or dissolved. Hemoglobin or red blood cells in the urine are not likely to be identified by the naked eye when there is less than one part of the blood per 1,000 parts of urine.

The presence of blood in the urine is referred to as *hemoglobinuria*. Hemoglobinuria is usually related to conditions outside the urinary tract and occurs when there is such extensive or rapid destruction (hemolysis) of circulating erythrocytes that the reticuloendothelial system cannot metabolize or store the excessive amounts of free hemoglobin.

When red blood cells or RBC casts are present in the urine, the term *hematuria* is used to indicate bleeding somewhere in the urinary tract. Usually both red blood cells and hemoglobin mark this disorder. Therefore, hematuria can be distinguished from hemoglobinuria by a microscopic examination of the sediment from a fresh urine specimen.

When urine gives a positive result for occult blood, but no red blood cells are seen in a microscopic examination of the sediment, *myoglobinuria* can be suspected. Myoglobinuria is the excretion of myoglobin, a muscle protein, into the urine as a result of (1) traumatic muscle injury such as may occur in automobile accidents, football injuries, or electric shock, (2) a muscle disorder such as an arterial occlusion to a muscle or muscular dystrophy, or (3) certain kinds of poisoning, such as carbon monoxide or fish poisoning.

Both hemoglobinuria and myoglobinuria are injurious to the kidney and can result in acute renal failure.

Procedure

A. *Hemoglobin in urine*
   1. Special chemically treated paper strips are dipped into the urine and the color change on the dipstick noted.
   2. The color of the strip is compared with a color chart.
   3. The color blocks indicate negative, small, moderate, and large amounts of hemoglobin.
B. *Hematuria*
   To identify red blood cells the urine is centrifuged and the sediment examined microscopically (See p. 139).

Clinical Implications

1. *Hematuria*
   One of the early indications of renal disease is the appearance of blood in the urine. This does not mean that blood will be present in every voided specimen in every case of renal disease. It does mean that in most cases of renal disease, occult blood appears in the urine with a reasonable degree of frequency.
2. Usually, when blood is present in urine, protein will also be present.
3. *Hemoglobinuria* is found in:
   (a) Extensive burns and crushing injuries
   (b) Transfusion reactions to incompatible blood
   (c) Febrile intoxication
   (d) Chemical agents and alkaloids (poisonous mushrooms, snake venom)
   (e) Malaria
   (f) Irrigation of operated prostatic bed with water

(g) Hemolytic anemias

(h) Paroxysmal hemoglobinuria (Large quantities of hemoglobin appear in urine at irregular intervals.)

4. Hematuria, hemoglobinuria, and myoglobinuria each result in a positive chemical test for blood in urine.

5. Drugs causing a positive result:
   (a) Drugs that are toxic to the kidneys (bacitracin and
   amphotericin)
   (b) Drugs that cause actual bleeding (coumarin)
   (c) Drugs that cause hemolysis of RBC's (aspirin)

Interfering Factors

1. High doses of ascorbic acid may give a false negative result
(Ascorbic acid may be a preservative for antibiotics such
as tetracycline).

2. Drugs that may give a false positive result include bromides,
copper, iodides, and oxidizing agents.

PROTEIN (ALBUMIN)

Normal Values

Negative 2–8 mg./dl.

Explanation of Test

Detection of protein in urine (proteinuria), combined with
the microscopic examination of urinary sediment, provides the
basis for differential diagnosis of renal disease.

In health, the urine contains no protein or only trace amounts
of protein, which consists of albumin (one third of normal urine
protein is albumin) and globulins from the plasma. Since
albumin is filtered more readily than the globulins, it is
usually very abundant in pathologic conditions. Therefore,
the term *albuminuria* is often used synonymously with
proteinuria.

Normally, the glomerules prevent passage of protein from

the blood to the glomular filtrate. Thus, the persistent presence of protein in the urine is the single most important indication of renal disease. Therefore, if more than a trace of protein is found in the urine, a quantitative 24-hour evaluation of protein excretion is necessitated.

Bence Jones Protein

Electrophoresis of urine can be used to demonstrate Bence Jones protein, a specific low molecular weight protein. This protein is found in:
  (a.) 40 per cent of multiple myeloma cases,
  (b.) tumor metastasis to the bone,
  (c.) chronic lymphocytic leukemia,
  (d.) amyloidosis,
  (e.) macroglobulinemia.

Procedure

A. *Collecting the Specimen*
   1. The patient is instructed to void at bedtime and discard the urine.
   2. The next morning a urine specimen is collected immediately after the patient awakes and has assumed a standing position.
   3. A second specimen is collected after the patient has been standing or walking for a period of time.
B. *Testing the Specimen*
   1. A reagent strip is dipped into a well-mixed sample of urine and the color changes compared immediately with the color charts provided.

Clinical Implications

1. A trace or one + reaction detects up to 20 mg. of protein and indicates significant proteinuria, implying an abnormally high excretion of protein and renal disease. Proteinuria is usually the result of increased glomerular filtration of

protein because of some kind of glomerular damage. A follow-up 24-hour urine test for protein is indicated.

2. Continued proteinuria of any amount in an apparently healthy person usually indicates minimal renal disease.

3. In pathologic states the level of proteinuria is rarely constant, and not every sample of urine will be abnormal in patients with disease.

4. Proteinuria occurs in the following renal diseases:
   (a) Nephritis
   (b) Nephrosis
   (c) Polycystic kidney
   (d) Tuberculosis and cancer of the kidney
   (e) Kidney stones
   (f) Ascites

5. Proteinuria may occur in the following nonrenal diseases:
   (a) Fever
   (b) Trauma
   (c) Severe anemias and leukemia
   (d) Toxemia
   (e) Abdominal tumors
   (f) Convulsive disorders
   (g) Hyperthyroidism
   (h) Intestinal obstruction
   (i) Cardiac disease
   (j) Poisoning from turpentine, phosphorous, mercury, sulfosalicylic acid, lead, phenol, opiates, and drug therapy.

6. Large numbers of leukocytes accompanying proteinuria usually indicate infection at some level in the urinary tract. Large numbers of both leukocytes and erythrocytes usually indicate a noninfectious inflammatory disease of the glomerulus.

7. Proteinuria does not always accompany renal disease. Pyelonephritis, obstructions, nephrolithiasis, tumors, and congenital malformations can cause severe illness without protein leakage.

8. Proteinuria is associated with the finding of casts on the sediment exam because protein is necessary for cast formation.

9. Postural proteinuria is the excretion of protein by patients

who are standing or moving in the day time. The proteinuria is intermittent and disappears when the person lies down. Postural proteinuria occurs in 3 to 5 per cent of healthy young adults.

Differentiation from other types of proteinuria is done by testing for protein in two urine specimens; one collected before and one collected after the person is erect. In postural proteinuria the first specimen contains no protein, the second is positive.

Interfering Factors

1. Functional, mild, and transitory protein in the urine, because of renal vasoconstriction, is associated with:
   (a.) violent exercise,
   (b.) severe emotional stress,
   (c.) cold baths
2. Increased protein in urine occurs:
   (a.) after eating large amounts of protein,
   (b.) in pregnancy or immediately following delivery,
   (c.) in newborn infants,
   (d.) in premenstrual state,
   (e.) in orthostatic proteinuria.
3. False or accidental proteinuria may be present because of a mixture of pus and red blood cells in urinary tract infections and the menstrual flow.
4. False positive results can occur from incorrect use and assessment out of the color strip test:
   (a.) prolonged dipping or allowing the strip to be held too long in the urine stream;
   (b.) failing to accurately match the reactive area with the color chart.
5. Alkaline urine can give a false positive test on the color strip test.
6. A very dilute urine may give a falsely low protein value.
7. Drugs that may cause false positive tests for uric protein include:
   (a.) gold,
   (b.) arsenic,
   (c.) sodium bicarbonate,

  (d.) acetazolamide, (c & d lab stix)
  (e.) massive doses of penicillin,
  (f) radiopaque contrast media for up to three days,
  (g.) sulfisoxazole,
  (h.) thymol
  (i.) chlorpromazine
  (j) turbidity test
8. See appendix for complete listing of drugs that affect tests for protein in urine.

PROTEIN (24-HOUR)

Normal Values
10–100 mg./24 hr.

Explanation of Test
Since the presence of protein in a screening test can have grave significance, it is important to confirm this finding by a 24-hour urine test, and hopefully, to arrive at a specific diagnosis. Increased renal excretion of protein has long been recognized as a sign of significant renal disease.

Procedure
1. A 24 hour-urine container is labeled with name of patient, test, and date.
2. Refrigeration of specimen is required.
3. General instructions for 24-hour urine collection are followed (p. 109).
4. Exact start and ending of collection are recorded on specimen container with patient's record. (Start 7:30 A.M. 2/6 and end 7:38 A.M. 2/7)

Clinical Implications
A. *Heavy Proteinuria*
  1. Above 400 mg./24 hrs.

2. Seen in:
    (a.) Glomerulonephritis
    (b.) Nephrotic syndrome
    (c.) Lupus nephritis
    (d.) Amyloid diseases
    (e.) Congestive heart failure

B. *Moderate Proteinuria*
1. Between 50 to 400 mg./24 hrs.
2. Seen in those conditions listed under Heavy Proteinuria, plus:
    (a.) Nephrosclerosis
    (b.) Pyelonephritis with hypertension
    (c.) Multiple myeloma
    (d.) Diabetic kidney disease
    (e.) Preeclampsia

C. *Minimal Proteinuria*
1. Less than 50 mg./24 hrs.
2. Found in:
    (a.) Intermittent glomerulonephritis
    (b.) Inactive phase of glomerular disease
    (c.) Polycystic kidney disease
    (d.) Renal tubular disease
    (e.) Benign postural proteinuria

Patient Preparation

1. Instruct patient about the purpose and collection of 24-hour specimen.
2. Food and fluids are permitted. Fluids should not be forced, for a very dilute urine can give a false negative value.

SUGAR (GLUCOSE)

Normal Values

Random specimen: negative
Quantitative 24-hour specimen: 100 mg./24 hrs.

Explanation of Test

Urine glucose tests are utilized in (1) screening to detect diabetes, (2) confirming a diagnosis of diabetes, or (3) monitoring the effectiveness of diabetic control.

Normally, urine does not contain a sufficient amount of sugar to react with any of the popular testing methods. Glucose is always present in the glomerular filtrate, but it is reabsorbed by the proximal tubule. However, should the blood glucose level exceed the reabsorption capacity of the tubules, glucose will be spilled into the urine.

The presence of sugar in the urine (*glucosuria* or *glycosuria*), as evidenced by positive tests, is not necessarily abnormal. For example, sugar may appear in urine after a heavy meal is eaten or in conjunction with emotional stress. In addition, for some people, a low tubular reabsorption rate may account for glycosuria occurring with normal blood glucose levels. This is a benign condition.

In the majority of cases, however, sugar in the urine is abnormal and is usually due to diabetes mellitus. Nonetheless, a positive test for urine sugar is not adequate for a diagnosis of diabetes. A single measurement of postprandial blood sugar gives more meaningful information in diabetes detection programs than does a urine sugar test. A urine sugar test accompanied by a blood sugar test gives more information than does a blood sugar test alone. Also, a postprandial urine sugar test is a more effective test for recognizing diabetes than a fasting urine sugar test.

Types of Glucose Tests

A. *Reduction Tests:* Benedict's, Clinitest, Galatest
   1. Are based on reduction of certain metal ions by glucose. When added to urine, a heat reaction takes place, resulting in precipitation and change in color of the urine.
   2. Are considered nonspecific for glucose for the reason that the reaction can be brought about by other reducing substances in the urine:
      (a) Uric acid, ascorbic acid
      (b) Other sugars, such as galactose, lactose, fructose, and maltose

B. *Enzyme Tests:* Clinistix, Diastix, Testape
    1. Are based on interaction between enzymes and glucose
       When dipped into urine the strip changes color according to the amount of glucose in the urine indicated by the manufacturer's color chart.
    2. All are specific for glucose.

Procedure

1. A freshly voided specimen should be used.
2. Directions on tablet or dipstick container must be followed exactly, and the color reaction compared to the closest matching color on the manufacturer's color chart.
3. Results are recorded on the patient's record.

CLINICAL ALERT
1. Determine exactly what drugs a diabetic is taking and whether the metabolites of these drugs affect the urine test.
2. Do not encourage patients to drink water between the first and second voidings since diluted urine may conceal glucose in the urine.
3. Always test for ketone bodies when the urine contains glucose.

Clinical Implications

1. Increased glucose in the urine is found in diabetes mellitus, brain injury, myocardial infarction, and when a lowered renal threshold is present.
2. A glucose tolerance test is indicated to confirm diabetes mellitus.
3. The greater the concentration of sugar in the urine, the greater the lack of control of the diabetes.

Interfering Factors

Note: Knowledge of manufacturer's guidelines on drugs known to affect test results must be continually updated. See appendix for complete listing.

1. Pregnancy and lactation may cause a false positive in Clintest. About 70 per cent of normal pregnant women show a temporary glucosuria that appears to be of no clinical significance.
2. Ascorbic acid, reg Gram, keflin, creatinine in concentrated urine, streptomycin, and homogentesic acid may cause a false positive reduction test; usually it will only be a trace reaction.
3. Stress, excitement, testing after a heavy meal, and following the administration of IV glucose may cause false positives of all tests. Usually it is a trace reaction.
4. Ascorbic acid in very large amounts may cause a false negative in the enzyme tests.
5. False negatives may be obtained if deteriorated or reagent strips have been used, or if directions are not followed exactly.

Patient Preparation

1. Instruct patient about the purpose of test, method of testing, and second voiding technique.
2. Patient voids, tests the specimen, and discards it.
3. 30 to 45 minutes later, the patient voids, if possible, and this specimen is tested. The second specimen reflects the immediate state of glucosuria more accurately than the first specimen which may be urine that has collected in the bladder over a period of hours.

KETONE BODIES (ACETONE)

Normal Values

Negative

Explanation of Test

Ketone bodies, resulting from the metabolism of fatty acid and fat, consist mainly of three substances: acetone, keta-hydroxybutyric acid and acetoacetic acid. The last two substances readily convert to acetone, making acetone, in essence, the main constituent being tested.

In healthy individuals, ketone bodies are formed in the liver and are completely metabolized so that only negligible amounts appear in the urine. However, when carbohydrate metabolism is altered, an excessive amount of ketones is formed (acetosis) on account of fat becoming the pre-dominant body fuel instead of carbohydrates. When the metabolic pathways of carbohydrates are disturbed, carbon fragments from fat and protein are diverted to form abnormal amounts of ketone bodies. The body's alkaline reserves thus become depleted, resulting in acidosis.

The excess production of ketones, (ketonuria) in the urine is mainly associated with diabetes. Testing for ketones in the urine of diabetics may provide the clue to early diagnosis of ketoacidosis and diabetic coma.

Indications for Ketone Testing

A. *General*

Screening for ketonuria is valuable in hospital admissions, presurgical patients, pregnant women, children and dia-betics.

B. *Glycosuria*

Testing for ketone bodies is indicated in any patients showing greater than normal excretion of sugar.

C. *Acidosis*

1. Ketone testing is used to judge the severity of acidosis and to follow the effects of treatment.
2. Blood ketone measurement frequently provides a more reliable estimate of acidosis than urine testing (Especially useful in emergency room situations).

D. *Diabetes*

1. Ketonuria may indicate ketoacidosis and possible diabetic coma.
2. When treatment is being switched from insulin to oral hypoglycemic agents, the development of keto-nuria within 24 hours after the withdrawal of insulin usually indicates a poor response to the oral hypo-glycemic agents.
3. The urine of diabetics treated with oral hypoglycemic

agents should be tested regularly for glucose and ketones, since oral hypoglycemic agents, unlike insulin, do not control diabetes when acute complications such as infection develop.

E. *Pregnancy*

In pregnancy, the early detection of ketones is essential since ketoacidosis is an important factor contributing to death in the uterus.

Procedure

1. Dip reagent strip in fresh urine, tap strip to remove excess urine, and compare to color chart after exactly 15 seconds.
2. The chart has four color blocks indicating negative, small, moderate, and large concentration of ketones.
3. A blood sample can also be tested using the color dip strips.

Clinical Implications

1. Ketosis and ketonuria may occur whenever increased amounts of fat are metabolized, carbohydrate intake is restricted, or the diet is rich in fat.
2. Ketonuria occurs in association with:
   (a) Fever
   (b) Anorexia
   (c) Gastrointestinal disturbances
   (d) Fasting
   (e) Starvation
   (f) Prolonged vomiting
   (g) Following anesthesia
3. In nondiabetics, ketonuria will frequently occur in acute illness. 15 per cent of hospitalized patients will have ketone bodies in their urine even though they do not have diabetes.
4. Children are particularly prone to developing ketonuria and ketosis.
5. Ketone bodies appear in the urine before there is any significant increase of ketone bodies in the blood.

Interfering Factors

1. A carbohydrate-free diet will cause ketonuria.
2. Drugs which may cause a false positive:

(a.) Levodopa
(b.) phthalein compound (B.S.P. or P.S.P.)
(c.) ether
(d.) insulin
(e.) isopropyl alcohol
(f.) metformin
(g.) paraldehyde
(h.) pyridium
(i.) Phenformin

Clinical Implications

1. A test for ketone bodies in the urine is helpful in differentiating between a diabetic coma and an insulin shock.
2. Any stressful situation which distorts the normal regulation of a diabetic can be recognized at an early point by a positive urine ketone test.
3. Urine ketones indicate caution, not a crisis situation, in either a diabetic or a nondiabetic patient.
   (a) In a diabetic patient the appearance of ketone bodies in the urine suggests that the patient is not adequately controlled, and that adjustments of either the medication or the diet should be made promptly.
   (b) In a nondiabetic, ketone bodies indicate a small amount of CHO metabolism and excessive fat metabolisms.

MICROSCOPIC EXAMINATION OF SEDIMENT

Background

Urinary sediment provides information useful for both prognosis and diagnosis. It constitutes a direct sampling of urinary track morphology. In renal parenchymal disease, the urine usually contains increased numbers of cells and casts discharged from an organ that is otherwise accessible only by biopsy or surgery.

In health, the urine contains small numbers of cells and other formed elements from the entire length of the genitourinary tract: casts and epithelial cells from the nephron; epithelial cells from the pelvis, ureters, bladder, and urethra; mucous threads and spermatozoa from the prostate; possibly some red or white blood cells and an occasional cast.

The sediment collected in the urine can be broken down into cellular elements (red and white blood cells and epithelial cells), casts, crystals, and bacteria.

These may originate anywhere in the urinary tract. Casts are formed in the renal tubules by precipitation and gelling of urinary mucoprotein secreted by the renal tubule. The interplay of high protein concentration, low pH, and high solute concentration frequently leads to a clumping of cellular material in the protein matrix, resulting in the formation of hyaline casts, red blood casts, and epithelial casts, among others. Normally there is not enough protein in the distal part of the nephron, where urine is acidified and concentrated, to provide more than an occasional cast. When casts do occur in the urine, the indication is one of tubular or glomerular disorders.

RED CELLS AND RED CELL CASTS

Normal Values

1 or 2 per low-powered field

Explanation of Test

In health, red cells and red cell casts are occasionally found in the urine, but the persistent findings of even small numbers of erythrocytes (RBC's) should be thoroughly investigated, since these cells come from the kidney and indicate serious renal disease.

Procedure

Urinary sediment is examined microscopically under low power.

Clinical Implications

A. *Red Cells*
1. The finding of more than two red cells per low-powered field is an abnormal condition and can indicate:
    (a) Renal or systemic disease
    (b) Trauma to the kidney
2. Increased red cells occur in:
    (a) Pyelonephritis
    (b) Lupus
    (c) Renal stones
    (d) Cystitis
    (e) Prostatitis
    (f) Tuberculosis and malignancies of the genitourinary tract
    (g) Hemophilia
3. Red cells in excess of WBC's indicate bleeding into the urinary tract as may occur in:
    (a) Trauma
    (b) Tumor
    (c) Aspirin ingestion
    (d) Anticoagulative therapy
    (e) Thrombocytopenia

B. *Red Cell Casts*
1. Casts composed largely of red blood cells indicate hemorrhage or desquamative conditions of the nephron.
2. Red blood casts indicate acute inflammatory or vascular disorders in the glomerulus.
3. May be only manifestation of:
    (a) Acute glomerulonephritis
    (b) Renal infarction
    (c) Collagen disease
    (d) Kidney involvement in subacute bacterial endocarditis

Interfering Factors

1. Increased numbers of red blood cells can be found

following violent exercise, a traumatic catheterization, passage of stones, or contamination by menstrual fluid.
2. Alkaline urine hemolyzes red cells and dissolves casts.
3. There are many drugs that can cause increased numbers of red blood cells to appear in the urine. See appendix under RBC or Hemoglobin.

WHITE CELLS AND WHITE CELL CASTS

Normal Values

WBC's: 3 or 4 per low-powered field
WBC casts: none—negative

Background

Leukocytes may come from anywhere in the genitourinary tract. White cell casts always come from the kidney tubules.

Procedure

Urinary sediment is examined microscopically under low power.

Clinical Implications

A. *Leukocytes*
1. Large numbers of white cells usually indicate bacterial infection in the urinary tract.
2. If the infection is in the kidney, the white cells tend to be associated with cellular and granular casts, bacteria, epithelial cells, and relatively few red cells.
3. Calls for a urine culture (p. 353).
B. *White Cell Casts*
1. White cell casts indicate renal parenchymal infection.
2. May be found in:
   (a) Acute glomerulonephritis
   (b) Nephrotic syndrome
   (c) Pyelonephritis
   (d) Interstitial inflammation of the kidney

3. Because pyelonephritis may remain completely asymptomatic even though renal tissue is being progressively destroyed, careful examination of urinary sediment for leukocyte casts is important.

Interfering Factors

Vaginal discharge can contaminate the specimen. A "clean-catch" specimen, or catheterized specimen, should be taken to rule out contamination.

EPITHELIAL CELLS AND EPITHELIAL CASTS

Normal Values

Occasional epithelial cell found.

Background

Epithelial cell casts are formed by cast-off tubular cells. Since the tubule is a living membrane, it is always replacing itself. For this reason, the finding of occasional epithelial cells or clumps is not remarkable.

Clinical Implications

The findings of many epithelial casts occur when the following diseases have damaged the tubular epithelium:
- (a) Nephrosis
- (b) Eclampsia
- (c) Amyloidosis
- (d) Poisoning from heavy metals and other toxins

HYALINE CASTS

Normal Values

Occasional hyaline casts are found.

Background

Hyaline casts are clear colorless,casts formed when protein within the tubules precipitates and gels. Their appearance within the urine depends on the rate of urine flow, urine, pH, and the degree of proteinuria.

Procedure

Urinary sediment is examined microscopically under low power.

Clinical Implications

1. Hyaline casts indicate possible damage to the glomerular capillary membrane which is permitting leakage of proteins through the glomerular filter.
2. Hyaline casts may be a temporary phenomenon due to:
   (a) Fever
   (b) Postural strain
   (c) Emotional exercise
   (d) Strenuous exercise
   (e) Palpation of the kidney
3. When large numbers of hyaline casts appear in the urine along with protein, nephrotic syndrome may be suggested.

GRANULAR CASTS

Normal Values

Occasional granular casts are found.

Background

Granular casts result from the disintegration of the cellular material in white and epithelial blood cells into coarse and then fine granular particles. A rare but final step in this process is the formation of waxy casts when urine flow is reduced.

Procedure

Urinary sediment is examined microscopically under low power.

Clinical Implications

1. Acute tubular necrosis
2. Advanced glomerulonephritis
3. Pyelonephritis
4. Malignant nephrosclerosis
5. Chronic lead poisoning

Waxy Casts

Found in:
1. Chronic renal disease
2. Indicate tubular inflammation and degeneration

FATTY BODIES AND FATTY CASTS

Background

In nephrotic syndrome, fat accumulates in the tubular cells and eventually sloughs off forming fat bodies. The coalescence of several fat bodies results in fatty casts.

Clinical Implications

Fatty casts are found in chronic renal disease and indicate tubular inflammation and degeneration.

CRYSTALS

Background

In a routine urinalysis, the presence of crystals is identified as a normal finding. The type and number of crystals vary with the pH of the urine.

Clinical Implications

A. *Normal Findings*
  1. Acid urine
      (a) Urates
      (b) Uric acid
      (c) Calcium oxalate (if numerous, may indicate hypercalcemia)
  2. Alkaline urine
      (a) Amorphous phosphates
      (b) Calcium phosphate
      (c) Ammonium biurate
B. *Abnormal Findings*
  1. Cystine
  2. Leucine or tyrosine (indicate protein breakdown)
  3. Cholestin
  4. Drug crystals (sulfonamides)

Interfering Factors

1. Drugs which may cause increased levels of crystals include:
    (a.) Acetazolamide
    (b.) Aminosalicylic acid
    (c.) Ampicillin
    (d.) Methenamine mandelate
    (e.) Sulfonamide
    (f.) Thiabendazole

SHREDS

Background

Shreds consists of a mixture of mucus, pus, and epithelial cells, and can be seen grossly.

Clinical Implications

1. When mucus predominates, the shreds float on the surface.
2. When epithelial cells predominate, the shreds occupy the mid zone.

3. When pus predominates, the shreds are drawn to the bottom of the specimen.

ADDIS COUNT

Normal Values

Will vary considerably among laboratories according to standards used:

ADULTS	*CHILDREN*
WBC—up to 1,000,000/12 hours and epithelial	WBC—up to 2,000,000/12 hours
RBC—up to 500,000/12 cells hours	RBC—up to 600,000/12 hours
Casts—up to 0–5,000/12 hours	Casts—up to 10,000/12 hours

Explanation of Test

An Addis count provides a quantitative evaluation of the cellular element present in the urinary sediment. It represents a method developed by Thomas Addis to count RBC's, WBC's, and casts collected in the urine over a 12-hour period after fluid has been restricted. The test is most valuable in judging the prognosis of renal disease, as well as the type and degree of the disease.

Procedure

1. A 12-hour urine container with preservative is labeled with the name of the patient, test, and date.
2. The 12-hour specimen is usually collected over the evening and night hours.
3. The specimen should have a specific gravity of 1.022 or higher. Therefore, the patient should have no liquid of any sort for 24 hours. In pediatric cases, a modified form of fluid restriction is advisable. Note: Some laboratories will permit up to 200 ml. fluid with each meal.

4. At about 8:00 P.M., the patient voids completely and discards the urine. The *exact time* of this voiding, as well as the date, should be recorded on the specimen container.

5. All urine obtained after 8:00 P.M., up to and including 8:00 A.M. the following morning, should be saved. If at all possible, the patient should not void again until exactly 12 hours have elapsed. At that time, the bladder should be completely emptied into the collection container.

6. The urine should be a clean, voided specimen.

7. The exact starting and ending of collection should be recorded on both the specimen container and the patient's record. For example: Start—8:03 A.M., 3/14; End—8:15 A.M., 3/15.

8. The container should be taken to the laboratory refrigerator as soon as the test is completed.

Note: It is believed that it is best to perform two separate Addis counts on successive days in order to obtain any degree of accuracy. If two successive counts are performed, the patient is allowed to eat a normal breakfast with liquids, but thereafter the instructions are followed closely, as on the first day.

Clinical Implications

1. Although there are many diseases in which the Addis count is typical, no specific count is diagnostic of any one disease.

2. WBC
   - (a) Increase in white blood cells is a response to bacterial infection.
   - (b) Clumping of leukocytes indicates presence of infection in the urinary tract or in an area having access to the tract.

3. RBC
   - (a) Increase in RBC count may be benign.
   - (b) If increased numbers are seen in repeated examination, or if they appear with protein, they are indicative of kidney disease.

Interfering Factors

1. A salt free diet may cause a falsely decreased red cell and cast count.

2. Dilute, alkaline urine is undesirable since these factors cause RBC's and casts to dissolve. For this reason, careful instructions must be given to patients.

Patient Preparation

1. Advise adult patient that he is not allowed any liquid of any sort for 24 hours. This will mean no fluids after a regular breakfast the day of the test until the following morning. Children will be given a modified form of liquid restriction.
2. Explain to patient that in the evening he will be taking a urine specimen at a specific time and will then be discarding this specimen.
3. Tell patient that he should try to avoid urinating for 12 hours (if at all possible).
4. Advise patient to avoid eating excessive quantities of fruit to prevent alkalinization of the urine.
5. If patient is to have two successive Addis counts, allow him to eat a normal breakfast with fluids on the second day, but to follow all other instructions adhered to on first day.

Patient Aftercare

As soon as test is over, provide patient with plenty of fluids, for he will be thirsty.

CLINICAL ALERT
Unless the specimen is properly collected, the times diligently noted, and the test carefully performed, the results are of no value

OTHER URINARY CONSTITUENTS TESTS

CHLORIDES (Cl); QUANTITATIVE (24 HOURS)

Normal Values

110–250 mEq./24 hrs.
10–20 gm. NaCl/24 hrs.

9 gm./l. (0.9 gm./ml.)

It is rather difficult to talk about "normal" and "abnormal" ranges, since the levels of urine chloride can vary as a result of salt intake and perspiration. The test findings have meaning only in relation to salt intake and output.

Explanation of Test

The amount of chloride excreted in the urine in a 24-hour period is an indication of the state of electrolyte balance. Chloride is most often associated with sodium and fluid change.

The measurement of urine chloride may be useful as a means of diagnosing dehydration or as a guide in adjusting fluid and electrolyte balance in postoperative patients. It also serves as a means of monitoring the effects of reduced salt diets which are of great therapeutic importance in patients with cardiovascular disease, hypertension, liver disease, and kidney ailment.

A patient on a restricted salt intake diet will usually not excrete more than 0.6 gm. per 100 ml. of NaCl in the urine, while a person on a normal salt diet would excrete 0.7 gm. per 100 ml. of NaCl or more.

Procedure

1. A 24-hour urine specimen is collected.
2. The exact times to start and complete the collection are recorded on the specimen container and on the patient's record.
3. When the specimen is completed, it should be sent to the laboratory for refrigeration.

CLINICAL ALERT

Because electrolyte and water balance are so closely related, appraise the patient's state of hydration by checking daily weight, accurate intake and output, and by observing and recording skin turgor and appearance of tongue and urine.

Clinical Implications

Results are significant only when considered in relation to other data such as state of health or illness, salt intake, and urine volume.

A. *Normal Findings*

Urinary excretion of chloride decreases to a very low level whenever the serum level is much below 100 mEq. per l.

B. *Decreased Levels*

1. In some conditions, urinary excretion of chloride increases even when the serum level is as low as 85 mEq. per l. or less. Occurs in Addison's disease when there is a deficiency of adrenal hormone that controls the excretion of sodium and chloride.
2. Decreased levels associated with:
   (a) Malabsorption syndrome
   (b) Pyloric obstruction
   (c) Prolonged gastric suction
   (d) Diarrhea
   (e) Diaphoresis
   (f) Congestive heart failure
   (g) Emphysema

C. *Increased Levels*

Associated with:
   (a) Dehydration
   (b) Starvation
   (c) Salicylate toxicity
   (d) Mercurial and chlorothiazide diuretics

Interfering Factors

1. Urinary chloride concentration varies with dietary salt intake and, to some degree, with urine volume.
2. False elevations may result if patient has taken bromides.

Patient Preparation

Instruct the patient about the purpose of the test and the method for collecting a 24-hour specimen.

SODIUM (Na); QUANTITATIVE (24 HOURS)

Normal Values

130–200 mEq./24 hrs.

Explanation of Test

This test measures electrolyte balance in the body by determining the amount of sodium excreted in 24 hours. It is indicated in the study of renal and adrenal disturbances and of water and acid-base imbalances.

Sodium is a primary regulator in the body's ability to retain or excrete water and maintain acid-base balance. The body has a strong tendency to maintain a total base content; only slight changes are found even under pathologic conditions. As the main base substance in the blood, sodium helps regulate acid-base balance due to its ability to combine with chloride and bicarbonate. Sodium also helps maintain the normal balance of electrolyte composition in intracellular and extracellular fluids by acting in conjunction with potassium (sodium-potassium pump). Sodium and potassium are important factors in nerve conduction, and they influence the irritability of the muscles, nerves, and heart.

Procedure

1. A 24-hour urine container is labeled with name of patient, test, and date.
2. Urine must be refrigerated.
3. General instructions for 24-hour urine collection are followed.
4. Exact start and ending of collection are recorded on specimen container and patient's record (start 7:05 A.M., 11/10; end 7:30 A.M., 11/11).
5. Send the specimen to the laboratory refrigerator when the test is completed.

Clinical Implications

Results are significant only when considered in relation to other data, such as a state of health or illness, salt intake, and urine volume.

A. *Increased Levels*
  1. Caused by:
     (a) Dehydration
     (b) Starvation
     (c) Salicylate toxicity
     (d) Adrenal cortical insufficiency
     (e) Mercurial and chlorothiazide diuretics
     (f) Chronic renal failure
     (g) Diabetic acidosis

B. Levels of Sodium associated with:
     (a) Malabsorption syndrome
     (b) Congestive heart failure
     (c) Pyloric obstruction
     (d) Diarrhea
     (e) Diaphoresis
     (f) Acute renal failure
     (g) Pulmonary emphysema
     (h) Aldosteronism
     (i) Cushing's disease

C. *Decreased Levels*
   Often accompanied by an equivalent loss of chloride

Interfering Factors

1. Dietary salt intake
2. Altered kidney function

Patient Preparation

1. Instruct patient about purpose of test, collection, and refrigeration of 24-hour urine specimen. Give a written reminder.
2. Food and fluids are permitted and encouraged.

CLINICAL ALERT
Since electrolyte and water balance are so closely related, determine the patient's state of hydration by checking daily weight, accurate intake and output, observation and recording of skin turgor, and appearance of tongue and urine.

POTASSIUM (K); QUANTITATIVE (24 HOURS)

Normal Values

40–80 mEq./24 hrs.

Explanation of Test

This test provides some insight into the electrolyte balance of the body by measuring the amount of potassium excreted in 24 hours. This measurement is useful in the study of renal and adrenal disorders and of water and acid-base imbalances. When a patient gives an obscure history in the presence of a known potassium deficit, evaluation of urinary potassium can be helpful in determining the origin of the deficit.

Potassium acts as a part of the body's buffer system; therefore, potassium balance serves a vital function in the body's overall electrolyte balance. Since the kidneys cannot conserve potassium, this balance is regulated by the kidney's excretion of potassium through the urine.

Procedure

1. A 24-hour urine container is labeled with name of patient, test, and date.
2. Urine must be refrigerated.
3. General instructions for 24-hour urine collection are followed.
4. Exact start and ending of collection are recorded on specimen container and patient's record (start 7:05 A.M., 11/10; end 7:30 A.M., 11/11).
5. Send the specimen to the laboratory refrigerator when the test is completed.

Clinical Implications

A. *Elevated Levels*
1. Found in:
    (a) Chronic renal failure
    (b) Diabetic and renal tubular acidosis

    (c) Dehydration
    (d) Starvation
    (e) Primary aldosteronism
    (f) Cushing's disease
    (g) Salicylate toxicity
    (h) Mercurial chlorothiazide, ammonium chloride, and Diamox diuretics

B. *Decreased Levels*
  1. Associated with:
    (a) Malabsorption syndrome
    (b) Diarrhea
    (c) Acute renal failure
    (d) Adrenal cortical insufficiency (can be normal or decreased)
    (e) Excessive mineralocorticoid activity (aldosterone)
      Since licorice contains a mineralocorticoid compound, people who consume large amounts of licorice may have lowered urinary potassium levels.
  2. In patients with potassium deficiency, regardless of the cause, the urine pH tends to fall. This fall occurs because hydrogen ions are secreted in exchange for sodium ions, inasmuch as both potassium and hydrogen are excreted by the same mechanism.

C. *Cautionary Findings*
  1. In excessive vomiting or stomach suctioning, the accompanying alkalosis maintains urinary potassium excretion at levels inappropriately high for the degree of actual potassium depletion.
  2. In diabetes insipidus, urinary potassium is normal.

Interfering Factors

Varies with dietary intake.

Patient Preparation

1. Instruct patient about purpose of test, collection and refrigeration of 24-hour urine specimen. Give a written reminder.
2. Food and fluids are permitted and encouraged.

CLINICAL ALERT
1. Since electrolyte and water balance are so closely associated, determine the patient's state of hydration by checking daily weight, accurate intake and output, and by observing and recording skin turgor and appearance of the tongue and urine.
2. Observe for signs of muscle weakness, tremors, and changes in electrocardiograms. The level of potassium increase or decrease at that which these symptoms become apparent, varies from patient to patient.

URIC ACID; QUANTITATIVE (24 HOURS)

Normal Values

0.4–1.0 gm./24 hrs. on normal diet
0.2–0.5 gm./24 hrs. on a purine-free diet
2.0 gm./24 hrs. on a high-purine diet

Uric acid formation occurs as a result of the metabolic breakdown of nucleic acids; purines are the principal source of this breakdown. The test is indicated in the investigation of metabolic disturbances to identify gout and diagnose kidney disease. It will also reflect the effect of uricosuric agents when these drugs are used, by indicating the total amount of uric acid excreted.

Procedure

1. A 24-hour urine container with preservative added is labeled with name of patient, test, and date.
2. General instructions for 24-hour urine collection are followed.
3. Exact start and ending of collection are recorded on specimen container and patient's record (start 7:30 A.M., 1/3, end 7:15 A.M., 1/4)
4. Send the specimen to the laboratory when the test is completed.

Clinical Implications

A. *Increased Levels* (uricosuria)
1. Found in:
   (a) Gout
   (b) Chronic myelogenous leukemia
   (c) Polycythemia vera
   (d) Liver disease
   (e) Febrile illnesses
   (f) Toxemias of pregnancy
   (g) Fanconi syndrome
2. Cytoxic drugs to treat lymphoma and leukemia often cause greatly increased urinary uric acid levels.
3. High uric acid concentration plus low urine pH may lead to uric acid stones in the urinary tract.

B. *Decreased Levels*
1. Found in kidney disease (chronic glomerulonephritis) because impaired renal function depresses uric acid excretion.

Interfering Factors

1. Drugs
   (a) Salicylates
   (b) Thiazide diuretics
   (c) Chronic alcohol ingestion
2. X-ray contrast media can markedly increase urine acid levels.
3. See appendix for complete listing of drugs that can interfere with test results.

Patient Preparation

1. Instruct patient about purpose of test, collection, and refrigeration of 24-hour urine specimen. Give written reminder.
2. Food and fluids are permitted and encouraged. In some diagnostic situations, a diet high or low in purines may be ordered during the test period.

CALCIUM; QUALITATIVE (SULKOWITCH TEST); QUANTITATIVE (24-HOUR)

Normal Values

24 hour levels   Sulkowitch
100–250 mg./average diet   1+ to 2+
150 mg./low calcium diet

Explanation of Test

The bulk of the calcium discharged by the body is excreted in the stool. However, there is a small quantity of calcium that is normally excreted in the urine, the amount increasing or decreasing as a result of changes in the quantity of dietary calcium ingested.

The Sulkowitch test is the most common test for urine calcium. It is a qualitative evaluation used primarily on random specimens to identify reduced or increased calcium excretion when calcium blood levels or certain signs and symptoms imply some related abnormality. To rule out hypercalcemia (and hypercalcinuria), an early morning specimen should be examined, since calcium excretion is lowest at that time. If hypocalcemia is suspected, the sample should be taken after a meal (when excretion is greatest). The test is also used to screen for suspected bone tumors, since calcium excretion is generally elevated in these instances.

The 24-hour test is most often ordered to determine the function of the parathyroid gland which maintains a balance between calcium and phosphorous via parathyroid hormone. Hyperparathyroidism is a generalized disorder of calcium, phosphate and bone metabolism that results from an increased secretion of parathyroid hormones and an increased excretion of urinary calcium. In hypoparathyroidism, the urinary calcium is decreased.

Procedure

1. A 24-hour urine container is labeled with name of patient, test, and date.

2. Usually no preservative or refrigeration is required if not ordered to be done with any other tests. Some laboratories will require a preservative.
3. General instructions for 24-hour urine collection are followed.
4. Exact start and ending of collection are recorded on specimen container and patient's record (start 7:05 A.M., 11/10; end 7:30 A.M, 11/11).
5. Send the specimen to the laboratory refrigerator when the test is completed.

Clinical Implications

A. *Increased Levels*
    1. Caused by:
        (a) Hyperparathyroidism (results in constant 3+ to 4+ Sulkowitch tests)
        (b) Sarcoidosis
        (c) Primary cancers of breast and lung
        (d) Metastatic malignancies
        (e) Myeloma with bone metastasis
        (f) Wilson's disease
        (g) Renal tubular acidosis
        (h) Glucocorticoid excess
    2. Increased urinary calcium almost always accompanies elevated blood calcium levels.
    3. Calcium excretion greater than intake is always excessive, and excretion above 400 to 500 mg. per 24 hours is reliably abnormal.
    4. Increased excretion of calcium occurs whenever calcium is mobilized from the bone, as in metastatic cancer and prolonged skeletal immobilization.
    5. When calcium is excreted in increasing amounts, a potential for nephrolithiasis or nephrocalcinosis is created.

B. *Decreased Levels*
    1. Caused by:
        (a) Hypoparathyroidism (Hypocalcemia caused by hypoparathyroidism is usually associated with a negative reaction.)

    (b) Vitamin D deficiency (Vitamin D is necessary for absorption of calcium.)

    (c) Malabsorption syndrome

Interfering Factors

A. *False Elevated Levels* are due to:
1. High sodium and magnesium intake
2. Very high milk intake
3. Level higher immediately after meals
4. Drugs
    (a) Androgens and anabolic steroids
    (b) Cholestyramine
    (c) Vitamin D
    (d) Parathyroid injection
    (e) Nandrolone, in some cancer patients

B. *False Negative Levels* are due to:
1. Increased dietary phosphates
2. Alkaline urine
3. Drugs
    (a) Sodium phytate
    (b) Thiazides
    (c) Viomycin

Patient Preparation

1. Instruct patient about purpose of test, collection of 24-hour urine specimen. Give a written reminder.
2. Food and fluids are permitted and encouraged.
3. If the urine calcium test is done because of a metabolic disorder, the patient should eat a low calcium diet and be on calcium medication restrictions for a one to three day period prior to collection of the specimen.
4. If the patient has a history of renal stone formation, a general diet will be prescribed.

CLINICAL ALERT
1. If a blood calcium determination is not available, this test can be used in an emergency, especially when hypercalcemia is suspected, since this can threaten life.

2. Observe patients with very low urine calcium levels for signs and symptoms of tetany.
3. The first sign of calcium imbalance may be the occurrence of pathological fracture which can be related to the problems of calcium excess.

FOLLICLE-STIMULATING HORMONE (FSH) AND LUTEINIZING HORMONE (LH)

Normal Values

10–50 Muu/24 hrs. (mouse uterine units)
In the laboratory the effect of this hormone is measured on an immature mouse or rat uterus.

Explanation of Test

This 24-hour urine test measures the gonadotropic hormones FSH and LH and may be helpful in determining whether a gonadal insufficiency is primary or due to insufficient stimulation by the pituitary hormones. Production of these gonadotropins is believed to be under control of the pituitary gland. In women, the follicle-stimulating hormone promotes maturation of the ovarian follicle, and the maturing follicle produces estrogens. As the levels of estrogen rise, luteinizing hormones are produced. Together, FSH and LH induce ovulation. In men, the follicle-stimulating hormone produces spermatogenesis, and the luteinizing hormone stimulates the secretion of androgens.

Procedure

1. A 24-hour urine container is labeled with name of patient, test, and date.
2. Urine is either collected with a preservative or refrigerated only.
3. A blood sample can also be obtained.
4. When all the urine is collected, the specimen is sent to the laboratory refrigerator.

Clinical Implications

A. *Decreased FSH Levels*
Decreased urinary FSH are found in feminizing and masulinizing ovarian tumors when production is inhibited as a result of increased estrogen.

B. *Increased FSH Levels*
  1. Turner's syndrome (ovarian dysgenesis)
     Approximately 50 per cent of patients with primary amenorrhea have Turner's syndrome.
  2. High in hypogonadism

Patient Preparation

Instruct patient about purpose of test and collection of 24-hour urine specimen. Give a written reminder.

PREGNANEDIOL

Normal Values

This test is difficult to standardize.
Proliferative phase:—0.5–1.5 mg./24 hr.
Luteal phase:—2–7 mg./24 hr.
Postmenopausal:—0.2–1.0 mg./24 hr.

Explanation of Test

This test is a measurement of ovarian and placental function. It is indicated when a deficiency of progesterone is suspected. Combined deficiency of estrogen and progesterone is evidenced by menstrual irregularities and difficulty in conceiving and maintaining a pregnancy. Specifically, it measures the hormone progesterone as its principal excreted metabolite, pregnanediol. Progesterone has its main effect in the endometrium by causing the endometrium to enter the secretory phase and become ready for implantation of the blastocyte if fertilization has occurred.

Procedure

1. A 24-hour urine container is labeled with name of patient, test, and date.
2. Refrigeration of specimen is required.
3. General instructions for 24-hour urine collection are followed.
4. Exact start and ending of collection are recorded on specimen container and patient's record. (start 7:06 A.M., 1/5; end 7:30 A.M., 1/6)
5. When all urine is collected, the specimen is sent to laboratory refrigerator.

Clinical Implications

A. *Increased Levels*
   1. Associated with:
      (a) Luteal cysts of ovary
      (b) Arrhenoblastoma of the ovary
      (c) Hyperadrenocorticism
B. *Decreased Levels*
   1. Associated with:
      (a) Amenorrhea
      (b) Sometimes in threatened abortion
      (c) Fetal death
      (d) Toxemia

Patient Preparation

1. Instruct patient about the purpose of test and collection of 24-hour urine specimen. Give a written reminder.
2. Food and fluids are permitted.

PREGNANETRIOL

Normal Values

4 mg./24 hrs.

Explanation of Test

Pregnanetriol is a compound substance reflecting one segment of adrenocortical activity. Pregnanetriol should not be confused with pregnanediol, despite the similarity of name. Pregnanetriol is a precursor in adrenal corticoid synthesis and arises from 17-hydroxyprogesterone, not from progesterone.

This 24-hour urine test is done to diagnose adrenogenital syndrome. The diagnosis of adrenogenital syndrome is considered in the following:

1. Adult females who show signs and symptoms of excessive endrogen production with or without hypertension.
2. Craving for salt
3. Sexual precocity in males
4. Infants who exhibit signs of failure to thrive
5. External genitalia in females (pseudohermaphrodism)

Procedure

1. A 24-hour urine container is labeled with name of patient, test, and date.
2. Refrigeration of specimen is required.
3. General instructions for 24-hour urine collection are followed.
4. Exact start and ending of collection are recorded on specimen container and patient's record. (start 7:06 A.M., 1/5; end, 7:30 A.M., 1/6)
5. When all urine is collected, the specimen is sent to laboratory refrigeratory.

Clinical Implications

Elevated pregnanetriol levels occur in:
1. Congenital adrenocortical hyperplasia
2. Stein-Leventhal syndrome

Patient Preparation

1. Instruct patient about the purpose of test and collection of 24-hour urine specimen. Give a written reminder.
2. Food are fluids are permitted.

5-HYDROXYINDOLACETIC ACID (5-HIAA)

Also known as
5 Hydroxy 3
Serotonin
Indolacetic Acid

Normal Values

Qualitative—negative
Quantitative—2–10 mg./24 hr.
60–100 mEq./24 hr.

Explanation of Test

The qualitative random sample test may be done for screening purposes, followed by a quantitative 24-hour test if need be, or the 24-hour test may be done initially.

The urine test is conducted to diagnose a functioning carcinoid tumor which is indicated by significant elevation of 5-hydroxyindolacetic acid (5-HIAA), a denatured product of serotonin. Serotonin is a vasoconstricting hormone normally produced by the argentaffin cells of the GI tract. The principle function of the cells is to regulate smooth muscle contraction and peristalsis.

Procedures

1. No bananas, pineapple, or avocados are to be eaten during the 24-hour test for the reason that they contain tryptophan (5-hydroxyindolacetic acid is a metabolic product of tryptophan).
2. A 24-hour urine container with preservative is labeled with name of patient, test, and date.
3. General instructions for 24-hour urine collection are followed.
4. Exact start and ending of collection are recorded on specimen container and patient's record (7:30 A.M., 11/17; end 7:06 A.M., 11/18).
5. Send the specimen to the laboratory refrigerator when the test is completed.

Clinical Implications

1. Levels over 100 mg. per 24 hours are indicative of large carcinoid tumor, especially when metastatic. However, this increase occurs in only 5 to 7 per cent of patients with carcinoid tumor.
2. Levels greater than 10 mg. but less than 100 mg. are found in:
   (a.) Hemorrhage
   (b.) Thrombosis
   (c.) Nontropical sprue
   (d.) Severe pain of sciatica or skeletal and smooth muscle spasm

Interfering Factors

A. *False Positive*
   1. Bananas, pineapples, plums, walnuts, eggplants, and avocados may increase the 5HAA level, for these foods contain serotonin.
   2. *Drugs that may cause false positives:*

(a) Acetanilid	(i) Methamphetamine
(b) Acetophenetidin	(j) Reserpine
(c) Caffeine	(k) Phenacetin solution
(d) Glycerylguaiacolate	(l) Lugol's solution
(e) Flourouracil (5-FU)	(preceding 3 days)
(f) Mephenesin	(m) Phenmetrazine
(g) Melphalan	(n) Methysergide maleate
(h) Methocarbamol	

B. *Drugs that may cause false negatives:*
   1. Drugs (depressing 5HAA)

(a) ACTH	(h) Methyldopa
(b) Chlorpromazine	(i) Phenothiazines
(c) Heparine	(j) Promethazine
(d) Imipramine	(k) p-Chlorophenylala-
(e) Isoniazid	nine
(f) MAO Inhibitor	
(g) Methenamine man-delate	

Patient Preparation

1. Instruct patient about purpose of test and collection of 24-hour urine specimen. Give a written reminder.
2. Food and water are permitted and encouraged. Bananas, pineapple, and avocados are not to be eaten during the test.

CLINICAL ALERT
Patient should take no drugs for 72 hours before the test, if at all possible.

VANILLYMANDELIC ACID (VMA)
(Catecholamines or 3 Methoxy-4 Methoxy Acid)

Normal Values

VMA up to 9 mg./24 hr.
Catecholamines:
 Epinephrine 100–230 µg/24 hrs.
 Norepinephrine 100–230 µg/24 hrs.
 Metanephrine 24–96 µg/24 hrs.
 Normetanephrine 12–288 mg./24 hrs.

Explanation of Test

This 24-hour urine test of adrenal medullar function is primarily done when a person with hypertension is suspected of having pheochromocytoma, a tumor of the chromaffin cells of the adrenal medulla (Less than 1 per cent of hypertensive patients have pheochromocytoma). The principal substances formed by the adrenal medulla and excreted in the urine include vanillymandelic acid, epinephrine, norepinephrine, metanephrine, and normatanephrine. These compounds contain a catechol nucleus and an amine group, and are thus referred to as catecholamines. The major portion of the hormones are changed into metabolites, the principal one being 3-methoxy 4-hydroxy mandelic acid, or VMA.

VMA is the main urinary metabolite of the catecholamine group, having a urine concentration much greater than the other amines (10–100 times). It is also easier to detect due to simpler laboratory methods than the methods which must be used for catecholamine determination. Testing for VMA is important in pheochromocytoma since these tumors secrete excessive amounts of catecholamine resulting in high urine levels of VMA.

Procedure

1. A 24-hour urine container with preservative is labeled with name of patient, test, and date.
2. General instructions for 24-hour urine collection are followed.
3. Exact start and ending of collection are recorded on specimen container and patient's record. (Start 10:06 A.M., 1/3; end 10:15 A.M., 1/4)
4. When all the urine is collected, the specimen is sent to laboratory refrigerator.

Clinical Implications

A. *Elevated VMA Levels*
    1. High levels found in pheochromocytoma
    2. Slight to moderate elevations in
        (a) Neuroblastomas
        (b) Ganglioneuromas
        (c) Ganglioblastomas

B. *Elevated Catecholamines*
    Found in:
        (a) Pheochromocytoma
        (b) Neuroblastomas
        (c) Ganglioneuromas
        (d) Ganglioblastomas
        (e) Progressive muscular dystrophy
        (f) Myasthenia gravis

Interfering Factors

A. *Increased levels of VMA* are caused by
    1. Starvation (For this reason, the test should *not* be scheduled while the patient is NPO)

2. Foods
   - (a) Tea
   - (b) Coffee
   - (c) Cocoa
   - (d) Vanilla
   - (e) Fruit, especially bananas
   - (f) Fruit juice
   - (g) Chocolate
   - (h) Cheese
   - (i) Cider vinegar
   - (j) Gelatin foods
   - (k) Salad dressing
   - (l) Carbonated drinks, except gingerale
   - (m) Jelly and jam
   - (n) Candy and mints
   - (o) Cough drops
   - (p) Chewing gum
   - (q) Foods containing artificial flavoring or coloring
   - (r) Foods containing licorice

3. Drugs causing increased VMA levels:
   - (a) Aspirin
   - (b) Bromsulphalein; (sodium sulfobromophthalein)
   - (c) Glyceryl guaiacolate
   - (d) Mephenesin
   - (e) Chlorpromazine
   - (f) Para-aminosalicylic acid (PAS)
   - (g) Methocarbamol
   - (h) Methylene Blue
   - (i) Nalidixic acid
   - (j) Oxytetracycline
   - (k) Penicillin
   - (l) Phenazopyridine
   - (m) Phenolsulfonphthalein (PSP)
   - (n) Sulfa drugs
   - (o) Isoproterenol
   - (p) Levodopa
   - (q) Lithium
   - (r) Nitroglycerin

B. *False Decreased Levels of VMA* are caused by
   1. Alkaline urine
   2. Uremia (causes toxicity and impaired excretion of VMA)
   3. Radiographic iodine contrast agents (For this reason, an IVP should not be scheduled prior to a VMA test.)
   4. Drugs causing decreased levels:
      - (a) Clofibrate
      - (b) Guanethidine drugs
      - (c) Imphamine
      - (d) Methyldopa
      - (e) Monoamine (MAO) Inhibitors
      - (f) Clonidine
      - (g) Reserpine
      - (h) Imipramine

C. *Interfering Factors in Determining Catecholamine Levels*
   1. Vigorous exercise may cause increase.
   2. Drugs:

(a) Ampicillin
(b) Ascorbic acid
(c) Chloral hydrate
(d) Epinephrine
(e) Erythromycin
(f) Hydralazine
(g) Methenamine
(h) Methyldopa
(i) Nicotinic acid
(j) Quinine
(k) Quinidine
(l) Tetracycline
(m) Vitamin B complex

Patient Preparation

1. Instruct patient about purpose of test and collection of 24-hour urine specimen. Give a written reminder.
2. Explain diet and drug restrictions
   (a) Restrictions will vary among laboratory policies, but coffee, tea, bananas, cocoa products, vanilla products, and aspirin are always excluded for three days (two days prior to testing and day of the test). Many laboratories require that all drugs be discontinued for three to seven days before testing.
3. Rest and adequate food and fluids are encouraged, and stress is to be avoided during the test.

Patient Aftercare

Restricted foods, drugs, and activity are permitted as soon as test is completed.

17-KETOSTEROIDS (17–KS)
17-KETOGENIC STEROIDS (17–KGS)
17-HYDROXYCORTICOSTEROIDS (17-OHCS)

Normal Values

17-ketosteroids (17 KS)
Male: 8–18 mg./24 hrs.
Female: 5–15 mg./24 hrs.

17-ketogenic steroids (17 KGS)
Male: 5.5–23 mg./24 hrs.
Female: 3–15 mg./24 hrs.

17-hydroxycorticosteroids (17 OHCS)
10 mg./24 hrs.

Explanation of Test

These 24-hour tests of adrenal function measure the excretion of urinary steroids and are indicated in the investigation of endocrine disturbances of the adrenals and testes.

Urinary steroids can be divided into three main groups:
17-ketosteroids (17 KS)
17-ketogenic steroids (17 KGS)
17-hydroxycorticosteroids (17 OHCS)

17-ketosteroids are composed of 19 carbon atoms with a ketone group at C-17. These steroids are composed of adrenal hormones and metabolites of testicular androgens. In men the adrenals produce two thirds of these hormones, while the testes produce the remainder. In women the adrenals produce all of the hormones.

17-ketogenic steroids are composed of glucocorticoid derivatives and pregnanediol, having 21 carbon atoms and a hydroxyl group at C-17. The level of ketogenic steroids gives a good reflection of the adrenal cortex activity.

17-hydroxycorticosteroids are composed of 21 carbons with hydroxyl groups at C-17 and C-21 and a ketone group at C-20. These steroids are also referred to as Porter-Silber chromogens.

Procedure

1. A 24-hour urine container with preservative is labeled with name of patient, test, and date.
2. General instructions for 24-hour urine collection are followed.
3. Exact start and ending of collection are recorded on specimen container and patient's record (start 8:06 A.M., 11/30; end 8:00 A.M., 12/1).
4. Send the specimen to the laboratory refrigerator when the test is completed.

Clinical Implications

1. There is a decrease in KGS and KS excretion in Addison's disease, hypopituitarism, Simmonds' disease, and cretinism.
2. There is an increase in KGS excretion in precocious puberty on account of adrenal hyperplasia, surgery, excessive burns, and infection.

3. Elevated 17 OHCS and KGS usually indicate hyperplasia of the adrenal cortex, tumor, cancer, or some variation of the adrenogenital syndrome.
4. Steroid levels are also elevated in Cushing's syndrome, eclampsia, acute pancreatitis, and ACTH therapy. If the beta alpha ratio is >0.4, it is indicative of adrenal carcinoma. Unless the total 17KS are increased, the beta:alpha ratio is not likely to be abnormal.

Interfering Factors

1. Severe stress will cause increased levels of KS and KGS.
2. KS levels are often increased in the third trimester of pregnancy.
3. Drugs:

    (a) *Increasing 17 KS levels*

Chloramphenicol	Oleandomycin
Chlorpromazine	Penicillin
Cloxacillin	Phenaglycodol
Dexamethasone	Phenazopyridine
Erythromycin	Phenothiazines
Ethinamate	Quinidine
Meprobamate	Secobarbital
Nalidixic acid	Spironolactone

    (b) *Decreasing 17 KS levels*

Chlordiazepoxide	Probenecid
Estrogen	Promazine
Meprobamate	Reserpine
Metyrapone	

    (c) *Increasing levels of 17 OHCS*

Acetazolamide	Digoxin
Ascorbic acid	Cortisone
Chloral hydrate	Ethinamate
Chloramphenicol	Etryptamine
Chlordiazepoxide	Glutethimide
Chlormerodrin	Meprobamate
Chlorpromazine	Hydralazine
Chlorthalidone	Oleandomycin
Colchicine	Paraldehyde
Cloxacillin	Quinine
Erythromycin	Quinidine
Digitoxin	Spironolactone

(d) *Decreasing levels of 17 OHCS*

Aminoglutethimide	Diphenylhydantoin
Estrogen	Dexamethasone
Calcium gluconate	Phenothiazines
Oral contraceptives	Mitotane
Corticosteroids	Reserpine

Patient Preparation

1. Instruct patient about the purpose of test and collection of 24-hour urine specimen. Give a written reminder.
2. Food and fluids are permitted and encouraged.

PORPHYRINS AND PORPHOBILINOGENS

Normal Values

Porphobilinogens: 2 mg./24 hr.
Porphyrins: 50–300 mg./24 hr.
DLA or ALA: 1.0–710 mg./24 hr.
Fluorescent: negative

Explanation of Test

Porphyrins are cyclic compounds formed from delta-aminoloevuli acid (DAL or ALA) which is important in the formation of hemoglobin and other hemoproteins that function as carriers of oxygen in the blood and tissues. In health insignificant amounts of porphyrin are excreted in the urine. However, in certain conditions such as porphyria (disturbance in metabolism of porphyrin), liver disease, lead poisoning, and pellagra, there is an increased level of porphyrins, as well as DAL and ALA in the urine. Disorders in porphyrin metabolism also result in porphobilinogen.

In acute attacks of porphyria, the patient may suffer skin lesions, abdominal pain, neuropathy, and mental disturbances. The urine of patients with this disease usually has a pinkish to reddish-black tinge and will become darker upon standing.

In the laboratory the urine is tested for the presence of porphyrins, porphobilinogen, and DLA or ALA. It is also given the black light screening test (porphyrins are fluorescent when exposed to black or ultraviolet light.)

Procedure

1. A 24-hour urine container with preservative is labeled with name of patient, test, and date.
2. No refrigeration is required.
3. General instructions for 24-hour urine collection are followed.
4. Exact start and ending of collection are recorded on specimen container and patient's record (start 7:05 A.M., 11/15; end 7:30 A.M., 11/16).
5. Send the specimen to the laboratory refrigerator when the test is completed.
6. Porphobilinogens are always done with the porphyrin test. Should a single, fresh voided specimen be ordered, only a porphobilinogen will be done.
7. Observe and record the color of urine. If porphyrins are present, the urine may have a grossly recognizable amber red or burgundy color. It may vary from pale pink to almost black. Some patients will excrete a urine of normal color which turns dark after standing in the light.

Clinical Implications

A. *Porphyria*
    1. In the porphyrias the urine contains increased amounts of porphyrins and porphobilinogens and may not contain increased quantities of DLA or ALA.
    2. ALA and DLA excretion is elevated in acute intermittent porphyria, an hepatic porphyria that is aggravated by alcohol, barbiturates, and other drugs affecting the liver.
B. *Lead Poisoning*
    1. ALA or DLA will be present in the urine.
    2. Porphyrins may or may not be present in the urine.

C. *Other Conditions with Increased Levels of Porphyrins*

1. Cirrhosis
2. Infectious hepatitis
3. Hodgkin's disease
4. Some cancers
5. Central nervous system disorders
6. Heavy metal poisoning
7. Carbon tetrachloride or benzine toxicity

Interfering Factors

1. During menstruation and pregnancy porphyrins may be normally increased.
2. Drugs causing false positive tests:
   - (a) Acriflavine
   - (b) Ethoxazene
   - (c) Phenazopyridine
   - (d) Sulfamethoxazole
   - (e) Tetracyclines
   - (f) Antipyretics
   - (g) Barbiturates
   - (h) Phenylhydrazine
   - (i) Sulfonamides

Patient Preparation

1. Instruct patient about purpose and collection of 24-hour urine specimen. Give a written reminder.
2. Food and fluids are permitted and encouraged.

CLINICAL ALERT

This test should not be ordered for patients receiving Donnatol and other barbiturate preparations. However, if suspected, intermittent porphyria is the reason for testing, the test should be done with the patient receiving these medications because these drugs may provoke an attack.

AMYLASE EXCRETION

Normal Values

35–260 somogyi units/hr.
260–950 somogyi units/24 hrs.

Explanation of Test

Amylase is an enzyme which changes starch to sugar. It is produced in the salivary glands, pancreas, liver, and fallopian tubes and normally is excreted in small amounts in the urine. If there is an inflammation of the pancreas or salivary glands, much more of the enzyme enters the blood and more amylase is excreted in the urine. Therefore, the timed urine amylase test (2 hours or 24 hours) is ordered to detect inflammation of the salivary glands or pancreas, to monitor treatment of acute pancreatitis, and to recognize recurrent attacks of acute pancreatitis in persons who exhibit severe abdominal pain.

The two hour amylase excretion in the urine is a more sensitive test than either the serum amylase or lipase test. In patients with acute pancreatitis the urine often shows a prolonged elevation of amylase as compared to the short-lived peak in the blood. However, urine amylase may be elevated when blood amylase is within normal range, and conversely, the blood amylase may be elevated when urine amylase is within normal range. The 24-hour level may be normal even when some of the one or two-hour specimens show increased values.

Procedure

1. A one-hour, two-hour, or 24-hour timed specimen will be ordered. A two-hour specimen is usually collected.
2. No preservative or refrigeration is required.
3. General instructions for a timed or 24-hour urine collection are followed.
4. Exact start and ending of collection are recorded on the specimen container and on the patient's record (8:06 A.M., 11/17; end 10:15 A.M., 11/17).
5. Send the specimen to the laboratory refrigerator when the test is completed.

Clinical Implications

1. Elevated levels of urine amylase are associated with acute pancreatitis and choledocolithiasis.

2. Patients with acute pancreatitis have values about 900 units per hour during the first two days of the attack.

Patient Preparation

1. Instruct the patient about purpose of test and collection of the urine specimen. Give a written reminder for 2-hour or 24-hour test.
2. Encourage fluids during test if fluids are not restricted for other medical reasons

PHENYLKETONURIA (PKU) IN BLOOD AND URINE

Normal Values

Blood <4 mg./100 ml.
   Urine: Negative-dipstick; no observed color change

Explanation of Test

Routine blood and urine tests are done on newborns to detect PKU, a genetic disease that can lead to mental retardation and brain damage if untreated. This disease is characterized by a lack of the enzyme which converts phenylalanine, an amino acid, to tyrosine, which is necessary for normal metabolic function. If tyrosine accumulates in the tissues, phenylpyruvic acid, a metabolite of phenylalanine, will be produced, resulting in brain damage. Phenylalanine can be detected in the blood of an abnormal child in four days. Phenylpyruvic acid appears in the urine of an abnormal child about two to eight weeks after birth. Current practice is to test for PKU either with a blood phenylalanine test or with a phenylpyruvic acid urine test.

Procedure (Collecting Blood Sample)

1. After the skin is cleansed with an antiseptic, the infant's heel is punctured with a sterile disposable lancet.

2. If bleeding is slow, it is helpful to hold the leg dependent for a short time before spotting the blood on the filter paper.
3. The circles on the filter paper must be completely filled. This can best be done by placing one side of the filter paper against the baby's heel and watching for the blood to appear on the front side of the paper and completely fill the circle.

Procedure (Collecting Urine Sample)

1. The reagent strip is either dipped into a fresh sample of urine or pressed against a wet diaper.
2. After exactly 30 seconds, the strip is compared to a color chart scaled at concentrations of 0, 15, 40, and 100 mg. phenylpyruvic acid.

Clinical Implications

1. In a positive test for PKU, the blood phenylalanine is greater than 15 mg. per 100 ml. Blood tyrosine is less than 5 mg. per 100 ml. It is never increased in phenylketonuria.
2. The urine test is positive in PKU.

Interfering Factors

1. Premature infants, infants weighing less than 11 kilograms (5 pounds), may have elevated phenylalanine and tyrosine levels without having the genetic disease. This is probably a result of delayed development of appropriate enzyme activity in the liver.
2. Large amounts of ketones in urine will produce an atypical color reaction.

Instructions to Mothers

1. Inform mother about the purpose of the test and the method of collecting the specimens.
2. Most parents would be interested in knowing that PKU (a genetic disease in which a defective gene is passed on from each parent) was first recognized about 40 years ago

by a young mother of two mentally retarded children. She was aware that the urine of these children had a peculiar odor, and on the basis of this was able to have a biochemist study the urine and identify phenylpyruvic acid. About 20 years ago the first successful dietary treatment (restriction of phenylalanine as in milk) of newborn babies identified as having PKU was started, resulting in normal mental development.

CLINICAL ALERT
1. The blood test must be performed at least three days after birth or after the child has had a chance to ingest protein for a period of 24 hours.
2. Urine testing is usually done at four or six week checkup if a blood sample was not obtained.
3. PKU studies should be done on all babies five pounds or more before they leave the hospital.

TUBULAR REABSORPTION PHOSPHATE (TRP)

Normal Values

>78% on normal diet
>85% on a low phosphate diet

Explanation of Test

This test is done to detect hyperparathyroidism. A fasting blood and a 24-hour or a 4-hour urine sample is obtained to determine the levels of phosphorus and creatinine. The results of the test are based on the ratio of creatinine clearance to phosphate clearance. TRP is a rough estimation of the level of parathyroid hormone in the blood. The test is based on the fact that excessive parathyroid hormone increases renal tubular re-absorption of phosphate. However, the test has a limited value, and a determination of increased calcium in the blood is still essential for the exact diagnosis of hyperparathyroidism.

Procedure

1. An overnight fast from food is usually necessary. Water is permitted.
2. A venous blood sample will be obtained the morning of the day the test is completed.
3. A 24-hour urine container (also used for 4-hour test) with preservatives is labeled with name of patient, test, and date.
4. General instructions for 24-hour or 4-hour urine collection are followed.
5. A good time to do this test is from noon to noon, although it is not necessary.
6. Exact start and ending of collection are recorded on specimen container and patient's record. (12 noon, 11/17; end 12:06 P.M., 11/18)
7. Send the specimen to the laboratory refrigerator when the test is completed.

Clinical Implications

1. In hyperparathyroidism, the reabsorption of phosphate is increased to less than 74 per cent on a normal diet and less than 85 per cent on a low phosphate diet
2. The TRP is decreased in hypoparathyroidism.

Interfering Factors

False positive results may occur in the presence of uremia, renal tubular disease, osteomalacia, and sarcoidosis.

Patient Preparation

1. Instruct patient about purpose of test, collection of 24-hour or 4-hour urine specimen, overnight fast if ordered, and blood sample. A normal or phosphate diet will be ordered. Give a written reminder.
2. If fasting is ordered encourage patient to drink water.

PHENOLSULFONPHTHALEIN (PSP) EXCRETION

Normal Values

15 min.—30–35% A normal 15 min. value indicates normal glomerular filtration rate.
30 min.—20–25% for a longer than 15 min. specimen
60 min.—10–15% for a longer than 30 min. specimen

Explanation of Test

This test of kidney function measures tubular secretions. It is a timed measurement of the rate of excretion of phenolsulfonphthalein dye by the kidney. This rate depends chiefly on the renal plasma flow. The dye is given in a single injection and is excreted most rapidly in the first few minutes. The rate of excretion is proportional to the amount presented to the kidney in the blood. Normally, 30 to 50 per cent of the dye will be excreted within 15 minutes of the injection. In reduced blood flow, the blood must be recirculated through the kidney over a longer period of time to excrete the same amount of dye. If given enough time, the damaged kidney will excrete the same amount of dye as the normal kidney, so decreased excretions may be apparent only during the first 15 minutes.

For many years, the rate of PSP excretion has been one of the most widely used tests for clinical evaluation of renal function.

Procedure

1. The test may be performed at any time of day.
2. Patient is asked to drink eight to ten glasses of water.
3. When patient indicates that he has the urge to void, 1 ml. (6 mg.) of PSP dye is injected intravenously.
4. Urine specimens are collected at 15 minutes, 30 minutes, and 60 minutes after injection.
5. All specimens are saved and sent to the lab.
6. The exact time of collection of specimens is recorded.

Clinical Implications

1. Decrease in the total per cent indicates either renal tubular disease or diminished renal plasma flow, as might occur in shock or heart failure.
2. The creatinine clearance test is probably a more reliable function test for clinical use.
3. During the course of renal failure, if effective plasma flow is reduced in rough proportion to the glomerular filtration rate, the PSP excretion should approximately parallel creatinine or urea clearance.
4. A delay in excretion with normal total values indicates urinary retention.
5. False positive results may occur in hepatic disease, multiple myeloma, and hypoalbuminuria.
6. Drugs that interfere with PSP excretion include
   - (a) salicylates,
   - (b) penicillin,
   - (c) some diuretic and formaldehyde-forming drugs,
   - (d) X ray contrast media.
7. See appendix for complete listing of drugs that may cause false positive or false negative results.

Interfering Factors

1. At least 24 hours must elapse between this test and a BSP (Bromsulphalein) test done for liver function.
2. Incomplete emptying of the bladder, inadequate urine volumes, and failure to inject an exact amount of dye are the most common causes of inadequate test results.

Patient Preparation

1. Instruct the patient about the purpose of the test, the drinking of water, the injection of dye, and the collection of specimens. Instruct patient to completely empty bladder at each voiding.
2. Inform patient that he may be ambulatory and that he need not fast.

3. Encourage fluid intake during the test so that the patient can void.
4. Instruct the patient that the dye may turn the urine color to red.
5. This test can be hazardous in severe renal insufficiency or heart failure because hydration is required prior to testing.

CLINICAL ALERT
1. Timing must be precise: a difference of a minute or two in the 15 minute specimen will alter the amount of dye excretion and give a falsely high or low result.
2. The test is worthless if the patient cannot void spontaneously. Before test is started, check with physician to determine if the bladder can be emptied by catheter if necessary.
3. Inject the dye only after the patient feels the urge to void.
4. Accurately inject exactly one ml., for the entire test depends upon a determination of the amount of dye excreted in the percentage of the amount injected.

BILIRUBIN

Normal Values

Negative—0.02 mg./dl.

Background

Bilirubin is formed in the reticuloendothelial cells of the spleen and bone marrow from the breakdown of hemoglobin. It is linked to albumin in the bloodstream and is transported to the liver. Bilirubin in the urine, however, indicates the presence of hepatocellular disease or intra or extra hepatic biliary obstruction. Urinary bilirubin excretion will reach significant levels in any disease process that increases the amount of conjugated bilirubin in the bloodstream (see blood chemistry). Normally, there is a small amount of urobilinogen, not bilirubin, in the urine.

Explanation of Test

This test should be done with a routine urinalysis. It should be performed when the color of the urine indicates the possibility of bilirubin (see p. 119). It is an aid in the diagnosis of hepatitis and liver dysfunction, and it is helpful in monitoring the course of treatment. In persons exposed to toxins and certain drugs, a positive test for bilirubinuria can be an early indication of liver damage.

Procedure

1. Examine urine within one hour of collection, because bilirubin is not stable in urine, especially when exposed to light.
2. *Strip testing*
   (a) Good lighting is necessary.
   (b) Close approximation to the color chart is an absolute must. Failure to make a close comparison is an important basis of failure to recognize bilirubin in urine.
   (c) The reagent strip is dipped in fresh urine, tapped to remove excess urine, and after a 20-second period, compared to the color chart on the reagent strip bottle.
   (d) The results are interpreted as negative and 1 to 3+ positive or as small, moderate, and large amounts of bilirubin.
3. *Tablets and test mats*
   (a) Place five drops of urine on the special test mat.
   (b) Place on Ictotest reagent bottle in moistened area of mat.
   (c) Flow two drops of water on table.
   (d) When elevated amounts of bilirubin are present in the urine, a blue to purplish color forms within 30 seconds. The rapidity and the intensity of the color formation and development are proportionate to the amount of bilirubin in the urine. Normal amounts of bilirubin in the urine give a negative test result.

Clinical Implications

1. Increased:
   (a) Liver disease due to infections or toxic agents
   (b) Obstructive biliary disease

Tests for Bilirubin

1. Reagent strips such as bili-Labstix, multistix, and N-multistix
2. Ictotest reagent tablets and special test mats

Interfering Factors

1. Drugs causing false positive reactions:
   - (a) Large doses of chlorpromazine (thorazine)
   - (b) Phenothiazines
   - (c) Acetophenazine
   - (d) Chlorprothixine
2. Drugs which interfere with testing procedures:
   - (a) Aspirin
   - (b) Pyridium
   - (c) Ponstel

D-XYLOSE ABSORPTION

Normal Values

Urine: more than 1.2 gm.
Blood: 25–40 mg./100 ml. in 2 hours.

Explanation of Test

This test is an indirect measure of intestinal absorption and is used in the differential diagnosis of steatorrhea. The usual problem is the differentiation of pancreatic from enterogenous steatorrhea. When d-xylose (which is not metabolized by the body) is administered orally, blood and urine levels are checked for absorption rates. Absorption is normal in pancreatic steatorrhea but will be impaired in interogenous steatorrhea.

Procedure

1. No food or liquids by mouth after midnight on the day of the test.
2. Have patient void between 8:00 and 9:00 A.M. Discard urine.

3. Then give five gm. of d-xylose orally. Dissolve 250 ml. (8 oz.) of water. Follow immediately with an additional 250 ml. of water. Note time and record on patient's record. No further fluids or food until test is completed.
4. Exactly two hours later, a venous blood sample of three ml. is obtained.
5. Patient must remain stationary until completion of test.
6. Have all urine voided during the test. Five hours after the test is started, have patient void. Add this urine to collected urine, if any. Send urine specimen to laboratory.

Clinical Implications

1. Decreased
   (a) Enterogenous steatorrhea
   (b) Malabsorption

Patient Preparation

Explain purpose and procedure of test and collection of urine specimen.

Patient Aftercare

Provide food and fluids and allow patient to be ambulatory.

CLINICAL ALERT
Nausea, vomiting, and diarrhea may occur as side effects of d-xylose, especially if more than five grains of drug are given.

AMINO ACID NITROGEN

Normal Values

50–200 mg./24 hours

Background

The renal threshold for amino acids in the blood is high, so that normally only small amounts of amino acids are found in urine. Amino acids are excreted by the glomeruli but are readily absorbed by the tubules. Amino acids that normally appear in the urine in larger quantities 25–200 mg. per 24 hours include:

1. Glycine
2. Taurine
3. Histidine
4. Glutamine

Amino acids that normally appear in urine in small amounts are (0–25 mg./24 hours):

1. Tryptophan
2. Tyrosine
3. Serine
4. Leucine
5. Cystine
6. Arginine
7. Phenylalanine

Explanation of Test

This test is done primarily to detect renal aminoaciduria due to defective tubular reabsorption of certain amino acids which leads to increased renal excretion.

Procedure

1. A 24-hour container with preservative is labeled with name of patient, test, and date.
2. Refrigeration of specimens is also required.
3. General instructions for 24-hour urine collection are followed.
4. Exact start and ending of collection are recorded on specimen container and patient's record (start 7:06 A.M., date; end 7:30 A.M., date)
5. When all urine is collected, the specimen is sent to laboratory refrigerator.

Clinical Implications

1. Increased in:
   - (a) Fanconi syndrome
   - (b) Cystinosis
   - (c) Wilson's disease
   - (d) Cystinuria
   - (e) Glycinuria
   - (f) Liver disease
   - (g) Megaloblastic anemias
   - (h) Lead poisoning
   - (i) Muscular dystrophies
   - (j) Leukemia
   - (k) Maple syrup urine disease
   - (l) Hartnup disease
   - (m) Phenylketonuria
   - (n) Oxalosis
   - (o) Tyrosinosis
   - (p) Pyridoxine deficiency
   - (q) Folic acid deficiency

Interfering Factors

1. Increased in premature and newborn infants.
2. Drugs which may cause increased levels include:
   - (a) ACTH
   - (b) Ampicillin
   - (c) Cortisone
   - (d) Sulfonamide
   - (e) Tetracycline
3. Drugs which may cause decreased levels include:
   - (a) Epinephrine
   - (b) Insulin

Patient Preparation

1. Instruct patient about the purpose of the test and collection of 24-hour urine specimen. Give a written reminder.
2. Food and fluids are permitted.

UROBILINOGEN (QUANTITATIVE AND ESTIMATED)

Normal Values

Estimation random specimen 0.3–3.5 mg/100 ml.
   2-hour specimen 0.3–1.0 Ehrlich units/2 hours
   24-hour specimen 1–4 mg./24 hours

Explanation of Test

This is one of the most sensitive of the tests used to determine impaired liver function. Determinations of urinary urobilinogen are a useful procedure in routine urinalysis since they serve as a guide in detecting and differentiating liver disease, hemolytic disease, and biliary obstruction. Sequential determinations also assist in evaluating progress of the disease and response to treatment. Although it is usually a 24-hour urine test, a single, freshly voided specimen or a timed two-hour urine specimen may be ordered.

Bilirubin, formed from the metabolism of hemoglobin entering the intestine in the bile, is transformed through the action of bacteria into urobilinogen. Part of the urobilinogen formed in the intestine is excreted with the feces; another portion is absorbed into the portal bloodstream and carried to the liver where it is metabolized and excreted in the bile. Traces of urobilinogen that escape removal from the blood by the liver are carried to the kidneys and excreted in the urine, the basis of the urine urobilinogen test.

Procedure

1. The estimation test must be performed on fresh urine.
2. General instructions for collection of a 24-hour, 2-hour, or random specimen collection are followed depending upon what has been ordered.
3. The 2-hour timed collection is best done from 1:00 to 3:00 P.M., or 2:00 to 4:00 P.M. Collect without preservatives. Record total amount of urine voided.
4. Color strip method of testing for urobilinogen:
    (a) The reagent color strip is dipped into urine, removed, and tapped free of excess urine.
    (b) The color reaction is compared to the color chart after exactly 60 seconds.
        1. The five color blocks provided on the chart range in color from light yellow to dark reddish brown, representing 0.1, 1, 4, 8, and 12 Ehrlich units per 100 dl. of urine

2. The first two color blocks 0.1 and 1 Ehrlich unit per dl. are within the normal range of values.
3. The remaining three color blocks indicate abnormally high values.
4. This test will not accurately detect a decrease or absence of urobilinogen.

CLINICAL ALERT
If any specimens are lost during the 24-hour urine collection, the test is nullified and should be restarted immediately. Notify laboratory and physician if this occurs.

Clinical Implications

1. Urinary urobilinogen is *increased* by any condition that causes an increase in the production of bilirubin and by any disease that prevents the liver from normally removing the reabsorbed urobilinogen from the portal circulation.
   (a) Increased urobilinogen is *increased* whenever there is excessive destruction of red blood cells as in:
      1. Hemolytic anemias
      2. Pernicious anemia
      3. Malaria
   (b) Values above normal also occur in:
      1. Infectious and toxic hepatitis
      2. Pulmonary infarct
      3. Biliary disease
      4. Cholangitis
      5. Hemolytic jaundice and anemia
      6. Chemical injury to liver due to chloroform and carbon tetrachloride poisoning
      7. Cirrhosis
      8. Congestive heart failure
      9. Infectious mononucleosis
   (c) An *increased* urobilinogen level is one of the earliest signs of acute liver cell damage.

2. Urinary urobilinogen is *decreased* or absent when normal amounts of bilirubin are not excreted into the intestinal tract. This usually indicates partial or complete obstruction of the bile ducts such as may occur in:
    (a) Cholelithiasis
    (b) Severe inflammatory disease
    (c) Cancer of the head of pancreas
        (1) During antibiotic therapy, suppression of normal gut flora may prevent breakdown of bilirubin to urobilinogen, leading to its absence in the urine.
        (2) Decreased values are also associated with:
            (a) Severe diarrhea
            (b) Renal insufficiency

Interfering Factors

1. Drugs and foods that may cause urobilinogen to be increased include:
    (a) Para-aminosalicylic acid (PAS)
    (b) Antipyrine
    (c) Bromsulphalein (BSP)
    (d) Cascara
    (e) Chloropromazine
    (f) Phenazopyridine
    (g) Phenothiazines
    (h) Sulfonamides
    (i) Drugs that cause hemolysis of RBC's (*e.g.,* aspirin)
    (j) Bananas
    Note: See appendix for complete listing of drugs that interfere with testing
2. Drugs that may cause decreased urobilinogen include those which cause cholestasis and those which reduce the bacterial flora in the gastrointestinal tract (*e.g.,* choloramphenicol and other antibiotics).
3. Peak excretion is known to occur from noon to 4:00 P.M. The amount of urobilinogen in the urine is subject to diurnal variation.
4. Strongly alkaline urine will show a higher value and strongly acid urine will show a lower level.

CREATININE CLEARANCE

Normal Values

115–120 ml./min. or 0.7–1.5 mg./ml. of blood in urine or blood.

Explanation of Test

This blood and urine test is a specific measurement ordered to determine kidney function, primarily glomerular filtration. It measures the rate at which creatinine is cleared from the blood by the kidney. Clearance of a substance may be defined as the imaginary volume (ml./min.) of plasma from which the substance would have to be completely extracted in order for the kidney to excrete that amount in one minute.

Creatinine is a substance that, in health, is easily excreted by the kidney. Creatinine is the by-product of muscle energy metabolism and is produced at a constant rate depending upon the muscle mass of the individual. Endogenous production of creatinine is constant as long as muscle mass remains constant. Since all the creatinine that is filtered in a given time interval appears in the urine, the creatinine is equivalent to the glomerular filtration rate (GFR). A disorder of kidney function prevents excretion of creatinine. More than 50 of the total kidney nephrons have to be altered to reflect change in the normal value.

Procedure

1. A 12 or 24-hour urine container is labeled with name of patient, test, and date.
2. No refrigeration is necessary.
3. General instructions for 24-hour urine collection are followed.
4. Exact start and ending of collection are recorded on specimen container and patient's record (Start 8:32 A.M./date; end 8:35 A.M./date)
5. Send specimen to the laboratory refrigerator when the test is completed.

6. A venous blood sample of seven ml. is obtained the morning of the day that the 12 or 24-hour collection will be completed.

Clinical Implications

1. A normal clearance cannot be used as a standard for a patient who is known to have existing renal disease.
2. A decreased clearance gives a reliable indication of impaired kidney function.
3. However, a normal blood creatinine does not always indicate unimpaired renal function.

Interfering Factors

Phenacetin will cause creatinine clearance to be decreased.

Patient Preparation

1. Instruct patient about the purpose of the test and collection of urine specimen. Give a written reminder.
2. Food and fluids are permitted. Encourage fluids so that voiding is easier because a large urine flow is best for greatest accuracy of the test.

OSMOLALITY

Normal Values

Dilute urine—less than 200 milliosmoles
urine—more than 850 milliosmoles

Background

Osmolality, a more exact measurement of urine concentration than specific gravity, depends on the number of particles of solute in a unit of solution, whereas specific gravity depends on both the quantity and precise nature of the particles in the unit. Protein, sugar, and IV dyes elevate urine specific gravity disproportionately more than the osmolality.

Explanation of Test

Whenever a more precise measurement than specific gravity is indicated in the evaluation of the concentration and diluting ability of the kidney, this test is done. The measurement of urine osmolality during water restriction is an accurate test of decreased kidney function. It is also used in the differential diagnosis of diabetes insipidus (compulsive water drinking).

Procedure

1. A high-protein diet is prescribed for three days.
2. On the evening before the test, a dry supper is eaten and no liquids drunk until the test is over.
3. At approximately 6:00 A.M., the patient empties the bladder and returns to bed. This urine is not saved.
4. The test urine specimen is collected at 8:00 A.M. and the sample is labeled and sent to the laboratory. Record on the patient's record. The test is then completed.

Clinical Implications

1. *Increased* in:
   (a) Post surgery
   (b) Hepatic cirrhosis
   (c) Congestive heart failure
   (d) Addison's disease
   (e) IV sodium
   (f) High protein diets
   (g) Inappropriate ADH secretion
2. *Decreased* in:
   (a) Aldosteronism
   (b) Diabetes insipidus
   (c) Hypokalemia
   (d) Hypercalcemia
   (e) Compulsive water drinking
   (f) IV 5 per cent dextrose and water

Patient Preparation

1. Explain the purpose and procedure of the test to patient.
2. No liquids are to be eaten with the evening meal before the

test. No food or liquids after the evening meal until test is completed.

Patient Aftercare

Provide patient with food and fluids as soon as 8:00 A.M. urine sample is obtained.

PREGNANCY TESTS AND PLACENTAL HORMONE TESTS

Normal Values

Negative, blood and urine

Background

From the earliest stage of development (nine days old), the placenta produces hormones, either on its own or in conjunction with the fetus. The very young placental trophoblast produces appreciable amounts of a hormone, human chorionic gonadotropin (HCG), that is excreted in the urine. HCG is not found in the urine of normal, young, nonpregnant women.

Explanation of Test

Increased urinary levels of HCG form the basis of most tests for pregnancy and trophoblastic tumors in men. All pregnancy tests are designed to detect HCG. HCG is present in blood and urine whenever there is living chorionic/placental tissue. HCG can be detected in the urine of pregnant women 26 to 49 days after the first day of the last menstrual period, or eight to ten days after the end of the last missed period. Pregnancy tests should be negative three to four days after delivery.

The tests using female rats or male frogs have been supplanted by immunologic tests which are more accurate, easier to perform, and do not require a laboratory to maintain animal facilities. Common urine tests for pregnancy are the Gravendex,

Placentex, Pregnosis, Pregnosticon. Biocept-5 is a common blood test for pregnancy.

Procedure (For Urine Tests)

1. An early morning urine specimen is collected. The first morning specimen generally contains the greatest concentration of HCG. However, specimens collected at any time may be used.
2. A 24-hour specimen is collected for quantitative studies. Then the general procedure for collection of 24-hour urine specimens is followed.

Procedure (For Blood Test)

1. A venous blood sample of ten ml. is obtained.

Clinical Implications

1. A positive result usually indicates pregnancy. Only two thirds of women with ectopic pregnancies will have positive pregnancy tests.
2. Positive results also occur in:
    - (a) Choriocarcinoma
    - (b) Hydatidiform mole
    - (c) Testicular tumors
    - (d) Chorioepithelioma
    - (e) Chorioadenoma destruens
    - (f) Conditions with a high ESR such as acute salpingitis

Interfering Factors

1. *False negative tests* and falsely low levels of HCG may be due to a dilute urine (low specific gravity) or from a specimen obtained too early in pregnancy.
2. *False positive tests* are associated with:
    - (a) Proteinuria
    - (b) Hematuria
    - (c) Presence of excess pituitary gonadotropin (HLH) as in menopausal women
    - (d) Drugs
        1. Anticonvulsants

2. Antiparkinson
3. Hypnotics
4. Tranquilizers

MORPHINE (ASSAY)

Normal Values

Negative

Explanation of Test

This test detects the presence of morphine and its analogs, detects drug overdose, and is used to identify a heroin or morphine drug user. Urine is the fluid most commonly sampled, but blood is also examined.

Procedure

1. A random sample or 24-hour urine sample may be ordered.
2. A venous blood sample is obtained.

Clinical Implications

1. The test is positive when heroin or morphine are present.
2. A positive result is also obtained when substances other than heroin or morphine are present as in:
   (a) An individual ingesting 20 mg. of codeine orally in cough syrup. This would be expected since codeine is closely related structurally to morphine.
   (b) Individuals consuming five to 15 gm. of poppy seeds.

REFERENCES

Collins, R. Douglas: ILLUSTRATED MANUAL OF LABORATORY DIAGNOSIS. 2nd Ed., Philadelphia, J. B. Lippincott Company, 1975.
Free, Alfred H. and Free, Helen M.: URODYNAMICS: CONCEPTS

RELATING TO ROUTINE URINE CHEMISTRY. Elkhart, Indiana, Ames Company, Division of Miles Laboratories, Inc. 1976.

Freeman, James, and Beeler, Myrton: LABORATORY MEDICINE-CLINICAL MICROSCOPY. Philadelphia, Lea & Febiger, 1974.

French, Ruth M.: GUIDE TO DIAGNOSTIC PROCEDURES. 4th Ed., New York, McGraw-Hill Book Company, 1975.

Garb, Solomon: LABORATORY TESTS IN COMMON USE. 6th Ed., New York, Springer Publishing Company, 1976.

Meyer, John S., et al.: REVIEW OF LABORATORY MEDICINE. St. Louis, The C. V. Mosby Company, 1975.

MODERN URINE CHEMISTRY: A GUIDE TO THE DIAGNOSIS AND METABOLIC DISORDERS OF URINARY TRACT DISEASES. Elkhart, Indiana, The Ames Company, Division of Miles Laboratories, Inc., 1976.

Tilkian, S. M., Conover, M. H., and Tilkian, A. G.: CLINICAL IMPLICATIONS OF LABORATORY TESTS. 2nd Ed., St. Louis, The C. V. Mosby Company, 1979.

URINE UNDER THE MICROSCOPE. Nutley, N.Y., Rocom Press, a Division of Hoffman-LaRoche, Inc., 1975.

Wallach, Jacques: INTERPRETATION OF DIAGNOSTIC TESTS—A HANDBOOK SYNOPSIS OF LABORATORY MEDICINE. 3rd Ed., Boston, Little, Brown and Company, 1978.

Widmann, Frances K.: Goodale's CLINICAL INTERPRETATION OF LABORATORY TESTS. 8th Ed., Philadelphia, F. A. Davis Company, 1978.

3 □□ FECAL STUDIES

INTRODUCTION: FORMATION AND COMPOSITION OF FECES

An adult excretes 100 to 300 grams of fecal matter a day, and of this, as much as 70 per cent may be water. The feces are what remains of the eight to ten liters of fluid that enter the intestinal tract each day. Food and fluid taken orally, saliva, gastric secretions, pancreatic juice, and bile contribute to the formation of feces.

Feces are composed of:
1. Waste residue of indigestible material in food
2. Bile (pigments and salts)
3. Intestinal secretions, including mucus
4. Leukocytes that migrate from the bloodstream
5. Sheded epithelial cells

6. Large numbers of bacteria which make up to one-third of total solids
7. Inorganic material (10–20%) which is chiefly calcium and phosphates
8. Digested food (present in very small quantities)

The output of feces depends on a complex series of absorptive, secretory, and fermentative processes. Normal function of the colon involves three physiologic processes: (1) absorption of fluid and electrolytes; (2) contractions which churn the contents, expose contents to the mucosa, and transport the contents to the rectum; and (3) defecation.

The small intestine is approximately 23 feet long, and the large intestine is 4 to 5 feet long. The small intestine degrades ingested fats, proteins, and carbohydrates to absorbable units and absorbs them. Pancreatic, gastric, and biliary secretions operate in the luminal contents to prepare them for active mucosal transport. Other active substances absorbed in the small intestine include fat-soluble vitamins, iron, and calcium. Vitamin B_{12} after complexing with intrinsic factors, is absorbed in the ileum. The small intestine also absorbs as much as 9.5 liters of water and electrolytes for return to the bloodstream. Small intestine contents (chyme) begin to enter the rectum as soon as two to three hours after a meal, but the process is not complete until six to nine hours after eating.

The large intestine performs less complex functions than the small intestine. The proximal or right colon absorbs most of the remaining water. Colonic absorption of water, sodium, and chloride is a passive process. Daily water excretion in the feces is only about 100 ml. The motility of the colon consists mainly of moving the luminal contents to and fro by seemingly random contractions of circular smooth muscle. More propulsive activity occurs after eating. Massive peristalsis usually occurs several times a day. Resultant distention of the rectum initiates the urge to defecate. In persons with normal motility and with a mixed dietary intake, transit time in the colon is 24 to 48 hours.

Normally evacuated feces reflect the shape and caliber of the colonic lumen. The normal consistency is somewhat plastic, neither fluid, mushy nor hard; the usual brown color results from bacterial degradation of bile pigments; the odor results from degradation of protein.

Appearance

Stool examination should include size, shape, consistency, color, odor, and presence or absence of blood, mucus, pus, tissue fragments, food residues, bacteria or parasites. (See Chapter 6 for a discussion of microbiological analysis of feces.) The gross appearance of feces should be done before administration of barium, laxatives, or enemas.

Patients and health personnel dislike examining, collecting and delivering feces for examination. But, this natural aversion must be overcome when considering the value of a feces examination in diagnosing many clinical conditions and diseases of the gastrointestinal tract.

RANDOM COLLECTION OF STOOL SPECIMENS

1. Feces should be collected in a dry, clean, urine-free container. The entire stool should be collected. The stool should be transferred to a container by using tongue blades. For the best results, stool specimens should be covered and delivered to the laboratory immediately after collection.
   (a) Warm stools are best for detecting ova and parasites.
   (b) Some coliform bacilli produce antibiotic substances that destroy enteric pathogens.
   (c) Refrigerate stool if it cannot be examined immediately. Never place a stool in an incubator.
2. A diarrheal stool will usually give good results.
3. A freshly passed stool is the choice specimen.
4. Preferably, stool specimens should be collected before antibiotic therapy is initiated, and as early in the course of disease as possible.
5. Only a small amount of stool is needed. A stool the size of a walnut is usually adequate. However, it is recommended that the entire passed stool be sent for examination. If mucus or blood is present, it should definitely be included with the specimen because parasites are more likely to be found in these substances.
6. Do not use a stool that has been passed into the toilet bowl.
7. Label all stool specimens with patient's name, date, and reason for testing.

Interfering Factors

1. Meat interferes with some tests and should usually be omitted from the diet for three days prior to test for blood.
2. Stool specimens from patients receiving barium, bismuth, oil, or antibiotics are not satisfactory for some testing methods.
3. Bismuth from paper towels and toilet tissue interferes with tests.

Patient Preparation

1. Explain purpose and procedure of test.
2. Instruct patient to defecate in a clean bedpan or large-mouthed container.
3. Instruction should be given to the patient that he is not to urinate into bedpan or collecting container.
4. Remind him that no toilet paper should be placed in a bedpan or container since it interferes with testing.
5. If the patient has diarrhea, newspaper (not paper towels, which contain bismuth) can be deposited into the toilet bowl and the diarrheal stool obtained above the water level of the toilet bowl. (Note: This method may be used if the patient collects the stool specimen at home.)

COLLECTION OF 24-, 48, and 72-HOUR STOOL SPECIMENS
(used with testing for fat and urobilinogen)

Special Instructions

1. Collect all stool specimens for one to three days. The entire stool should be collected.
2. Label specimens as to Day #1, Day #2, Day #3, time of day, patient's name, and purpose of examination.
3. Submit individual specimens to laboratory as soon as collected.

Interfering Factors

Mineral oil, laxatives, and enemas interfere with quantitative fat testing and should not be administered during the three-day collection period.

CONSISTENCY, SHAPE, AND FORM

Normal Values

Plastic, soft, formed; soft and bulky on a high vegetable diet; small and dry, on a high meat diet; seeds and vegetable skins present

TABLE 3-1. NORMAL VALUES IN STOOL ANALYSIS

Macroscopic Examination	Normal
1. Color	Brown
2. Odor	Varies with pH stool and dependent on bacterial fermentation and putrefaction
3. Consistency	Plastic; not unusual to see suds and vegetable skins; soft and bulky in a high vegetable diet; small and dry in a high meat diet.
4. Size, shape	Formed
5. Gross blood	None
6. Mucus	None
7. Pus	None
8. Parasites	None

Microscopic Examination	Normal
1. Fat	Colorless, neutral fat (18%), and fatty acid crystals and soaps
2. Undigested food; meat fibers, starch, trypsan	None to small amount
3. Eggs and segments of parasites	None
4. Yeasts	None

Chemical Examination	Normal
1. pH	Neutral or weakly alkaline
2. Occult blood	Negative

Explanation of Test

Normally evacuated feces reflect the shape and caliber of the colonic lumen as well as the colonic motility. The bowel habits of healthy persons vary widely. For this reason, the words "diarrhea" and "constipation" have little meaning except when viewed as a change from the customary individual pattern. Detailed information is important in evaluating either abnormality.

Procedure

See "Random Collection of Stool Specimens," p. 210.

Clinical Implications

1. The consistency of feces may change in various disease states:
   - (a) Diarrhea mixed with mucus and blood is associated with:

1. Typhus	4. Amebiasis
2. Typhoid	5. Large-bowel cancer
3. Cholera	

   - (b) Diarrhea mixed with mucus and pus is associated with:

1. Ulcerative colitis	3. Shigellosis
2. Regional enteritis	4. Salmonellosis

   - (c) "Pasty" stool is associated with a high fat content:
     1. A significant increase of fat is usually detected grossly.
     2. In obstruction of the common bile duct, the fat gives a puttylike appearance to the stool (acholic).
     3. In sprue and celiac disease, the appearance of the stool often suggests radiator paint due to fatty acid.
     4. In cystic fibrosis, the increase of neutral fat gives a greasy "butter stool" appearance.
2. Alterations in size or shape indicate altered motility or abnormalities in the colonic wall.
   - (a) A narrow ribbon-like stool suggests the possibility of spastic bowel or rectal narrowing or stricture, decreased elasticity, or a partial obstruction.

   (b) Excessively hard stools are usually due to increased absorption of fluid as a result of prolonged contact of luminal contents with the mucosa of the colon because of delayed transit time.

   (c) A very large caliber stool indicates dilatation of the viscus.

   (d) Small, round, hard stools accompany habitual, moderate constipation.

   (e) Severe fecal retention can produce huge impacted masses with a small amount of pasty stool as overflow.

Assessment of Diarrhea and Constipation

1. When patients complain of diarrhea and constipation it is important to obtain and record:
   (a) An estimate of volume and frequency of fecal output
   (b) Consistency, blood, pus, mucus, oiliness and bad odor. Obtain through direct examination.
   (c) Reduction or increase in frequency of defecation
   (d) Sensations of rectal fullness with incomplete evacuation of stools
   (e) Painful defecation due to hard stools
2. Assess the patient's emotional status. In many instances, the onset of psychologic stress is the major reason for altered bowel habits.

ODOR AND pH

Normal Values

Characteristic odor varies with the pH of stool.
   Normal pH neutral or weakly alkaline

Explanation of Test

The odor of feces varies with the pH of the stool. The pH is dependent on bacterial fermentation and putrefaction in the bowel.

   Substances called indole and skatole, formed by intestinal

putrefaction and fermentation, are primarily responsible for the odor of normal stools.

An observation should be made about the odor of feces.

Interfering Factors

1. Carbohydrate fermentation changes the pH to acid.
2. Protein breakdown changes the pH to alkaline.

COLOR

Normal Values

Brown

Explanation of Test

The color of the feces should be noted for the reason that it can provide information on pathologic conditions, organic dysfunction, bleeding, diet, and intake of drugs. An abnormality in color may aid the clinician in selecting appropriate diagnostic chemical and microbiological tests of stool.

The brown color of normal feces is probably due to stercobilin, a bile pigment derivative, which results from the action of reducing bacteria in bilirubin.

Procedure

See "Random Collection of Stool Specimens," p. 201

Clinical Implications

1. The color of feces changes in disease states:
    (a) Yellow to yellow-green—severe diarrhea
    (b) Green—severe diarrhea
    (c) Black—usually the result from bleeding into the upper gastrointestinal tract.
    (d) Tan or clay-colored—associated with blockage of the

common bile duct as well as pancreatic insufficiency which produces a pale, greasy, "acholic" stool. In these instances, reduced quantities of bile pigments enter the intestine because of intrinsic hepatobiliary disease or obstruction.

(e) Red—possible result of bleeding from the lower gastrointestinal tract.

2. Grossly visible blood always indicates an abnormal state:

(a) Blood streaked on the outer surface usually indicates hemorrhoids or anal abnormalities.

(b) Blood present in stool can also arise from abnormalities higher in the colon. If transit time is sufficiently rapid, blood from the stomach or duodenum can appear as bright or dark red in stool.

Interfering Factors

1. Stool darkens on standing.
2. Color is influenced by diet, food dyes, certain foods, and drugs.

(a) Yellow to yellow-green occurs in the stool of breast-fed infants who lack normal intestinal flora. It also occurs in sterilization of bowel by antibiotics.

(b) Green occurs in diets high in chlorophyll-rich vegetables and with use of the drug calomel.

(c) Black or very dark brown may be due to drugs such as iron, charcoal, and bismuth, to foods such as cherries, or to an unusually high proportion of meat in the diet.

(d) Light-colored with little odor may be due to diets high in milk and low in meat.

(e) Claylike color may be due to a diet with excessive fat intake.

(f) Red may be due to a diet high in beets or drugs such as Bromsulphalein (sodium sulfabromophthalein).

(g) Certain color changes may result from drugs, summarized below:

Black—iron salts, bismuth salts, charcoal
Green—mercurous chloride, indomethacin, calomel
Green to blue—dithiazanine

Brown staining—anthraquinones
Red—phenolphthalein, pyrvinium pamoate, tet-
racyclines in syrup, Bromsulphalein
Yellow—santonin
Yellow to brown—senna
Light—sitosterols
Whitish discoloration—antacids
Orange-red—phenazopyridine
Pink to red to black—anticoagulants, excessive dose
and salicylates causing internal bleeding

CLINICAL ALERTS
A good dietary and drug history will help to differentiate significant
abnormalities from interfering factors.

BLOOD IN STOOL

Normal Values

Negative

Explanation of Test

Passage of more than 2.8 ml. of blood in 24 hours is an
important sign of gastrointestinal disease. Blood is most commonly seen when hemorrhoids and anal fissures are present.
Drugs such as salicylates, steroids, indomethacin, colchicine,
iron (when used in massive therapy) and rauwolfia derivatives
are associated with increased gastrointestinal blood loss in
normal persons, and with even more pronounced bleeding
when disease is present. Gastrointestinal bleeding can also
follow parenteral administration of these drugs.

Procedure

Chemical Test for Occult Blood in Stool
Detection of occult blood in the stool is very useful in detecting
or localizing disease of the gastrointestinal tract. The common

tests for detecting blood in feces use substances that depend on peroxidase content as an indication of hemoglobin content to cause a color change in the stool specimen that is tested. The reagent substances used differ in sensitivity. Tests to detect occult blood:

1. Orthotoluidine (Occultest) is one to ten times more sensitive than benzidine.
2. Benzidine is ten to 1,000 times more sensitive than the guaiac test.
3. Guaiac is the least sensitive of the three tests.

Clinical Implications

1. A dark red to black tarry appearance to the stool is indicative of a loss of 0.50 to 0.75 ml. of blood from the upper gastrointestinal tract. Smaller quantities of blood in the gastrointestinal tract can produce similar stools or appear as bright red blood.
2. A stool should be considered grossly bloody only after chemical testing to prevent confusing bloody stool with coloring from diet or drugs (see "Color of Stool").
3. Blood in the stool is abnormal and should be reported and recorded.
4. Gross or occult blood in the stool may indicate chronic nonspecific ulcerative colitis, or carcinoma of the colon.
5. Stool specimens may be positive for blood in diaphragmatic hernia.
6. Occult blood may appear in stool in diverticulitis, gastric carcinoma, and gastritis.

Interfering Factors

1. Meat in the diet contains hemoglobin and enzymes that can give false positive tests for up to four days after eating. The guaiac method does not require a meat-free diet.
2. Vitamin C taken in quantities greater than 500 mg. per day may cause a false negative test for occult blood in the stool.
3. Drugs which may cause a false positive test for occult blood include:
   (a) Boric acid

(b.) Bromides
(c.) Colchicine
(d.) Iodine
(e.) Iron, inorganic
(f.) Oxidizing agents

Patient Preparation

1. If the patient is to have either the orthotoluidine test or the benzidine test, he must be instructed to have a meat-free diet for at least three days prior to test.

PUS IN STOOL

Normal Values

Negative

Explanation of Test

Recognizable pus is seldom seen in stools unless there is a draining rectal infection or ulcerating or fungating process.

Procedure

See "Random Collection of Stool Specimens," p. 201.

Clinical Implications

1. Large amounts of pus accompany:
   (a) Chronic ulcerative colitis
   (b) Chronic bacillary dysentery
   (c) Localized abscesses
   (d) Fistulas to sigmoid rectum or anus
2. Large amounts of pus seldom accompany amebic colitis. Its presence is evidence against this diagnosis.
3. Pus in the stool is abnormal and should be reported and recorded.

MUCUS IN STOOL

Normal Values

Negative

Explanation of Test

The mucosa of the colon secretes mucus in response to parasympathetic stimulation. Mucus in the stool appears in conditions of parasympathetic excitability.

Procedure

See "Random Collection of Stool Specimens," p. 201.

Clinical Implications

1. Presence of recognizable mucus in a stool specimen is abnormal and should be reported and recorded.
2. Translucent gelatinous mucus clinging to the surface of formed stool occurs in:
   (a) Spastic constipation
   (b) Mucous colitis
   (c) Emotionally disturbed patients
   (d) Excessive straining at stool
3. Bloody mucus clinging to the feces is suggestive of neoplasma or inflammation of rectal canal.
4. In villous adenoma of colon, copious quantities of mucus may be passed (up to three to four liters in 24 hours).
5. Mucus with pus and blood is associated with:
   (a) Ulcerative colitis
   (b) Bacillary dysentery
   (c) Ulcerating cancer of colon
   (d) Acute diverticulitis } rarely
   (e) Intestinal tuberculosis

FAT IN STOOL

Normal Values

In a normal diet, the stool can contain up to 18 per cent colorless fatty acid crystals and soaps.

Explanation of Test

Normal stool does not contain free neutral fats. The presence of free fat is indicative of interference with normal fat absorption, or with bile or pancreatic excretion.

Procedure

1. Collect a random stool specimen or a 72-hour specimen. If a 72-hour specimen is required, each individual stool specimen is collected and identified with name of patient and time and date and sent immediately to laboratory.
2. Follow procedure for collection of random or 72-hour specimen (pp. 201–202).

Clinical Implications

1. Increases in fecal fat and fatty acids are associated with:
   (a) Enteritis and pancreatic diseases when there is a lack of lipase
   (b) Surgical removal of a section of the intestine
   (c) Malabsorption syndromes
2. A stool specimen high in fat content will have a pasty appearance and can be detected by gross examination.
3. A low fat value is indicative of steatorrhea.

Interfering Factors

Increased neutral fat may occur under the following conditions:
1. With use of rectal suppositories
2. With ingestion of castor oil and mineral oil
3. With ingestion of dietetic low-calorie mayonnaise

Patient Preparation

1. Explain purpose of test and procedure for collection of specimen.
2. If a 72-hour stool collection is ordered, a diet containing 100 grams of fat per day is ordered during testing. Follow procedure for collection of 72-hour stool specimen.

REFERENCES

Bauer, John, Ackerman, Philip, and Toro, Gelsen: CLINICAL LABORATORY METHODS. 8th Ed., St. Louis, The C. V. Mosby Company, 1974.

Berkow, Robert (ed.): THE MERCK MANUAL OF DIAGNOSIS AND THERAPY. 13th Ed., Rahway, N.J., Merck Sharp & Dohme Research Laboratories, 1977.

Collins, R. Douglas: ILLUSTRATED MANUAL OF LABORATORY DIAGNOSIS. 2nd Ed., Philadelphia, J. B. Lippincott Company, 1975.

Gillies, R. R.: LECTURE NOTES ON MEDICAL MICROBIOLOGY. 2nd Ed., Oxford, Blackwell Scientific Publications, 1978.

Wallach, Jacques: INTERPRETATION OF DIAGNOSIC TESTS—A HANDBOOK OF LABORATORY MEDICINE. 3rd. Ed., Boston, Little, Brown and Company, 1978.

4 □ CEREBROSPINAL FLUID STUDIES

DESCRIPTION, FORMATION, AND COMPOSITION OF CSF

Background

Cerebrospinal fluid (CSF) is a clear, colorless liquid formed within the cavities of the brain (the lateral and fourth ventricles) by the choroid plexus and diffused blood plasma. Approximately 150 ml. of the fluid is formed per day.

Circulating slowly from the ventricular system into the spaces surrounding the brain and spinal cord, the CSF serves as a hydraulic shock absorber diffusing the force from a hard blow to the skull that might otherwise cause severe injury. The CSF also works as a hydrostatic barrier between the brain and spinal cord and the bony protection of the skull and vertebrae.

Most constituents of the CSF are present in the same or lower concentrations as in the blood plasma, except for chloride concentrations which are usually higher. Thus, like blood plasma, CSF contains few cells and little protein. Disease, however, can cause elements ordinarily restrained by the blood brain barrier to enter the spinal fluid. Erythrocytes and leukocytes can enter the CSF from the rupture of blood vessels or from meningeal reaction to irritation, and bilirubin, normally not present, can be found in the spinal fluid after intracranial hemorrhage. In such cases the arachnoid granulations and the nerve root areas will reabsorb the fluid; and although normal CSF pressure will consequently be maintained by the absorption of CSF in amounts equal to production, this will not be a source of nourishment to the central nervous system, for the CNS is mainly nourished by the blood circulatory system's carotid arteries to the brain. Of the many factors that regulate the level of CSF pressure, venous pressure is the most important since the reabsorbed fluid ultimately drains into the venous system.

Despite the continuous production and reabsorption of CSF and the exchange of substances between the CSF and the blood plasma, considerable pooling occurs in the lumbar sac. The lumbar sac at L3 to L4 is the usual site for puncture since damage to the nervous system is unlikely to occur in this area which is occupied solely by the filum terminale. In children the spinal cord persists more caudally than in adults and a low lumbar puncture should be made.

In some instances, such as head injury, a question may arise about the nature of small amounts of clear liquid draining from the nose and/or ear. When such drainage occurs, a test-tape for glucose such as clinistix (Ames Company) can be inserted into the nose or ear and left there for five minutes. A positive glucose reaction of 2+ to 3+ suggests that the fluid is most likely CSF.

CLINICAL ALERT
Thirty per cent of the tests reported with this test-tape technique for detection of CSF leakage show *false positive* results.

Explanation of Test

Cerebrospinal fluid is usually obtained by lumbar puncture. A lumbar puncture is done for several reasons:

1. Examination of the spinal fluid, as in cases of suspected meningitis and intracranial hemorrhage.
2. Determination of level of CSF to document impairment of CSF flow or to lower the pressure by removal of a volume of fluid. Fluid removal can be dangerous; the brain stem could be dislocated.
3. Diagnosis of organic central nervous system disease
4. Introduction of anesthetics, drugs, and X ray contrast media
5. Evaluation of certain electrolyte disturbances
6. Removal of blood or exudate from the subarachnoid space

Examination of CSF

Certain observations are made every time lumbar puncture is performed:

1. General appearance, consistency, and tendency to clot are noted.
2. Pressure is measured.
3. Cell count is performed in laboratory to distinguish types of cells present.
4. Protein, chloride and sugar concentrations are determined.
5. Other clinical serologic and bacteriologic tests are done when the patient's condition warrants such as tests for aerobes and anaerobes, tuberculosis, VDRL, fungal studies, and colloidal gold test.

Note: Blood levels should always be measured simultaneously with CSF.

PROCEDURE FOR STERILE LUMBAR PUNCTURE (SPINAL TAP)

1. The patient is usually placed in a side-lying position with head flexed onto the chest and knees drawn up to the abdomen to bow the back. This position helps to increase the space between the lower lumbar vertebrae so that the spinal needle can be inserted with ease between the spinal proc-

esses. However, a sitting position (patient straddles a straight-backed chair) with head flexed to chest can be used. The patient is helped to relax with soothing words and instructed to breathe slowly and deeply with mouth open.

2. The puncture site is selected, usually between L3-L4 or L4-L5 or lower. The site is thoroughly cleansed with an antiseptic solution, and the surrounding area is draped with sterile towels.
3. A local anesthetic is injected slowly into the puncture site.
4. A spinal needle with stylet is inserted into the midline between the spines of the third and fourth lumbar space. The spinal cord is avoided; the needle is to enter the subarachnoid space. The patient may feel the prick of the needle and a feeling of pressure. Patient should be helped to slowly straighten his legs.
5. The stylet is removed and a manometer is attached to the needle to record opening CSF pressure.

    Note: If the initial pressure is normal and a subarachnoid block is suspected, the Queckenstedt test is done. In this test, pressure is placed on both jugular veins to temporarily occlude them and to produce an acute rise in CSF fluid. Normally pressure rapidly returns to average levels. Total or partial spinal block is diagnosed if the lumbar pressure fails to rise when both jugular veins are compressed or if the pressure requires more than 20 seconds to fall after compression is released.
6. A specimen of five to ten ml. of CSF is removed and usually is collected in three tubes. Tubes are labeled "1," "2," and "3" in correct order of collection. A closing pressure reading is done and the needle is withdrawn.
7. A small sterile dressing or adhesive bandage is applied to the puncture site.
8. Tubes should be correctly labeled with number (#1, 2, or 3), patient's name and date. CSF specimens must be delivered immediately to laboratory personnel. The spinal fluid should never be placed in the refrigerator provided for other specimens. Refrigeration will alter test results if bacteriological and fungal studies are done. Analysis should be started immediately.

Patient Preparation

1. Explain purpose of test; give a step-by-step description of procedure.
2. Help patient to be as relaxed as possible. Breathing slowly and deeply with mouth open may help patient to relax.

Patient Aftercare

1. Patient should lie flat, usually for four to eight hours, on back or abdomen to help prevent headache. Turning from side to side is permitted.
2. Female patients will have difficulty in voiding in this position. The use of a "fracture bedpan" may help to alleviate voiding problems.
3. Fluids are encouraged to help in prevention and relief of possible headache.
4. Observe patients for change in neurological state, such as elevated temperature, increase in blood pressure, irritabilily, as well as numbness and tingling sensations in lower extremities.
5. If headache should occur, administer ordered sedatives and analgesics and encourage longer period of bedrest.

CLINICAL ALERT

1. Extreme caution should be used in lumbar puncture when intracranial pressure is elevated, especially when papilledema is present. In some cases of increased intracranial pressure, however, such as with a comatose patient, intracranial bleeding, or suspected meningitis, the need to establish a diagnosis is absolutely essential and outweighs the danger of the procedure.
2. Other contraindications to lumbar puncture are:
   (a) Serious spinal deformities
   (b) Extreme age
   (c) Infection or severe dermatologic disease in the lumbar area may result in spinal fluid infiltration and infectious complications.
   (d) Severe personality problems or chronic back pain in neurotics

TABLE 4–1. NORMAL CSF VALUES IN ADULTS

Volume	90–150 ml.
	clear as water
Pressure	75–150 mm. H_2O
Total cell count	0–5/cc. mm.
	(All cells are lymphocytes PMN's and RBC's absent)
Specific gravity	1.006–1.008
Osmolality	280–290 mOsm/kg.
Clinical Tests	
Glucose	45–85 mg./dl.
Protein	15–45 mg./dl. (lumbar)
	15–25 mg./dl. (cisternal)
	5–15 mg./dl. (ventricular)
A/G ratio (albumin to globulin)	8:1
Chloride	118–132 mEq./L.
Urea nitrogen	6–16 mg./dl.
Creatinine	0.5–1.2 mg./dl.
Cholesterol	0.2–0.6 mg./dl.
Uric acid	0.5–4.5 mg./dl.
Bilirubin	0 None
Electrolytes and pH	
pH	7.30–7.40
Chloride	118–132 mEq./L.
Sodium	144–154 mEq./L.
Potassium	2.0–3.5 mEq./L.
CO_2 content	25–30 mEq./L. (m. mol)
PCO_2	42–53 mm. Hg.
PO_2	40–44 mm. Hg.
Calcium	2.1–2.7 mEq./L.
Magnesium	2.4–3.1 mEq./L.

COLOR

Normal Value

Crystal clear and colorless, like water

Background

A slight color change may be difficult to detect and CSF should be compared with a test tube of distilled water held against a white background. If there is no turbidity, a newspaper can be read through the tube.

TABLE 4–2. COLOR CHANGES IN CSF SUGGESTIVE OF DISEASE STATES*

Appearance	Condition
Opalescent, slightly yellow with delicate clot	Tuberculous meningitis
Opalescent to purulent, slightly yellow with coarse clot	Acute pyogenic meningitis
Slightly yellow; may be clear or opalescent with delicate clot	Acute anterior poliomyelitis
Bloody; purulent; may be turbid	Primary amebic meningoencephalitis
Generally clear, but may be xanthochromic	Tumor of brain or cord
Xanthochromic	Toxoplasmosis

*Color and clot changes are only *very general* indications of disease states. They must not be thought of as specific indicators.

Clinical Implications

1. Abnormal colors are due to:
   - (a) Blood (the blood is evenly mixed in all three tubes in subarachnoid and cerebral hemorrhage)
   - (b) Bilirubin, as in bilirubinemia (conjugated in adults; unconjugated in infants)
   - (c) Yellow pigments (xanthochromia) usually signify previous bleeding as in subarachnoid hemorrhage. The xanthochromia grading range is 1+ to 4+.
   - (d) Dark yellow with a tendency to clot usually indicates subarachnoid block
   - (e) If the CSF protein is more than 100 mg. per dl., an abnormal color will result.
   - (f) Carotene, as in carotenemia
   - (g) Melanin, from meningeal melanosarcoma.
2. Turbidity usually signifies considerable numbers of leukocytes, especially neutrophils. In acute meningitis it may vary from slight cloudiness to almost pure pus. In a cryptococcal infection, tubidity is due to the presence of yeast cells.
3. Clear CSF fluid does not rule out intracranial hemorrhage.

Interfering Factors

1. If the blood in the specimen is due to trauma during lumbar puncture, the fluid in the third tube is usually lighter in color.

2. Contamination of the specimen with a disinfectant such as merthiolate will cause an abnormal color.
3. A traumatic tap will cause an abnormal color. Resulting specimen may appear similar to that obtained in subarachnoid hemorrhage.

MICROSCOPIC EXAMINATION OF CELLS; TOTAL CELL COUNT; DIFFERENTIAL CELL COUNT OF CSF

Normal Values

0 to 8 cu. mm. (all small lymphocytes)

Background

CSF is essentially free of cells. When the cells are counted they are identified by cell type, and the percentage of cell type is compared to the total number of white cells present.

Clinical Implications

A. Cell Counts
1. An increase in the number of cells in CSF is termed *pleocytosis*, which may be classified as follows:
   (a) 5–10 cells: borderline or slight pleocytosis
   (b) 25–50 cells: elevated or moderate pleocytosis
   (c) Over 50 cells: severe pleocytosis
2. Disease processes may lead to abrupt increases or decreases (shift to the right or left) of otherwise normal cells (see p. 19) and the appearance of cells not usually found in the CSF.
   (a) White cell counts above 500 usually arise from a purulent infection and are predominantly granulocytes.
   (b) White cell counts of 300 to 500 with predominantly monocytic (lymphocytes or monocytes) clear cells are indicative of:
      1. Viral infections, such as poliomyelitis and aseptic meningitis

2. Syphilis of CNS
3. Tuberculous meningitis
4. Multiple sclerosis
5. Tumor or abscess

(c) White cell counts with 40 per cent or more monocytes are seen after subarachnoid hemorrhage.

B. Abnormal Cells
1. Malignant cells (lymphocytes and/or histiocytes) are present with primary and metastatic brain tumors
2. Lymphocytoid and plasmacytoid cells are present in:
   (a) Subacute and chronic inflammatory processes
   (b) Multiple sclerosis
   (c) Leukoencephalitis
   (d) Delayed hypersensitivity responses
   (e) Subacute viral encephalitis
   (f) Meningitis (tuberculous or fungal)
   (g) Some brain tumors
   These cells (#a–f, above) are responsible for an increase in IgG and for altered patterns in immunoelectrophoresis (see p. 426).
3. Macrophages are present in traumatic and ischemic cranial infarcts.
4. Glial, ependymal, and plexus cells may be present after surgical procedures or trauma to the central nervous system.

PROTEIN IN CSF

Normal Values

15–45 mg./dl. (lumbar)
15–25 mg./dl. (cisternal)
5–15 mg./dl. (ventricular)

Background

CSF normally contains very little protein, because the protein in blood serum is in the form of large molecules that do not

TABLE 4-3. PROTEIN LEVELS IN CSF IN VARIOUS DISEASES*

Disease	Level of Protein (mg./dl.)
Congenital toxoplasmosis	≤ 2000
Cerebral hemorrhage	≤ 2000
Tumor of spinal cord	≤ 3500 (may be normal in 15% of patients)
Subarachnoid hemorrhage	≤ 1000
Cryptococcal meningitis	≤ 500
Tuberculous meningitis	45–500
Acute anterior poliomyelitis	20–350

*Based on figures in Wallach, J.: *Interpretation of Diagnostic Tests* 3rd Ed., Boston, Little, Brown and Co., 1978 pp. 240–243.

cross the blood-brain barrier. However, the proportion of albumin to globulin is higher in CSF than in the blood plasma, since the albumin molecule is significantly smaller and can more easily cross the blood-brain barrier. Increased permeability of the blood-brain barrier to protein occurs in infections.

Clinical Implications

1. Moderate to marked increases in total protein levels and alterations in the ratio of albumin to globulin (A/G ratio) occur in:
   (a.) Purulent meningitis
   (b.) Guillain-Barré syndrome
   (c.) Froin's syndrome
   (d.) Tuberculous meningitis
   (e.) Aseptic meningitis
   (f.) Syphilis
   (g.) Brain tumors and abscesses
   (h.) Subarachnoid hemorrhage
2. In most diseases any changes in CSF cell count and protein are parallel. For example, as the CSF cell count rises, the CSF protein level also rises.

Interfering Factors

1. Drugs which may cause increased levels include:
   (a.) Anesthetics (local) contaminant
   (b.) Chlorpromazine
   (c.) Salicylates
   (d.) Streptomycin
   (e.) Sulfanilamide
   (f.) Tryptophan

2. Drugs which may cause decreased levels include
    (a.) Albumin   (b.) Acetophenetidin

CLINICAL ALERT
Neurosyphilis is characterized by an increase in protein, a reactive VDRL, and an increase in number of lymphocytes.

PRESSURE OF CSF

Normal Values
75–150 mm. H_2O

Background
CSF fluid pressure is directly related to pressure in the jugular and vertebral veins, which connect with the intracranial dural sinuses and spinal dura. In conditions such as congestive heart failure and obstruction of the superior vena cava CSF pressure is increased, but in circulatory collapse it is decreased.

Removal of CSF produces a fall in CSF pressure (5–10 mm. drop for every ml. of fluid removed from the lumbar sac). For example, if ten ml. is removed, the closing pressure should be 50 to 100 mm. less than the opening pressure.

Clinical Implications
1. Increases in pressure can be a significant finding in:
    (a) Intracranial tumors
    (b) Purulent or tuberculous meningitis
    (c) Low-grade inflammatory processes
    (d) Encephalitis
    (e) Neurosyphilis
2. Decreases in pressure can be a significant finding in:
    (a.) Tumor of spinal cord (CSF pressure could also be normal in this condition)

(b.) Bloody tap (pressure could be normal)

(c.) Diabetic coma

3. Variations in opening and closing CSF pressures are significant in:

    (a) Tumors or spinal block when there is a large pressure drop indicative of a small CSF pool.

    (b) Hydrocephalus when there is a small pressure drop that is indicative of a large CSF pool.

Interfering Factors

1. Slight elevations of pressure may occur in the anxious person who holds his breath or tenses his muscles.

2. If an obese person's knees are flexed too firmly against his abdomen, venous compression will cause an elevation in pressure.

CHLORIDE IN CSF

Normal Values

118–132 mEq./l.

Background

Any condition that alters the blood plasma chloride level will also affect the CSF level. Chlorides in CSF are higher (1.2 to 1) than in blood plasma. The measurement of CSF chloride is most useful in the diagnosis of tuberculous meningitis.

Clinical Implications

1. *Decreased* levels are associated with:

    (a) Tuberculous meningitis

    (b) Bacterial meningitis

Interfering Factors

1. Concurrent IV administration of chloride will invalidate test results.

2. Test values are invalidated if blood, as in a traumatic tap, is mixed with the specimen.

GLUCOSE IN CSF

Normal Values

45–85 mg./dl. (20 mg./dl. less than blood level)

Background

The CSF glucose level varies with the blood glucose levels. CSF is usually 50 to 80 per cent of blood glucose. A blood glucose specimen should be obtained at least 30 to 60 minutes prior to lumbar puncture for comparison. Any changes in blood sugar are reflected in the CSF after one to 3 hours.

Clinical Implications

1. *Decreased* levels are associated with:
   - (a) Pyogenic, tuberculous, and fungal meningitis
   - (b) Toxoplasmosis
   - (c) Sarcoidosis
   - (d) Subarachnoid hemor- rhage
   - (e) Primary brain tumors
   - (f) Lymphomas
   - (g) Leukemia
   - (h) Melanoma
   - (i) Viral meningo- encephalitis

   Note: (*All types* of organisms consume glucose, and decreased glucose reflects bacterial activity)
2. *Increased* levels are associated with:
   - (a) Mump encephalitis
   - (b) Cerebral trauma
   - (c) Brain tumors accompanied by increased intracranial pressure
   - (d) Hypothalamic lesions
3. CSF glucose levels are usually normal in some viral infections of the brain and in meninges and aseptic meningitis

Interfering Factors

1. CSF glucose is decreased in hypoglycemia.
2. CSF glucose is increased in diabetes.

CALCIUM IN CSF

Normal Values

2.1 to 2.7 mEq./l.
  The CSF contains only half as much calcium as the blood. CSF calcium is usually 50 per cent of the blood serum calcium. When the CSF protein increases, the CSF calcium also increases. CSF calcium tends to reflect ionized calcium levels in serum.

Clinical Implications

Increases are associated with tuberculous meningitis.

UREA IN CSF

Normal Values

7 to 15 mg./dl.

Background

The urea levels in CSF and blood are approximately equal. Urea is sometimes administered intravenously to reduce cerebral edema. This will cause an induced uremia that will result in a shifting of fluid from the brain to the spinal fluid. 24 to 48 hours after urea administration, urea levels should return to normal.

Clinical Implications

Increased urea levels are associated with uremia.

REFERENCES

Bauer, John D., Ackermann, Philip, and Toro, Gelson, *Clinical Laboratory Methods.* 8th Ed., St. Louis, C. V. Mosby Company, 1974.

Davidson, Israel, and Henry, John Bernard, Todd-Sanford, *Clinical Diagnosis by Laboratory Methods.* 15th Ed., Philadelphia, W. B. Saunders Company.

Meyer, John S., *et al. Review of Laboratory Medicine.* 2nd Ed., St. Louis, C. V. Mosby Company, 1975.

Widmann, Frances. *Clinical Interpretation of Laboratory Tests.* 8th Edition, Philadelphia, F. A. Davis Company, 1979.

5 □ □ BLOOD CHEMISTRY AND ELECTROLYTE ANALYSIS

INTRODUCTION

Blood chemistry is a means of identifying many of the body's chemical constituents found in the blood. Although the relation of the abnormal levels of these constituents to disease can be evaluated, unfortunately, very few diseases show a single abnormality in body chemistry. Thus, it is often necessary to measure several body chemicals to establish a pattern of abnormalities characteristic of a particular disease. The quantity of blood that is drawn for samples will vary, depending on the method used in testing and the available machines or equipment.

A wide range of tests falls into the category of blood chemistry. Several can be grouped under the broad headings of enzymes, electrolytes, blood sugar, protein or protein by-products, and toxicity. Others have no such common denominator.

From the numerous tests included here, selected tests serve as screening devices in general patient care. Most of these tests constitute the patient profile that is obtained from the autoanalyzer printout indicated below.

Use of the Autoanalyzer

The use of autoanalyzers in a laboratory setting has made it possible to conduct a wide variety of chemical tests on a single sample of blood. Analyzers such as the Technicon SMA 12/60 System (Sequential Multiple Analyzer) (see Fig. 5–1) and the MSSP (Multiple Sequential Screening Panel) require approximately eight minutes to process a single sample through about 12 basic chemical analyses. The results of these tests are automatically recorded on a strip chart on which the chemical tests are listed horizontally and the numerical ranges vertically. The normal ranges are shaded in gray so that any abnormal readings will be easily noticed.

Because of the speed of the autoanalyzer and the number of tests it can process in a short period of time, it has become a major means of screening patients during hospital admission. Not only does it provide a baseline for future comparison while the patient is in the hospital, but it also uncovered unsuspected diseases in 4 per cent of patients admitted, allowing for early diagnosis of diseases whose symptoms are either vague or absent.

Text continues on p. 241.

Fig. 5–1 (A–I). *Results of a multiparameter test for multiparameter testing, provided by the Technicon SMA 12/60 System, a multichannel system that can perform 12 blood chemistry analyses simultaneously. Certain patterns of increases and decreases in blood constituents are associated with particular disease entities. The normal range for each constituent tested is indicated by a vertical shaded strip. (Used with permission of Technicon Instruments Corporation, Tarrytown, New York.)*

Figure appears on pages 232 to 240.

12/60

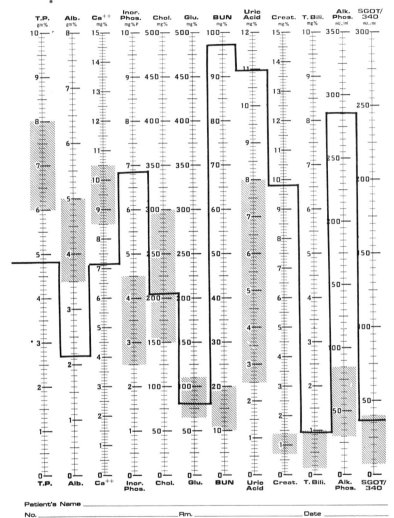

Patient's Name _____

No. _____ Rm. _____ Date _____

Fig. 5-1(A). *Chronic glomerulonephritis.*
Calcium: low
Inorg. phos.: high
Alk. phos.: high
BUN: high
Uric acid: high
Creatinine: high
Total protein: low
Albumin: low

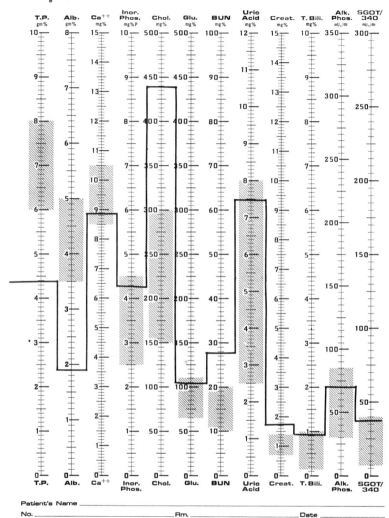

Fig. 5–1 (B).   *Nephrotic syndrome.*
Cholesterol: high
Total protein: very low
Albumin: low
BUN: moderately elevated

S M A 12/60

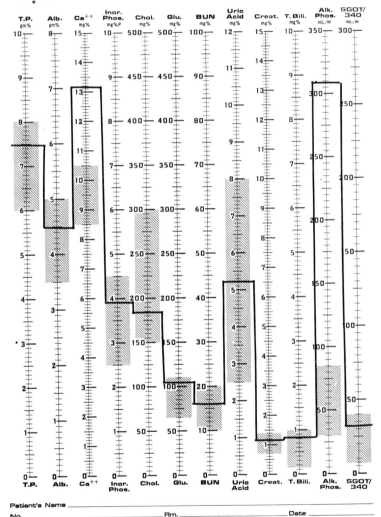

Patient's Name _____

No. _____ Rm. _____ Date _____

Fig. 5-1 (C).   *Metastatic carcinoma of bone.*
Calcium: high
Osteoblasts proliferate
Alkaline phosphatase: dramatically increases

234

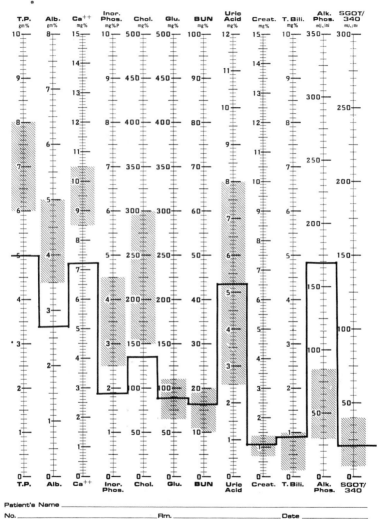

S M A 12/60

Fig. 5–1 (D). Severe malabsorption syndrome.
Serum calcium: low
Alkaline phosphatase: high
Total protein, albumin, cholesterol: reduced
Metastatic carcinoma of liver.

235

12/60

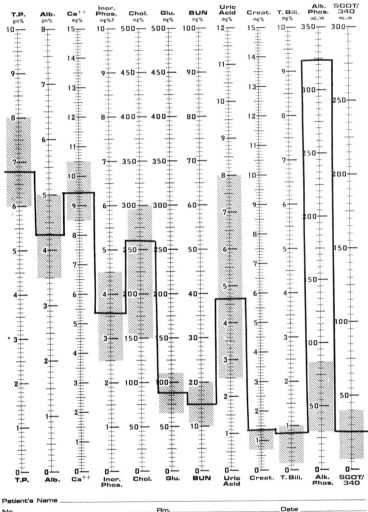

Patient's Name _____

No. _____ Rm. _____ Date _____

Fig. 5-1 (E). *Isolated elevation of alkaline phosphatase.*
Metastatic carcinoma of liver.

236

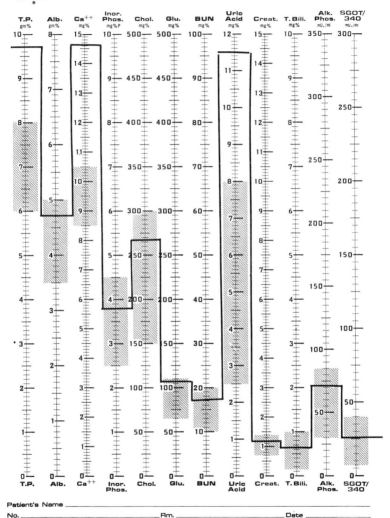

Fig. 5–1 (F).   *Multiple myeloma.*
Calcium: elevated
Alkaline phosphatase: normal
Uric acid: elevated
Total protein: markedly elevated

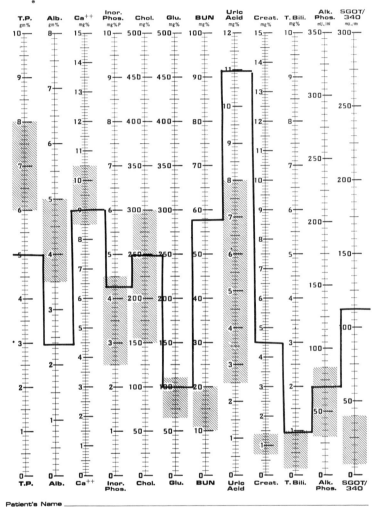

Patient's Name _____

No. _____ Rm. _____ Date _____

Fig. 5–1 (G). *Acute eclampsia.*
BUN: elevated
Uric acid: elevated
Creatinine: elevated.
SGOT: elevated
Albumin: decreased
Total protein: decreased

S M A 12/60

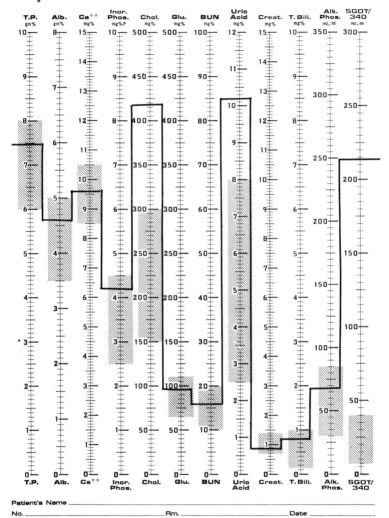

Fig. 5-1 (H).   *Myxedema.*
Cholesterol: elevated
Uric acid: elevated
SGOT: elevated

239

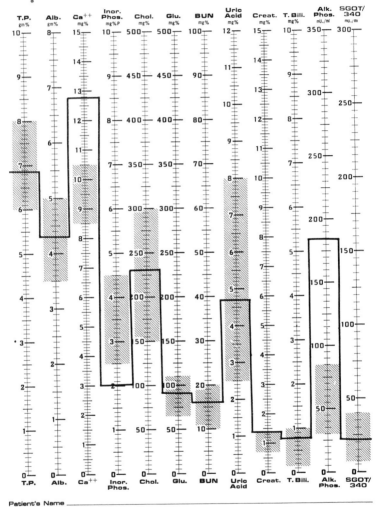

Patient's Name _____

No. _____ Rm. _____ Date _____

Fig. 5-1 (I). *Primary hyperparathyroidism.*
Calcium: elevated
Alkaline phosphatase: elevated
Inorganic phosphorus: decreased

The blood chemistries usually recorded include:

Total Protein (T.P.)	Uric Acid
Albumin	Creatinine
Calcium (Ca++)	Total Bilirubin
Inorganic Phosphorus	Alkaline phosphatase
Cholesterol	Serum Glutamine oxaloacetic
Glucose	transaminase. (SGOT/340)
Blood Urea Nitrogen (BUN)	

Various combinations of these chemical values provide insight into liver function, kidney disease, cardiovascular and pulmonary disorders, hematologic and reticuloendothelial dysfunction, and possible cancerous conditions.

CALCIUM (Ca++)

Normal Values

Total	Ionized
9.0–10.6 mg./dl.	4.2–5.2 mg./dl.
4.5–5.3 mEq./l.	2.1–2.6 mEq./ l.

Explanation of Test

This test measures the concentration of calcium in the blood and is used as a measure of parathyroid function and calcium metabolism.

The bulk of body calcium (98–99%) is stored in the skeleton and teeth, which act as huge reservoirs for maintaining the blood levels of calcium. About 50 per cent of the blood calcium is ionized; the rest is protein-bound. However, only ionized calcium can be used by the body in such vital processes as muscular contraction, cardiac function, transmission of nerve impulses, and blood clotting. Yet the ionized calcium cannot be measured independent of the total calcium levels. Therefore, the 50 per cent ratio is only estimated and can fluctuate depending on general acid-base balance: in acidosis, the ionized calcium will be higher than 50 per cent; in alkalosis, it will be lower.

The amount of protein in the blood will also affect calcium

levels since 50 per cent of the blood calcium is protein-bound. Thus a decrease in serum albumin would result in a concomitant decrease in total serum calcium.

A patient suffering from a deficiency of ionized calcium will show signs of tetany accompanied by muscular twitching and eventual convulsions (a neuromuscular response to the decreased calcium at the nerve junctions).

Factors Influencing Calcium Levels

A. *Parathyroid Hormone*
   1. Blood calcium is regulated by parathyroid hormone which exerts a direct effect on bone to release calcium into the blood.
   2. Parathyroid hormone also acts on both the intestines, increasing absorption of calcium, and the kidneys, causing calcium to be reabsorbed by the proximal tubules.
B. *Calcitonin*
   This hormone lowers blood calcium levels by increasing calcium clearance by the kidneys.
C. *Vitamin D*
   Stimulates calcium absorption by the intestines
D. *Estrogens and Androgens*
   1. Estrogens increase calcium deposits in the bones. (Osteoporosis, following menopause, may respond to estrogen therapy.)
   2. Androgens—Hyperfunction of the adrenal cortex or thyroid may result in hypocalcemia and bone decalcification.
E. *Carbohydrates and Lactose*
   1. Carbohydrates increase intestinal absorption of calcium.
   2. Addition of lactose to the diet increases the absorption and retention of calcium.

Clinical Implications

A. *Normal Levels of Calcium Combined with Other Findings*
   1. Normal calcium levels with overall normal findings in other tests indicate that there are no problems with calcium metabolism.

2. Normal calcium and abnormal phosphorus indicate impaired calcium absorption due to alteration of parathyroid hormone activity or secretion. In rickets, the calcium level may be normal or slightly lowered and the phosphorus level is depressed.

3. Normal calcium and elevated BUN indicates:
   (a.) Possible secondary hyperparathyroidism
   Initially a lowered serum calcium results from uremia and acidosis. The lower calcium level stimulates the parathyroid to release parathyroid hormone which acts on bone to release more calcium.
   (b.) Possible primary hyperparathyroidism
   Excessive amounts of parathyroid hormone cause elevation in calcium levels, but secondary kidney disease would cause retention of phosphate and concomitant lower calcium.

4. Normal calcium and decreased serum albumin
   This is indicative of hypercalcemia since there should be a decrease in calcium when there is a decrease in albumin because of the 50 per cent of serum calcium that is protein-bound.

B. *Hypercalcemia* (Increased calcium levels)
   Hypercalcemia is associated with many disorders, but its greatest clinical importance rests in its association with *cancer,* including multiple myeloma, parathyroid tumors, nonendocrine tumors producing a parathyroid-like substance, and cancers metastasizing to the bone.
   Increased calcium levels are caused by or associated with:
   1. Hyperparathyroidism due to:
      (a.) Parathyroid adenoma ⎫ Associated with
      (b.) Hyperplasia of para- ⎬ hypophosphatemia
           thyroid glands   ⎭
   2. Cancer
      (a.) Metastatic cancers involving bone
           Cancers of lung, breast, thyroid, kidney, and testes may metastasize to bone
      (b.) Hodgkin's disease and other lymphomas
      (c.) Multiple mytiple myeloma in which there is extensive bone destruction

(d.) Lung and renal cancers may produce parathyroid hormone resulting in symptoms of hypercalcemia.

(e.) Sarcoidosis

(f.) Leukemia

3. Addison's disease

4. Hyperthyroidism

5. Paget's disease of bone (also accompanied by high levels of alkaline phosphatase)

6. Prolonged immobilization

7. Bone fractures combined with bedrest

8. Excessive intake of vitamin D

9. Prolonged use of diuretics, thiazides

10. Respiratory acidosis

11. Milk-alkali syndrome (history of peptic ulcer could indicate excessive intake of milk and antacids)

C. *Hypocalcemia* (decreased calcium levels)

Commonly caused by or associated with:

1. Pseudohypocalcemia

Actually what looks like hypocalcemia is really a reflection of reduced albumin (as revealed by a serum protein electrophoresis). It is the reduced protein which is responsible for the low calcium, since 50 per cent of the calcium total is protein-bound.

Note: Excessive use of IV fluids will decrease albumin levels and thus decrease the amount of calcium.

2. Hypoparathyroidism

May be due to accidental removal of parathyroid glands during a thyroidectomy.

3. Chronic renal failure results in increased phosphate levels.

4. Malabsorption

Due to sprue, celiac disease, pancreatic dysfunction (fatty acids combine with calcium and are precipitated and excreted in the feces.)

5. Acute pancreatitis

6. Alkalosis (calcium ions become bound to protein)

7. Osteomalacia
8. Diarrhea
9. Rickets

CLINICAL ALERT
1. Thiazide diuretics may lead to impairment of urinary calcium excretions and consequent hypercalcemia.
2. In patients with renal insufficiency who are undergoing dialysis, a calcium-ion exchange resin is sometimes used for hyperkalemia. The use of this resin may lead to increased calcium levels.
3. Increased intake of magnesium and phosphates and the excessive use of laxatives may lower the blood calcium level. This occurs because of the increased intestinal loss of calcium these elements produce.
4. When decreased calcium levels are due to magnesium deficiency, as in poor absorption from the bowel, the administration of magnesium will correct the calcium deficiency.

Interfering Factors

There are many drugs which may cause increased or decreased levels of calcium. See appendix for complete listing.

PHOSPHATE/INORGANIC PHOSPHORUS (P) (PO₄)

Normal Values

Adult: 2.5–4.8 mg./dl.
Child: 3.5–5.8 mg./dl.

Explanation of Test

Approximately 85 per cent of the body's total phosphorus content is combined with calcium in the bone. The remainder is located within the cells. Most of the phosphorus in the blood exists as phosphates or esters.

Phosphate is required for generation of bony tissue and

functions in the metabolism of glucose and lipids, in the maintenance of acid-base balance, and in the storage and transfer of energy from one site in the body to another. It is for these reasons that blood phosphate levels must be controlled within reasonably constant limits.

Phosphate levels are always evaluated in relation to calcium levels for the reason that there is an inverse relationship between the two. When calcium levels are decreased, phosphorus levels increase. When phosphorus levels decrease, calcium levels increase. An excess in serum levels of one causes the kidneys to excrete the other. Many of the causes of elevated calcium are also causes of lower phosphorus levels. As with calcium, the controlling factor is parathyroid hormone.

Clinical Implications

A. *Hyperphosphatemia* (Increased phosphorus levels)

The most common causes of elevated blood phosphate levels are found in association with kidney dysfunction and uremia. This is because of the retention of phosphorus tending to contribute to the acidosis associated with uremia and because of the diseased kidneys inability to excrete phosphorus.

Increased phosphorus levels are associated with:

(a.) Renal insufficiency and severe nephritis (accompanied by elevated BUN and elected creatine)

(b.) Hypoparathyroidism (accompanied by elevated phosphorus, decreased calcium and normal renal function)

(c.) Hypocalcemia

(d.) Excessive intake of alkali (possible history of peptic ulcer)

(e.) Excessive intake of vitamin D

(f.) Fractures in the healing stage

(g.) Bone tumors

(h.) Addison's disease

(i.) Acromegaly

B. *Hypophosphatemia* (decreased phosphorus levels)

Decreased phosphorus levels may be associated with:

(a.) Hyperparathyroidism (accompanied by elevated calcium; no renal disease)

(b.) Rickets (childhood) or osteomalacia (adult)
(c.) Diabetic coma because of increased carbohydrate metabolism
(d.) Insulin administration, phosphorus used in metabolism of glucose
(e.) Continuous administration of intravenous glucose in a non-diabetic patient.

Interfering Factors

1. Normally high in children
2. Falsely increased by hemolysis of blood
3. Drugs causing possible elevation:

   (a.) Diphenylhydantoin (phenytoin)
   (b.) Heparin
   (c.) Pituitrin
   (d.) Vitamin D
   (e.) Methicillin
   (f.) Tetracyclines
   (g.) Alkaline antacids
   (h.) Lipomol

4. The use of laxatives or enemas containing large amounts of sodium phosphate will cause increased phosphorus levels. With the oral intake of the laxative, the blood level may increase as much as five mg per dl two to three hours after the dose. This increased level is only temporary (5–6) hours, but this factor should be considered when abnormal levels are seen that cannot otherwise be explained.
5. Drugs causing possible decreases

   (a.) Aluminum hydroxide
   (b.) Epinephrine (Adrenaline)
   (c.) Insulin
   (d.) Mannitol
   (e.) Mithramycine
   (f.) Parathyroid injection

MAGNESIUM (Mg⁺⁺)

Normal Values

1.8–3.0 mg./dl.
or
1.5–2.5 mEq./l.

Background

Since all natural foods are rich in magnesium, magnesium deficiency is rare, in a normal diet. Ingestion of magnesium increases not only the amount of magnesium absorbed, but also the amount of calcium absorbed. On the other hand, a high phosphate diet suppresses both magnesium and calcium absorption.

Magnesium is required for the utilization of adenosine triphosphate (ADP) as a source of energy. It is therefore necessary for the action of numerous enzyme systems such as:

1. Carbohydrate metabolism
2. Protein synthesis
3. Nucleic acid synthesis
4. Contraction of muscular tissue

Along with sodium, potassium, and calcium ions, magnesium also regulates neuromuscular irritability. In addition it is needed in the clotting mechanism.

Magnesium and calcium are intimately tied together in their body functions, and deficiency of either one has a marked effect on the metabolism of the other. This is because of magnesium's importance in absorption of calcium from the intestines and in calcium metabolism. A magnesium deficiency will result in the draft of calcium out of the bones, possibly resulting in abnormal calcification in the aorta and the kidney in the absence of a calcium pump mechanism. This condition responds to administration of magnesium salts.

Normally 95 per cent of the magnesium that is filtered through the glomerulus is reabsorbed in the tubule. When there is decreased kidney function, greater amounts of magnesium are retained, resulting in increased blood serum levels.

Explanation of Test

Measurement of magnesium levels is used as an index to metabolic activity in the body and to renal function.

The bulk of total magnesium in the body is concentrated in the bone, cartilage, and within the cell itself.

Procedure

A venous blood sample of ten ml. is obtained.

Clinical Implications

A. *Reduced Magnesium Level*

Causes of *reduced* magnesium levels include:

(a.) Chronic diarrhea   (i.) Hyperaldosteronism

(b.) After hemodialysis   (j.) Toxemia of pregnancy

(c.) Chronic renal disease   (k.) Hyperparathyroidism

(d.) Hepatic cirrhosis   and hypoparathyroidism

(e.) Chronic pancreatitis   (l.) Excessive lactation

(f.) Use of diuretics   (m.) Cirrhosis of liver due to

(g.) Aldosteronism   alcohol and other causes

(h.) Ulcerative colitis

B. *Increased Magnesium Level*

Causes of *increased* magnesium levels include:

(a.) Renal failure

(b.) Diabetic coma before treatment

(c.) Hypothyroidism

(d.) Addison's disease

(e.) After adrenalectomy

(f.) Controlled diabetes in older people

(g.) Use of antacids containing magnesium (milk of magnesia)

(h.) Dehydration

(i.) Use of thiazides

(j.) Use of ethracynic acid

Interfering Factors

1. Prolonged salicylate therapy, lithium, and magnesium products will cause falsely increased magnesium levels.

2. Calcium gluconate can interfere with testing methods and cause falsely decreased results. Other drugs that will cause decreased results include

(a.) Amphotericin B   (e.) Insulin

(b.) Aldosterone   (f.) Mercurial diuretics

(c.) Ethracynic acid   (g.) Neomycin

(d.) Ethanol

CLINICAL ALERT
1. Treatment of diabetics in coma will often result in low plasma magnesium levels. This is because of magnesium moving with potassium into the cells after insulin administration.
2. Magnesium deficiency may cause apparently unexplained hypocalcemia and hypokalemia. In these instances, patients may have neurologic and G. I. symptoms.
3. Signs and symptoms of magnesium *deficiency* may mimic hypocalcemia or indicate *severe neuromusclar irritability* Such signs should be observed, reported and recorded:
   (a) Hyperflexia
   (b) Tremor in extremities
   (c) Carpopedal spasms
   (d) Positive Chvostek and Trosseau signs
   (e) Tachycardia
   (f) Hypertension
   Patients exhibiting these signs are very susceptible to auditory, mechanical, and visual stimuli.
4. Increased magnesium levels can act as a sedative as reflected in the following signs and symptoms:
   (a) depression of cardiac activity
   (b) depression of neuromuscular activity

BILIRUBIN; ICTERUS INDEX

Normal Values

Total bilirubin: 0.3–1.3 mg./dl.
Direct conjugated: 0.1–0.4 mg./dl.
Free indirect unconjugated: 0.2–0.18 mg./dl.
   (total minus nonconjugated)
Newborn: 1–12 mg./dl.
Icterus Index
   Normal serum levels 4–6 units

Background

Bilirubin, resulting from the breakdown of hemoglobin in the red blood cells, is a by-product of hemolysis (red blood cell destruction). Removed from the body by the liver, which excretes it into the bile, it gives the bile its major pigmentation.

Usually a small amount of bilirubin is found in the serum. A rise in serum levels will occur if there is an excessive destruction of red blood cells or if the liver is unable to excrete the normal amounts of bilirubin produced.

There are two forms of bilirubin in the body: (1) indirect or unconjugated bilirubin (which is protein bound), and (2) direct or conjugated bilirubin which circulates freely in the blood until it reaches the liver, where it is conjugated with glucuronide and then excreted into the bile. An increase in protein-bound bilirubin (unconjugated bilirubin) is more frequently associated with increased destruction of red blood cells (hemolysis); an increase in free-flowing bilirubin is more likely seen in dysfunction or blockage of the liver.

A routine examination measures only the total bilirubin. A normal level of total bilirubin rules out any significant impairment of the excretory function of the liver or excessive hemolysis of red cells. Only when the levels are elevated will there be a call for differentiation of the bilirubin according to the conjugate and unconjugate levels.

Jaundice/Icterus

Excessive amounts of bilirubin eventually seep into the tissues which then assume a yellow hue. The yellow color is a clinical sign of jaundice. In newborns, signs of jaundice may indicate hemolytic anemia or congenital icterus. If the bilirubin levels reach a critical point in the infant, damage to the central nervous system may occur in a condition known as kinicterus. Therefore, in these infants, it is the level of bilirubin which is the deciding factor in the decision to do an exchange transfusion.

Explanation of Test

Bilirubin

The measurement of bilirubin is important in evaluating liver function, hemolytic anemias, and hyperbilirubinemia (in newborns).

Icterus Index

The icterus index does not measure bilirubin directly but instead offers an approximate measure of the degree of jaundice by comparing the degree of yellowness of the sternum to a standard yellow compound. This comparison is based on the unit ranges of a colorimeter.

The normal range of blood is four to six units.

Clinical jaundice is usually evident at approximately 15 units.

Procedure

1. A venous sample of ten ml. is obtained before patient eats breakfast.
2. The sample must be protected from bright light.
3. Air bubbles and unnecessary shaking of the sample are to be avoided while blood is collected.
4. If the specimen cannot be examined immediately, then it should be stored in a refrigerator.
5. In infants, blood must be collected from a heel puncture. Two full micro blood sampling tubes are collected.

Clinical Implications

A. *Bilirubin elevations accompanied by jaundice* may be due to hepatic, obstructive, or hemolytic causes.

1. *Hepatocellular jaundice* results from injury or disease of the parenchymal cells of the liver and can be caused by:
   - (a.) Viral hepatitis
   - (b.) Cirrhosis
   - (c.) Infectious mononucleosis
   - (d.) Reactions of certain drugs such as chlorpromazine,

2. *Obstructive jaundice* is usually the result of obstruction of the common bile or hepatic ducts due to stones or neoplasms. The obstruction produces high conjugated bilirubin levels due to bile regurgitation.

3. *Hemolytic jaundice* is due to overproduction of bilirubin resulting from hemolytic processes that produce

high levels of unconjugated bilirubin. Hemolytic jaundice can be found in

(a.) Erythroblastosis fetalis
(b.) Pernicious anemia
(c.) Sickle cell anemia
(d.) Transfusion reactions
(e.) Crigler-Najjar syndrome (a severe disease that results from a genetic deficiency of a hepatic enzyme needed for the conjugation of bilirubin)

B. *Elevations of* **non-conjugated** *bilirubin levels occurs in*
   1. Hemolytic anemias
   2. Trauma in the presence of a large hematoma
   3. Hemorrhagic pulmonary infarcts
   4. Crigler-Najjar syndrome (rare)
   5. Gilbert's disease (rare)

C. *Elevated* **conjugate** *bilirubin levels occur in:*
   1. Cancer of the head of pancreas
   2. Choledocholithiasis
   3. Dubin-Johnson syndrome

D. *Elevation of* **both conjugate and nonconjugate** *levels (with the conjugate levels more elevated) occurs in:*
   1. Hepatic metastasis
   2. Hepatitis
   3. Lymphoma
   4. Cholestasis secondary to drugs
   5. Cirrhosis

Interfering Factors

1. A one-hour exposure of the specimen to sunlight or high intensity artificial light at room temperature will decrease the bilirubin content.
2. Contrast media 24 hours prior to measurement may cause an altered reaction.
3. A high fat meal may cause decreased bilirubin levels by interfering with the clinical reactions.
4. Air bubbles and shaking of the specimen may cause decreased levels.
5. Foods (carrots, yams) and drugs which increase the yellow hue in the serum.
6. Refer to the appendix for a listing of the many drugs which may interfere with testing for bilirubin.

GLUCOSE; FASTING BLOOD SUGAR (FBS)

Normal Values

Fasting serum: 70–110 mg./dl.

Fasting whole blood: 60–100 mg./dl.

Explanation of Test

The purpose of this test is to detect any disorder of glucose metabolism, mainly diabetes. Glucose is formed from the digestion of carbohydrates and the conversion of glycogen by the liver. Two hormones directly regulate blood glucose: glucagon and insulin. Glucagon accelerates the breakdown of glcogen in the liver, causing blood glucose to rise. Insulin increases the permeability of cellular membranes to glucose, transports glucose into cells for metabolism, and further stimulates formation of glucogen and reduces blood glucose levels. Other hormones that contribute to glucose metabolism are ACTH, adrenocorticosteroids, epinephrine, and thyroxine.

Therefore, the test for blood sugar is used as a screening procedure to detect disorders of metabolism which may be the result of one of several causes:

1. Inability of the islet cells of the pancreas to produce insulin
2. Inability of the intestines to absorb glucose
3. Inability of the liver to accumulate and break down glycogen
4. The presence of increased amounts of hormones (*i.e.,* ACTH).

In most cases, any degree of elevated blood sugar (hyperglycemia) indicates diabetes. At the same time, it is important to remember that in mild cases of diabetes, the blood sugar may be within normal ranges. Therefore, in any suspected cases of diabetes, a glucose tolerance test is in order (see p. 258).

While diabetes is the most readily suspected disorder in the presence of hyperglycemia, other diseases may be responsible for the elevated blood sugar and therefore should not be dismissed. (see below)

Procedure

A venous blood sample of seven ml. is drawn while patient is in a fasting state. If patient is a known diabetic, blood should be drawn before insulin or oral hypoglycemics are given.

Clinical Implications

A. *Elevated blood sugar (hyperglycemia)*
   1. Diabetes
     Values over 120 mg. per dl. on several testings may indicate diabetes mellitus. Except for diabetes, the FBS rarely exceeds 120 mg. per 100 ml.
   2. Other possible conditions
     (a.) Cushing's disease (increase in glucocorticoids causes increase in blood sugar)
     (b.) Acute stress (such as in MI or severe infections, *i.e.*, meningitis, encephalitis)
     (c.) Pheochromocytoma
     (d.) Pituitary adenoma (growth hormone leads to elevated blood sugar)
     (e.) Hyperthyroidism
     (f.) Adenoma of pancreas (may result in production of glucagon which counteracts insulin)
     (g.) Pancreatitis
     (h.) Brain trauma and brain damage
     (i.) Chronic liver disease
B. *Lower glucose levels (hypoglycemia)*
   1. Overdose of insulin (most frequent cause)
   2. Addison's disease (hypoglycemia is accompanied by elevated potassium and decreased sodium and elevated BUN)
   3. Bacterial sepsis
   4. Islet cell carcinoma of pancreas (secretes excessive amount of insulin)
   5. Hepatic necrosis
   6. Hypothyroidism
   7. Glycogen storage disease
   8. Psychogenic causes

Interfering Factors

1. Many drugs such as ACTH, physostigmine, steroids, and diuretics. See appendix for complete listing.
2. Pregnancy (normally a slight elevation in glucose)
3. Anesthesia (sometimes in excess of 200 mg. per 100 ml.)

Patient Preparation

1. Since fasting blood sugar is being tested, the patient must fast for 12 hours.
2. Water is permitted.

Patient Aftercare

Patient may eat or drink as soon as blood sample is drawn.

TWO-HOUR POSTPRANDIAL BLOOD SUGAR (2 HR. P.P.B.S.)

Normal Values

Less than 145 mg. per dl.

Explanation of Test

A "postprandial" test, a test taken *after* a meal, is an excellent screening test for diabetes. Glucose concentration in a fasting blood specimen obtained two hours after a meal is rarely elevated in normal individuals, but is significantly increased in diabetic patients.

Procedure

1. For best results, a high carbohydrate diet should be taken two to three days prior to testing.
2. After an overnight fast (water is permitted) the patient eats a high carbohydrate breakfast. Meal should include orange juice, cereal with sugar, toast, and milk.

3. Two hours after the patient finishes eating breakfast, a venous blood sample of 7 ml. is obtained.
4. Record time breakfast is completed and notify laboratory.

Clinical Implications

Values above 145 mg. per dl. are abnormal. This figure strictly applies to adults under 50 years of age. The level should be raised to 160 mg. per dl. for those in their sixties, and to as much as 180 mg. per dl. for older people.

A. *Increased Levels* occur in many stressful or serious conditions:

1. Malnutrition
2. Advanced cirrhosis of liver
3. Cushing's syndrome
4. Acromegaly
5. Hyperthyroidism
6. Pheochromocytoma
7. Lipoproteinemias
8. Myocardial or cerebral infarction
9. Some malignancies
10. Pregnancy
11. Anxiety states

B. *Decreased Levels* occur in:

1. Anterior pituitary insufficiency
2. Islet cell adenoma
3. Steatorrhea
4. Addison's disease

Interfering Factors

Smoking may raise the blood glucose level.

Patient Preparation

1. Instruct the patient about the purpose of the test and the procedure: (a) fast from food overnight; at least eight hours, and permission (b) to drink water but no other liquids.

Patient Aftercare

After blood sample is drawn, patient may eat and drink normally.

CLINICAL ALERT
1. Values greater than 145 mg. per dl. warrant the use of the glucose tolerance test.
2. Test results are reliable only if patient is properly prepared.

GLUCOSE TOLERANCE

Normal Values

FBS (Fasting Blood Sugar)	below 100 mg./100 ml.
30 minutes	155 mg./100 ml.
1 hour	165 mg./100 ml.
2 hours	140 mg./100 ml.
3 hours	80 mg./100 ml.

All urines are negative for glucose.

Explanation of Test

This timed test of blood and urine is done to rule out diabetes by determining the rate of removal of a concentrated dose of glucose from the bloodstream. In the healthy individual, the insulin response to a large oral dose of glucose is almost immediate, peaking in 30 to 60 minutes and returning to normal within three hours.

Testing is usually done in the morning after an overnight fast. The glucose tolerance test is indicated when there is sugar in the urine or when the fasting blood sugar or two-hour postprandial blood sugar is more than slightly elevated. The glucose tolerance test is more definite than a two-hour postprandial blood sugar test in diagnosing hypoglycemia and malabsorption syndrome. It is also ordered in a questionable diagnosis of Cushing's syndrome or acromegaly.

Indications for Test

The *glucose tolerance* test rather than the *two-hour postprandial blood* sugar test should be done on certain patients.

(a.) Family history of diabetes

(b.) Obesity

(c.) Unexplained episodes of hypoglycemia

(d.) History of recurrent infections such as boils and abscesses.

(e.) In women, a history of delivery of large infants, stillbirths, neonatal death, premature labor, and abortions.

(f.) Transitory glycosuria or hyperglycemia in pregnancy, surgery, trauma, stress, myocardial infarction, ACTH administration.

Tolerance tests can also be performed for pentoses, lactose, galactose, and D-xylose.

Procedure

This is a timed test.

1. A diet containing at least 300 grams of carbohydrate should be eaten for three days prior to test.

2. Drugs which may influence the test should be discontinued for three days before the test.

   (a.) Hormones, including oral contraceptives

   (b.) Salicylates

   (c.) Diuretid agents

   (d.) Hypoglycemic agents

3. Insulin or oral hypoglycemics should not be given until after test is completed.

4. A sample of seven ml of venous blood is drawn after an overnight fast. At least three other blood samples will be obtained (dependent on physician's order and laboratory practice).

5. Patient is given a drink of very sweet commercial preparation liquid, containing 1.75 gm. of glucose per kg. of body weight. He is encouraged to drink it all quickly. All of the solution must be taken.

6. Blood and urine samples are usually obtained at intervals of 30 minutes, one, two, and sometimes three hours after ingestion of glucose and tested for glucose.

7. Inclusion of the fourth hour specimens of both blood and urine is valuable in detecting hypoglycemia.

Clinical Implications

1. In maturity onset diabetes, the secretion of insulin is delayed, followed by a slightly higher than normal glucose level at two hours. Blood glucose is elevated until the two-hour point.
2. In overt diabetes, there is no secretion of insulin, resulting in above normal glucose levels throughout the test.

   Diabetes is diagnosed when the fasting or two-hour levels or both are greater than 120 mg. per dl. and the glucose tolerance level is greater than 165 mg. per dl.

3. In hypoglycemia, the blood glucose is below normal after the two-hour point and up to 4 to 5 hours because of high insulin levels. Tolerance tests can also be performed for pentoses, lactose, galactose, and D-xylose.

Interfering Factors

1. Smoking will increase glucose level.
2. Inadequate diet (such as a weight reducing diet) prior to testing can diminish carbohydrate tolerance and suggest a false diabetes.
3. Levels intend to increase normally in older people; the maximum can reach 200 mg. per 100 ml.
4. Prolonged administration of oral contraceptives will give significantly higher glucose levels in the second hour or in later blood specimens.
5. Bed rest over a lengthy period of time will influence glucose tolerance. For this reason the test should be performed on ambulatory patients, not on patients whose condition requires bed rest.
6. Infectious diseases and surgery will affect tolerance. Several days of recovery should be allowed before the test.
7. Certain drugs will impair glucose tolerance:

   (a.) Insulin
   (b.) Oral hypoglycemias
   (c.) Large doses of salicylates
   (d.) Thiazide diuretics
   (e.) Oral contraceptives
   (f.) Corticosteroids
   (g.) Estrogens
   (h.) Ferrous ascorbinate
   (i.) Nicotonic acid

(j) Phenothiazines   (l) Metapyrine
(k) Lithium

Patient Preparation

1. Instruct the patient about the purpose and procedure of the test and leave him a written reminder.
   - (a.) Stress a normal diet with high carbohydrates (300 gms.) for three days preceding the test.
   - (b.) He must fast for eight to 12 hours before the test.
   - (c.) Water is permitted and encouraged.
2. Determine his weight and record.
3. Collect urine and blood specimens and test for glucose, recording exact time of collection. Have the patient empty his bladder for each specimen.
   - (d.) No liquids can be taken other than water. Have the patient empty his bladder for each urine specimen.
   - (e.) No food is to be eaten during the test periods.
   - (f.) No alcohol should be taken the previous evening.
   - (g.) Encourage patient to stay in bed or rest quietly during the test period (weakness or feeling faint may occur during test).
   - (h.) No smoking is allowed during the test.

Patient Aftercare

1. The patient may eat and drink normally as soon as the test is over.
2. Administer insulin or oral hypoglycemias to diabetics as soon as the test is complete.

CLINICAL ALERT
1. This test is contraindicated in patients who have had a recent history of surgery, myocardial infarction, labor, and delivery, for these conditions can cause erroneous results (altered carbohydrate tolerance).
2. Record and report any reactions during the test. Weakness, faintness, and sweating may occur between the second and third hours. This is a normal response as the blood sugar falls to normal limits and is transitory unless hyperinsulinism is involved.

CORTISONE GLUCOSE TOLERANCE

Normal Values

At 1 hour: blood glucose 160 mg./dl.
At 2 hours: blood glucose 140 mg./dl.
(Add an additional 18 mg. per dl. at age 40 and for each
decade over 40 years)

Explanation of Test

This is a glucose tolerance test based on the fact that cortisone increases blood glucose. The test is also known as the "steroid challenge" test for the reason that cortisone acetate is given before the standard glucose tolerance test is begun.

Indications for Test

1. When the results of the standard glucose tolerance test are doubtful and altered carbohydrate metabolism is strongly suspected
2. In patients with suggestive signs of vascular or neurological disease
3. In persons with a strong family history of diabetes
4. In women whose pregnancies were complicated by glycosuria and delivery of large infants.

Procedure

The procedure is the same as for the glucose tolerance test with the following exceptions:
1. An oral dose of cortisone acetate is given eight hours before glucose ingestion, and again two hours before glucose is given.
2. A venous blood sample is obtained after the second dose of cortisone.

Clinical Implications

If the two-hour level is above 140 mg. per dl., a person is considered to be prediabetic and should be followed closely for the development of diabetes.

Interfering Factors

See *Glucose Tolerance Test.*

CORTISOL HYDROCORTISONE

Normal Values

7:00 A.M. to 10:00 A.M.   5–25 μg/dl.
5:00 P.M. to 8:00 P.M.   2–18 μg/dl.

Background

Cortisol, compound F, is a glucocorticosteroid of the adrenal cortex and affects metabolism of proteins, carbohydrates, and lipids. Cortisol (hydrocortisone) is the most potent of the glucocorticoids and inhibits the affect of insulin. Cortisol stimulates glucogenesis by the liver and decreases the rate of glucose utilization by the cells. In the healthy individual, the secretion rate of cortisol is higher in the early morning (6–8 A.M.) and lower in the evening (4–6 P.M.)

Explanation of Test

This is a test of adrenal hormone function.

Procedure

Venous blood samples of 0.5 ml. are obtained in the morning and evening.

Clinical Implications

Extreme elevation in the morning and no variation later in the day suggest carcinoma.
A. *Decreased levels* are expected in:
    1. Liver disease
    2. Addison's disease
    3. Anterior pituitary hyposecretion
    4. Hypothyroidism

B. *Increased levels* are found in:
1. Hyperthyroidism
2. Stress
3. Obesity
4. Cushing's syndrome

Interfering Factors

Pregnancy and oral contraceptives will cause an increased value.

CAROTENE

Normal Values

50–300 mg./100 ml.

Background

Carotene is a fat soluble vitamin and is the precursor of vitamin A. Since absorption of the fat soluble vitamins is impaired when fat is poorly absorbed, a low carotene serum level is indicative of the fat malabsorption syndrome. The level in the blood is influenced by the amount of carotene in the diet.

Explanation of Test

This is a very useful screening test for the fat malabsorption syndrome.

Procedure

A fasting (preferred) venous blood sample of ten ml. is obtained.

Clinical Implications

A. *Decreased Carotene Levels* are associated with:

1. Fat malabsorption
   syndrome
2. Steatorrhea

3. Febrile illnesses
4. Liver disease
5. Poor dietary intake

B. *Increased Carotene Levels* are associated with:

1. Myxedema
2. Diabetes mellitus
3. Hypothyroidism
4. Chronic nephritis

5. Hyperlipidemia
6. Excessive dietary intake, especially carrots

Patient Preparation

1. Patient must be fasting and receiving no vitamin A or foods containing vitamin A or carotene for 24 to 48 hours before testing. Check with laboratory procedure.
2. Water is permitted.

GASTRIN

Normal Values

92–275 pg./ml.

Background

Gastrin is a hormone secreted by the mucosa of the pylorus of the stomach. The gastrin is absorbed into the blood and returned to the stomach where it stimulates the secretion of gastric acid. Excessive production of gastrin, then, can result in hypersecretion of gastric acid. Hydrochloric acid, one of the gastric secretions, in turn inhibits the secretion of gastrin.

Explanation of Test

Although elevated levels of gastrin are found in disorders such as pernicious anemia, measurement of serum gastrin is generally used to diagnose a stomach disorder.

Procedure

A fasting venous blood sample of ten ml. is obtained.

Clinical Implications

Increased Gastrin Levels are found in:

1. Stomach cancer because of significant reduction of gastric acid secretion
2. Gastric and duodenal ulcers
3. Zollinger-Ellison syndrome
4. Pernicious anemia (low secretion of hydrochloric acid results in elevated gastrin levels)
5. End-stage renal disease (gastrin is metabolized by the kidneys)
6. In elderly patients because of reduced secretion of HCL acid.

Patient Preparation

1. Patient should be in a fasting state for 12 hours preceding the test.
2. Water is permitted.

TOTAL BLOOD PROTEINS; ALBUMIN AND GLOBULIN; A/G RATIO

Normal Values

Total Protein	6 to 8 gm./dl.
Albumin	4 to 4.5 gm%
Globulin	1.5 to 3 gm.%
Albumin globulin ratio (A/G)	1.5:1 to 2.5:1

Explanation of Test

Proteins and nucleic acids, the structural components of a cell, serve as biocatalysts (enzymes), regulators of metabolism (hormones), and preservers of genetic make-up (chromosomes). Amino acids are the building blocks of protein.

Much clinical information is obtained by examining and measuring proteins because of the involvement of proteins in so many functions. The three major categories of protein are tissue or organ proteins, plasma proteins, and hemoglobin. Because of its large size, muscle mass provides the greatest amount of protein in conditions of deprivation. Tissue protein in muscle mass has the largest buffering capacity of the protein sites.

Plasma proteins serve as a source of nutrition for the body tissues and function in body buffering ability by combining with hemoglobin to exert an effect comparable to that of bicarbonate and other inorganic blood buffer systems.

Albumin and Albumin/Globulin Ratio

Albumin is a protein which is formed in the liver and which helps to maintain normal distribution of water in the body (colloidal osmotic pressure) as well as the transport of blood constituents such as ions, pigments, bilirubin, hormones, fatty acids, enzymes, and certain drugs. Approximately 52 to 60 per cent of total protein is albumin, the rest is globulin, which functions in antibody formation, and other plasma protein (fibrinogen and prothrombin) functioning in coagulation.

Although the serum globulins function mainly as immunologic agents, they also play a part in maintaining the osmotic pressure of the blood; they are less effective than the serum albumin in this role because the globulin molecule is so much larger than the albumin molecule. Normally, the capillary walls are impermeable to the plasma protein, but in certain diseases the albumin will "seep through". The larger globulins, however, remain within the bloodstream and assume the major function in maintaining osmotic pressure. Because of the globulin's inability to function as effectively as the albumin, the osmotic pressure may be below normal even though the total protein is retained at normal levels. Thus the ratio of albumin to globulin becomes an important indicator of certain disease states.

Procedure

A venous blood sample of at least 0.5 ml. is obtained.

Clinical Implications

A. *Decreased albumin levels*
    1. Severe hypoalbuminemia is often associated with

edema and decreased transport function such as hypocalcemia.

2. Decreased albumin levels are caused by many different conditions:
   (a.) Inadequate iron intake
   (b.) Severe liver diseases
   (c.) Malabsorption
   (d.) Diarrhea
   (e.) Eclampsia
   (f.) Nephrosis
   (g.) Exfoliative dermatitis
   (h.) Third-degree burns
   (i.) Starvation
   (j.) Excessive administration of IV glucose in water

B. *Increased albumin levels* are generally not observed.
C. *Increase in Total Protein* (hyperproteinemia)
   1. May be due to hemoconcentration as a result of dehydration from loss of body fluid and may occur in vomiting, diarrhea, wound drainage, or poor kidney function.
      (a.) Both albumin and globulins increase in the same proportions so that A/G ratio is unchanged.
      (b.) This is the only instance in which an increase in albumin is found.
   2. When the total protein increases and the albumin is unchanged or slightly decreased while globulins increase, the A/G ratio falls markedly.
      Caused by:
      (a.) Lupus erythematosus
      (b.) Rheumatoid arthritis and other collagen diseases
      (c.) Chronic infections
      (d.) Acute liver disease
      (e.) Multiple myeloma, sarcoidosis and other malignant tumors
D. *Decrease in Total Protein* (Hypoproteinemia)

1. Associated with low albumin and small change in globulin, resulting in low A/G ratio.
2. Due to
    (a.) Increased loss of albumin in urine
    (b.) Decreased formation in liver
    (c.) Insufficient protein intake
    (d.) Severe hemorrhage when the plasma volume is replaced more rapidly than the protein level.
3. Associated conditions
    (a.) Severe liver disease
    (b.) Malabsorption
    (c.) Nephrotic syndrome
    (d.) Diarrhea
    (e.) Exfoliative dermatitis
    (f.) Severe burns
    (g.) Dilution by excessive IV administration of glucose in water

    Note: The liver is so crucial to protein metabolism that liver disease is frequently associated with alterations in proteins and disturbances of protein metabolism. For example, in undernutrition and liver disease, the albumin level may be decreased by inadequate synthesis.

Interfering Factors

1. Low levels of albumin occur normally in all trimesters of pregnancy.
2. Bromosulphalein may cause a false elevation. Therefore a serum protein test should not be done within 48 hours following a BSP test.
3. See appendix for complete listing of drugs that interfere with total protein levels.

CLINICAL ALERT
Observe, report, and record signs and symptoms of possible accompanying edema or hypocalcemia. (See tests on calcium, p. 241.)

MUCOPROTEINS (SEROMUCOID)

Normal Values

83–203 mg./l.
Average 135 mg./l.

Background

Mucoproteins are amino compounds whose action in the body is undetermined. It is known that in diseases such as cancer, infections, and inflammations, there is an increase of mucoproteins in the blood. In cancer, the more widespread the condition, the greater the increase in mucoproteins.

Explanation of Test

This test has its greatest value as a guide to the successful treatment of cancer indicated by a decrease in mucoproteins and in the differential diagnosis of liver diseases.

Procedure

A venous blood sample of ten ml. is obtained.

Clinical Implications

A. *Increased Levels* are found in:
1. Cancer
2. Rheumatoid arthritis
3. Infections
4. Ankylosing spondylitis
B. *Decreased Levels* are found in:
1. Infectious hepatitis
2. Infectious cirrhosis

BLOOD UREA NITROGEN (BUN)

Normal Values

10–15 mg./100 ml.

Explanation of Test

Urea is formed in the liver and constitutes the major nonprotein nitrogenous end product of protein catabolism. The urea is then carried to the kidneys via the blood to be excreted in the urine.

The test for BUN, measuring the nitrogen portion of urea, is used as a gross index of glomerular function and the production and excretion of urea. Rapid protein catabolism and impairment of kidney function will result in an elevated BUN. The rate at which the BUN rises is influenced by the degree of tissue necrosis, protein catabolism, and the rate at which the kidneys excrete the urea nitrogen.

The nonprotein nitrogen (NPN) is a similar test for measuring kidney function; however, the BUN is considered more reliable.

Procedure

A venous blood sample of at least 0.5 ml. is obtained. The amount drawn is dependent upon the method and type of equipment used.

Clinical Implications

A. *Increased BUN*
   1. The most common cause of increased BUN level is inadequate excretion due to kidney disease or urinary obstruction, frequently occurring in cases of prostate.
      (a.) An increased BUN of 50 to 150 mg. per 100 ml. indicates serious impairment of renal function.
      (b.) An increased BUN of 150 to 250 mg. per 100 ml. is definitive for severely impaired renal failure.
   2. Increased BUN levels are associated with:

(a.) Impaired renal function	(g.) Some malignancies
(b.) Shock	(h.) Acute myocardial infarction
(c.) Dehydration	(i.) Chronic gout
(d.) GI hemorrhage	(j.) Excessive protein intake or protein catabolism
(e.) Infection	
(f.) Diabetes	

   Increases of 50 mg. per 100 ml. per day in the BUN have occurred in previously healthy people who have undergone *severe crusing injuries* or are suffering from *overwhelming infection.*

B. *Decreased BUN*

Associated with:

(a.) Liver failure
(b.) Negative nitrogen balance as may occur in malnutrition, excessive use of IV fluids, and physiologic hydremia of pregnancy
(c.) Impaired absorption as in celiac disease
(d.) Occasionally in nephrotic syndrome
(e.) Overhydration
A decreased further BUN of 6 to 10 mg. per 100 ml. is possible in overhydration.

Interfering Factors

1. A combination of a low protein and a high carbohydrate diet can cause a decreased BUN level.
2. The BUN is normally lower in children and women because they have a smaller muscle mass than adult men.
3. Increased BUN values normally occur in late pregnancy and infancy because of increased utilization of protein.
4. Older people may have an increased BUN when their kidneys are not able to concentrate urine adequately.
5. Decreased BUN values may normally occur earlier in pregnancy because of physiologic hydremia.
6. There are many drugs which may cause increased BUN levels. See appendix for complete listing.
7. Drugs which may cause decreased BUN levels include
    (a.) Dextrose in fusions
    (b.) Phenothiazines
    (c.) Thymol

CLINICAL ALERT
1. If a patient is confused, disorientated, or has convulsions, the BUN should be checked. If the level is high, it may help to explain these signs and symptoms.

2. In patients with an elevated BUN, fluid and electrolyte regulation may be impaired.
3. Excessive IV fluids can result in lowered BUN levels.

AMMONIA

Normal Values

40–110 mg./100 mg.
There is a great deal of variation in reported values because of methods used.

Background

Ammonia, one of the end products of protein metabolism, is formed from the action of bacteria on proteins in the intestines and from hydrolysis of glutamine in the kidneys. The liver normally removes most of the ammonia from the portal vein blood flow and converts ammonia to urea. Since any appreciable level of ammonia in the blood would affect acid-base balance and brain function, an adequate mechanism for its removal is essential. The liver accomplishes this by synthesis of urea for excretion by the kidney.

Explanation of Test

Measurement of blood ammonia levels is used to evaluate metabolism as well as the progress of severe liver disease and response to treatment.

Procedure

1. A fasting venous blood sample of three cc. is obtained.
2. If blood sample cannot be examined immediately, sample is placed in an iced container.

3. Laboratory should be notified of all antibiotics patient is receiving because of the possibility of these drugs lowering ammonia levels.

Clinical Implications

Increased Ammonia Levels—occur in:

1. Liver disease
2. Hepatic coma due to:
   (a.) Cirrhosis
   (b.) Severe hepatitis
3. Severe heart failure
4. Azotemia
5. Cor pulmonale
6. Erythroblastosis fetalis
7. Pulmonary emphysema
8. Acute bronchitis
9. Pericarditis
10. Myelocytic and lymphatic leukemia

Patient Preparation

1. Instruct patient to fast for eight hours before the blood test.
2. Water is permitted.

Interfering Factors

1. Ammonia levels vary with protein intake.
2. Exercise may cause an increase in ammonia levels.
3. There are many drugs that may affect blood ammonia levels. See appendix for complete listing of drugs.

CLINICAL ALERT
In patients with impaired liver function demonstrated by elevated ammonia levels, the blood level can be lowered by reduced protein intake and by use of antibiotics to reduce intestinal bacteria counts.

CREATININE

Normal Values

0.2 to 0.5 mg./dl.

Explanation of Test

Creatinine is a by-product in the breakdown of muscle creatine phosphate resulting from energy metabolism. It is produced at a constant rate depending upon the muscle mass of the individual and is removed from the body by the kidneys. Production of creatinine is constant as long as muscle mass remains constant. A disorder of kidney function reduces excretion of creatinine, resulting in increased levels of blood creatinine.

The test is used to diagnose impaired renal function. It is a more specific and sensitive indicator of kidney disease than the BUN, although in chronic renal disease, the BUN correlates more accurately with symptoms of uremia than does the blood creatinine.

Procedure

A venous blood sample of two ml. is obtained. The minimum amount needed is 0.5 ml.

Clinical Implications

A. *Increased Creatinine levels* occur in:
1. Impaired renal function
2. Chronic nephritis
3. Obstruction of the urinary tract
4. Muscle disease
   (a.) Gigantism
   (b.) Acromegaly
B. *Decreased Creatinine levels* occur in:
   Muscular dystrophy

Interfering Factors

1. PSP dyes in the blood from previous tests will give a falsely increased level; BSP dyes may give a falsely decreased level.
2. High levels of ascorbic acid can give a falsely increased level.
3. Drugs influencing kidney function (diuretics and dextran), chloral hydrate, marijuana, acetohexamide, guanethidine,

furosemide, chloramphenicol, sulfonamides can cause a change in the blood creatinine.
4. A diet high in roast meat will cause increased levels.
5. Many drugs may cause a change in the blood creatinine. See appendix for complete listing.

CLINICAL ALERT
A normal blood serum creatinine does not always indicate unimpaired renal function. A normal value cannot be used as a standard for a patient who is known to have existing renal disease.

URIC ACID

Normal Values

Women: 3.0–7.5 mg./100 ml.
Men: 7–8.5 mg./100 ml.

Explanation of Test

Uric acid is formed from the breakdown of nucleonic acids and is an end product of purine metabolism. The basis for this test is that an overproduction of uric acids occurs in conditions in which there is excessive cell breakdown and catabolism of nucleonic acids (as in gout), excessive production and destruction of cells (as in leukemia), or an inability to excrete the substance produced (as in renal failure).

Measurement of uric acid is used most commonly in the evaluation of renal failure, gout, and leukemia. In hospitalized patients, renal failure is the most common cause of elevated uric acid levels, and gout is the least common cause. This test is also valuable in assessing the prognosis of eclampsia because of the uric acid level's ability to reflect the extent of liver damage in toxemia of pregnancy.

Procedure

A venous blood sample of 20 ml. is obtained.

Clinical Implication

A. *Elevated Levels* (Hyperuricemia)

1. Increased levels of blood uric acid levels are associated with nitrogen retention and with increases in urea, creatinine, and other nonprotein nitrogenous substances of the blood. These findings are usually interpreted as another indication of decreased *kidney function*.

2. Increased levels are found in *gout*, but the increase may be slight in the early stages of the disease. The amount of increase is not directly related to the severity of disease.

3. Other conditions associated with elevated uric acid level

(a.) Leukemia
(b.) Acute stages of infectious diseases such as infectious mononucleosis
(c.) Lymphomas
(d.) Metastatic cancer
(e.) Severe eclampsia
(f.) Starvation
(g.) Shock
(h.) Alcoholism
(i.) Chemotherapy for cancer
(j.) Excessive x-rays
(k.) Multiple myeloma
(l.) Metabolic acidosis
(m.) Diabetic ketosis
(n.) Lead poisoning

B. *Decreased Levels*

Values lower than normal are not significant. However, the blood uric acid level should fall in patients who are treated with uricosuric drugs such as allopurinol, probenecid, and sulfinpyrazone.

Interfering Factors

1. Stress will cause increased levels.
2. Drugs which may cause *increased* blood levels include:
   (a.) Thiazide diuretics
   (b.) Prolonged low doses of salicylates
   (c.) Methyldopa
   (d.) Dextran
   (e.) Levodopa
   (f.) Ascorbic acid

3. Drugs which may cause *decreased* blood levels include:
   - (a.) Coumarin
   - (b.) Clofibrate
   - (c.) Cinchophen
   - (d.) ACTH
   - (e.) Phenothiazines
   - (f.) Marijuana
4. Refer to appendix for complete listing of drugs that will cause increased or decreased levels of uric acid.

AMYLASE

Normal Values

60–200 Somogyi units/100 ml.

Background

Amylase is an enzyme which changes starch to sugar. It is produced in the salivary glands, pancreas, liver, and fallopian tubes. If there is an inflammation of the pancreas or salivary glands, much more of the enzyme enters the blood. Amylase levels in the urine reflect blood changes by a time-lag of six to ten hours. (See p. 175, *Amylase in Urine*).

Explanation of Test

This test is used to diagnose and monitor treatment of acute pancreatitis and to detect inflammation of salivary glands.

Procedure

A venous blood sample of ten ml. is obtained.

Clinical Implications

A. *Increased Levels*
   1. Greatly increased in acute nonhemorrhagic pancreatitis early in course of disease. Increase begins in three to six hours after onset of pain.
   2. Increases also occur in:
      - (a.) Acute exacerbation of chronic pancreatitis

    (b.) Partial gastrestomy
    (c.) Obstruction of pancreatic duct
    (d.) Perforated peptic ulcer
    (e.) Alcohol poisoning
    (f.) Mumps
    (g.) Obstruction or inflammation of salivary duct or gland
    (h.) Acute cholecystitis
    (i.) Intestinal obstruction with strangulation
    (j.) Ruptured tubal pregnancy
    (k.) Ruptured aortic aneurysm

B. *Decreased Levels* occur in:

1. Acute pancreatitis subsidence
2. Hepatitis
3. Cirrhosis of liver
4. Toxemia of pregnancy
5. Severe burns
6. Severe thyrotoxicosis

SERUM GLUTAMIC OXALOACETIC TRANSAMINASE (SGOT); ASPARTATE TRANSAMINASE (AST)

Normal Values

5–40 Sigma Frankel μ/ml.
0–36 IU./l., lower in females

Explanation of Test

SGOT is an enzyme present in tissues of high metabolic activity. It occurs in decreasing concentration in the heart, liver, skeletal muscle, kidney, brain, pancreas, spleen, and lungs. The enzyme is released into the circulation following the injury or death of cell. Any disease that causes change in these highly metabolic tissues will result in a rise in SGOT/AST. The amount of SGOT in the blood is directly related to the number of damaged cells and the amount of time that passes between injury to the tissue and the test. Following severe cell damage, the blood SGOT level will rise in 12 hours and remain elevated for about five days.

Procedure

A venous sample of five ml. is obtained. Hemolysis during the procedure should be avoided.

Clinical Implications

A. *Increased Elevations*
    1. Myocardial Infarction
        (a.) In MI, the SGOT/AST level may be increased 4 to 10 times the normal values.
        (b.) The SGOT level reaches a peak in 24 hours and returns to normal by the third or fourth day. Secondary rises in SGOT levels suggest extension or recurrence of MI.
        (c.) The SGOT/AST curve in MI parrallels that of CPK (see p. 287).
        (d.) Elevated SGOT/AST levels do not always indicate MI in suspected patients. Severe arrhythmias and severe angina can also cause elevation.
    2. Liver Disease
        (a.) SGOT/AST is always elevated in cirrhosis of the liver.
        (b.) In liver disease, the SGOT/AST level may be ten to 100 times normal.
        (c.) Liver diseases associated with elevated SGOT levels:
            (1.) Acute hepatitis
            (2.) Active cirrhosis
            (3.) Infectious mononucleosis with hepatitis
            (4.) Hepatic necrosis
    3. Other diseases associated with elevated SGOT levels:
        (a.) Acute pancreatitis
        (b.) Trauma and irradiation of skeletal muscle
        (c.) Acute hemolytic anemia
        (d.) Acute renal disease
        (e.) Severe burns
        (f.) Cardiac catheterization and angiography
        (g.) Recent brain trauma with brain necrosis
        (h.) Crushing injuries
        (i.) Progressive muscular dystrophy

B. *Decreased Levels*

Causes of reduced levels of SGOT/AST include:
1. Beriberi
2. Uncontrolled diabetes mellitus with acidosis
3. Occasionally, liver disease may cause a decrease instead of the expected increase.

Interfering Factors

1. Slight decreases occur during pregnancy when there is abnormal metabolism of pyridoxine.
2. Drugs which can cause elevated levels are:

(a.) Aspirin	(h.) Meperidine
(b.) Codeine	(i.) Hydralazine
(c.) Cortisone	(j.) Erythromycin
(d.) Cholinergics	(k.) Morphine
(e.) Theophylline	(l.) Tolbutamide
(f.) Vitamin A	(m.) Guanethidine
(g.) Large doses of	analogs
nicotinic acid	(n.) Grisseofulvin

3. See appendix for complete listing of all drugs which can cause falsely elevated levels.
4. Salicylates may cause falsely decreased or increased SGOT levels.

SERUM GLUTAMIC PYRUVIC TRANSAMINASE (SGPT); ALANINE TRANSAMINASE (ALT)

Normal Values

5–35 Sigma Frankel μ/ml.
0–48 IU./l.

Explanation of Test

While high concentrations of SGPT/ALT are found in the liver, heart, muscle, and kidney, the test of SGPT levels is done primarily to diagnose liver disease to monitor the course of treatment for hepatitis, active postnecrotic cirrhosis, or the effects of drug treatment that might be toxic to the liver. It is also used to differentiate between hemolytic jaundice and jaundice due to liver disease. In comparison to SGOT, the SGPT test is more specific for liver malfunction.

Procedure

1. A five ml. sample of venous blood is obtained.
2. Hemolysis should be avoided during collection of specimen.

Clinical Implications

A. *Increased Levels* found in:
   1. Hepatocellular disease (moderate to high increase)
   2. Active cirrhosis (mild increase)
   3. Metastatic liver tumor (mild increase)
   4. Obstructive jaundice/biliary obstruction (mild to moderate increase)
   5. Infection or toxic hepatitis
   6. Liver congestion
   7. Pancreatitis (mild increase)
   8. Hepatic injury in myocardial infarction complicated by shock
B. *SGOT/SGPT comparison*
   1. Although the SGOT level is always increased in acute myocardial infarction, the SGPT level does not always increase proportionately.
   2. The SGPT is usually increased more than the SGOT in acute extrahepatic biliary obstruction.

Interfering Factors

1. There are many drugs which may cause falsely increased SGPT levels. See appendix for complete listing.
2. Salicylates may cause decreased or increased levels.

LACTIC ACID DEHYDROGENASE (LD, LDH)

Normal Values

80–120 Wacker Units
120–340 IU./l.
150–450 Wroblewski Units

Background

Lactic acid dehydrogenase is an intracellular enzyme that is widely distributed in the tissues of the body, particularly in the kidney, heart, skeletal muscle, brain, liver, and lungs. Increases in the reported value usually indicate cellular death and leakage of the enzyme from the cell.

Explanation of Test

Although elevated levels of LDH are nonspecific, this test is useful in confirming myocardial or pulmonary infarction when viewed in relation to other test findings. It is also a diagnostic test for extensive cancer, and it may be used to monitor the course of cancer chemotherapy (A good response to therapy is followed by decreasing LDH levels). It is also helpful in the differential diagnosis of muscular dystrophy and pernicious anemia. More specific findings may be found by breaking down the LDH into the five isoenzymes which constitute LDH (When LD values are reported or quoted *total* LDH is meant).

Procedures

1. A venous blood sample of five ml. is obtained.
2. Avoid hemolysis in obtaining blood sample.

Clinical Implications

A. *Myocardial Infarction*
   The elevation of LDH that follows a myocardial infarction is characteristic in that there are:

      (a.) High levels within a few hours of infarction (6–12 hours)

      (b.) Elevations that may continue for six to ten days. For this reason, LDH determinations may be useful in the late diagnosis of myocardial infarction.

B. *Pulmonary Infarction*

In pulmonary infarction, there is usually an increased LDH within 24 hours of the onset of pain. The pattern of normal SGOT and elevated LDH that levels one to two days after an episode of chest pain provides evidence for pulmonary infarction.

C. *Conditions in General and According to Degree of Increase in Levels*

    1. *Elevated* levels of LDH are observed in a variety of conditions:

      (a.) Acute myocardial infarction

      (b.) Acute leukemia

      (c.) Hemolytic anemias

      (d.) Acute pulmonary infarction

      (e.) Malignant neoplasms

      (f.) Acute renal infarctions and chronic renal disease

      (g.) Hepatic disease

      (h.) Skeletal muscle necrosis

      (i.) Sprue

      (j.) Shock with necrosis of minor organs

      (k.) Mxyedema

    2. The *greatest increase* (2–40 times) of LDH are seen in:

      (a.) Megaloblastic anemias

      (b.) Extensive cancer

      (c.) Shock and anoxia

    3. *Moderate* increase (2–4 times) of LDH are seen in:

      (a.) Myocardial infarction

      (b.) Pulmonary infarction

      (c.) Granulocytic or acute leukemia

      (d.) Hemolytic anemia

      (e.) Infectious mononucleosis

      (f.) Progressive muscular dystrophy

    4. *Slight* increases occur in:

      (a.) Delirium tremens   (c.) Obstructive jaundice

      (b.) Hepatitis   (d.) Cirrhosis

Interfering Factors

1. Strenuous exercise and the muscular exertion involved in childbirth will cause increased levels.
2. Skin diseases can cause falsely increased levels.
3. Hemolysis or red blood cells due to freezing, heating, or shaking the blood sample will cause falsely increased levels.
4. Drugs which may cause increased levels include:
   - (a.) Codeine
   - (b.) Clofibrate
   - (c.) Mepheridine
   - (d.) Mithramycin
   - (e.) Morphine
   - (f.) Procainamide
5. Oxalate is a drug known to cause decreased levels.

CLINICAL ALERT

Since many diseases increase LDH levels, it is important notify the laboratory of each disease the patient has.

ELECTROPHORESIS OF LDH (LD)

Normal Values

Amer./Europ. LDH 1/5	Amer./Europ. LDH 2/4	Amer./Europ. LDH 3
29%	38%	19%

Amer./Europ. LDH 4/2	Amer./Europ. LDH 5/1
8%	5%

Variations of 2 to 4 per cent are usually considered normal.

Explanation of Test

Electrophoresis or separation of LDH identifies the five isoenzymes or fractions of LDH, each with its own characteristic physical and electrical properties. (Note: The American nomenclature differs from the European. Be certain which standards are used when attempting to identify elevated fractions.) Fractionating the LDH activity sharpens its diagnostic value since LDH is found in many organs.

TABLE 5-1. CLASSIFICATION OF LDH ISOENZYMES AND ORGANS WHERE CONCENTRATED.*

European Nomenclature	American Nomenclature	Organs or Tissue Where Concentrated
LDH_1	LDH_5	Liver, skeletal muscle and kidney, lung
LDH_2	LDH_4	Liver, skeletal muscle, brain, and kidney, lung
LDH_3	LDH_3	Lung, spleen, pancreas, thyroid, adrenal lymph glands, brain, and kidney
LDH_4	LDH_2	Lung, myocardium, brain, red blood cells, and kidney
LDH_5	LDH_1	Myocardium, brain, kidney and red blood cells, lung

*Isoenzyme should be evaluated in terms of patterns established, not on basis of a single isoenzyme.

The five isoenzyme fractions of LDH show different patterns in various disorders. Abnormalities in the pattern suggest which tissues have been damaged and help to diagnose the following three diseases:
1. Myocardial infarction
2. Pulmonary infarction
3. Liver disease (This test is sensitive enough to detect increased hepatic fraction in infectious hepatitis before clinical jaundice appears.)

Procedure

A venous blood sample of ten ml. is obtained.

Clinical Implications

1. Increased LD_1 and LD_2 indicate myocardial infarction.
2. Increased LDH_3 indicates pulmonary infarction.
3. Increased LDH_4 and LDH_5 indicate liver disease.

CREATINE PHOSPHOKINASE (CPK);
CREATINE KINASE (CK)

Normal Values

0–12 Sigma units/ml.
Male: 5–35 ug./ml.; 20–140 IU./l.
Female: 5.25 ug. per ml.; 10–100 IU./l.
MB isoenzyme: Less than 3 IU./l.

Explanation of Test

CPK/CK is found in high concentrations in the heart and skeletal muscles and in much smaller concentrations in the brain tissue. Since CPK exists in relatively few organs, this test is used as a specific index of injury to myocardium and muscle. Thus it is important in the diagnosis of myocardial infarction and as a reliable measure of a skeletal muscle disease such as muscular dystrophy. In fact, CPK levels can prove helpful in recognizing muscular dystrophy before clinical signs appear. It is also of value in following the course of inflammatory muscle disease.

CPK/CK Isoenzymes

CPK can be divided into three isoenzymes: MM, BB, and MB. The isoenzyme studies help distinguish whether the CPK originated from the heart (MB) or the skeletal muscle (MM). Thus, elevation of MM levels is an indication of skeletal muscle injury. Elevation of MB, the cardiac enzyme, provides a more definitive indication of myocardial cell damage or death than total CPK alone.

Procedure

A blood sample of at least two ml. is obtained by venipuncture. If a patient has been receiving multiple I.M. injections, this fact should be noted on the laboratory requisition.

Clinical Implications

A. *Myocardial Infarction*
   1. Rise starts soon after an attack (about four hours) and reaches a peak of 10 to 25 times normal within 36 hours.
   2. Rise of CPK parallels that of SGOT, but persists longer than SGOT.
   3. Level returns to normal two to four days after infarction. Thus, if patient is seen within this period following an infarction, the CPK levels can help determine that an infarction did occur.
   4. If the CPK rise is extensive, then the indication is that the infarcted area is extensive and the prognosis is thus unfavorable.

B. *Other Diseases*
   1. Progressive muscular dystrophy (levels may reach 300 to 400 times normal
   2. Dermatomyositis (involves muscle inflammation and neurons)
   3. Delirium tremors and chronic alcoholism (an episode of acute intoxication may be accompanied by CPK/CK levels comparable to those found in MI.)
   4. Electric shock
   5. Myxedema
   6. Cardiac surgery
   7. Cardiac defibrillation
   8. Electromyography
   9. Convulsions, cerebral infarction, or subarachnoid hemorrhage
   10. Hypokalemia
   11. Hypothyroidism (mild elevations may occur)
   12. Acute psychosis
   13. Central nervous system trauma
   14. Pulmonary infarction or edema (raise in CPK levels is unexplainable)

Interfering Factors

1. Strenuous exercise (up to three times normal) and surgical procedure that damage skeletal muscle may cause increased levels.

2. High doses of salicylates may cause increased levels.
3. Athletes have a higher value because of greater muscle mass.
4. Multiple intramuscular infections may cause increased levels.
5. Drugs which may cause increased levels include:
   (a.) Amphotericin B
   (b.) Ampicillin, I.M.
   (c.) Carbenicillin, I.M.
   (d.) Chlorpromazine, I.M.
   (e.) Clofibrate

ALKALINE PHOSPHATASE

Normal Values

1.5–4.5 μ/dl. (Bodansky method)
4.3 μ/dl. (King-Armstrong method)
0.8–2.3 y./nk. (Bessey-Lowry method)
15.35 μ/ml. (Shinowar-Jones-Reonhart)

Explanation of Test

Alkaline phosphatase is an enzyme originating mainly in the bone, liver, and placenta, with some activity in the kidney and intestines. It is called alkaline since it functions best at a pH of 9.

This enzyme test is used chiefly as an index of liver and bone disease when correlated with other clinical findings. In bone disease, the enzyme rises in proportion to new bone cell production resulting from osteoblastic activity and deposit of calcium in the bones. In liver disease, the blood level rises when excretion of this enzyme is impaired as a result of obstruction in the biliary tract.

Procedure

A venous blood sample of ten ml. is obtained.

Clinical Implications

A. *Elevated Levels*

   1. Liver Disease (correlates with abnormal liver function tests)

      An elevation of alkaline phosphatase is often associated with elevated SGOT/AST and elevated bilirubin.

      (a.) Marked Increases

         (1.) Obstructive jaundice (gall stones obstructing major biliary ducts; accompanies elevated bilirubin)

         (2.) Space-occupying lesions of the liver such as cancer and abscesses

         (3.) Hepatocellular cirrhosis

         (4.) Biliary cirrhosis

      (b.) Moderate Increases

         (1.) Hepatitis

         (2.) Cirrhosis of liver

   2. Bone Disease

      (a.) Marked Increases

         (1.) Paget's disease

         (2.) Metastatic bone disease

         (3.) Osteitis deformans

      (b.) Moderate Increases

         (1.) Osteomalacia (elevated levels help differentiate between osteomalacia and osteoporosis, in which there is no elevation)

         (2.) Rickets

   3. Other Diseases

      (a.) Hyperparathyroidism (accompanied by hypercalcemia)

      (b.) Infectious mononucleosis

B. *Reduced Levels*

   1. Hypophosphatasia (markedly reduced)

   2. Malnutrition

   3. Hypothyroidism

   4. Pernicious anemia

   5. Scurvy

   6. Milk-alkali syndrome

   7. Placental insufficiency

Interfering Factors

1. A variety of drugs producing mild to moderate elevations of alkaline phosphatase are:

   (a.) Phenothiazine tranquilizers   (g.) Tolbutamide
   (b.) Methyltestosterone   (h.) Isoniazid
   (c.) Oral contraceptives   (i.) PAS
   (d.) Allopurinol   (j.) Erythromycin
   (e.) Methyldopa   (k.) Oxacillin
   (f.) Procainamide   (l.) Ergosterol
        See appendix for complete listing of drugs that increase levels

2. Young children, pregnant women in the third trimester, and all females have physiologically high levels of alkaline phosphatase.
3. The level is slightly increased in older people.
4. After IV administration of albumin there is sometimes a marked increase lasting for several days.
5. Drugs which may cause decreased levels include:

   (a.) Fluorides   (d.) Placebo
   (b.) Oxalates   (e.) Propranolol
   (c.) Phosphates   (f.) Vitamin D

ACID PHOSPHATASE

Normal Values

1.0–4.0 King Armstrong μ/dl.
0.5–2.0 Bodansky or Gutman μ/dl.
0–1.1 Shinowara μ/ml.
0.1–0.73 Bessey Lowry μ/nk.

Explanation of Test

Acid phosphatases are enzymes that are widely distributed in tissue, including the bone, liver, spleen, kidney, red blood cells and platelets. However, its greatest importance is found in the prostate gland where acid phosphatase activity is 100 times higher than in other tissue.

For this reason, the test of acid phosphatase levels is used to diagnose metastatic cancer of the prostate and to follow the effectiveness of treatment. It is known that elevated levels of acid phosphatase are seen in patients with prostate cancer that has metastasized beyond the capsule to other parts of the body, especially the bone. It is believed that once the carcinoma has spread, the prostate starts to release acid phosphatase resulting in an increase in blood level.

Procedure

A venous blood sample of ten ml. is obtained.

Clinical Implications

1. A significantly elevated value nearly always is indicative of metastatic cancer of the prostate. If the tumor is successfully treated, this enzyme level will drop within three to four days after surgery or three to four weeks after estrogen administration.
2. Moderately elevated values also occur in the absence of prostate disease in :
   - (a.) Paget's disease
   - (b.) Gaucher's disease
   - (c.) Hyperparathyroidism
   - (d.) Multiple myeloma
   - (e.) Any cancer that has metastasized to the bone.
   - (f.) Hepatitis
   - (g.) Obstructive jaundice
   - (h.) Acute renal impairment.
   - (i.) Sickle cell crisis
   - (j.) Excessive destruction of platelets

Interfering Factors

1. Drugs which may cause *increased levels* include:
   - (a.) Androgens in females
   - (b.) Clofibrate
2. Drugs which may cause *decreased levels* include:
   - (a.) Fluorides
   - (b.) Oxalates
   - (c.) Phosphates

Y-GLUTAMYL TRANSPEPTIDASE (YGT); Y-GLUTAMYL TRANSFERASE (YGT); Y-GAMMA-GLUTAMYL TRANSFERASE (YGGT)

Normal Values

Men: 11–38 IU/l.
Women: 7–25 IU/l.

Background

The enzyme Y-glutamyl transpeptidase transferase is present mainly in the liver, kidney, prostate, and spleen. The liver is considered the source of normal serum activity, despite the fact that the kidney has the highest level of the enzyme. This enzyme is believed to function in the transport of amino acids and peptides into the cell across the cell membrane, and to be involved in glutathione metabolism.

Explanation of Test

This test is used to determine liver cell dysfunction and to detect alcohol-induced liver disease. It is also an efficient way to screen for the consequences of chronic alcoholism. YGT activity is elevated in all forms of liver disease. This test is much more sensitive than either the alkaline phosphatase test or the the transaminase test in detecting obstructive jaundice, cholangeitis, and cholecystitis.

Procedure

A venous blood sample of ten ml. is obtained.

Clinical Implications

1. *Increased* YGT levels are associated with:
    (a.) Cholecystitis
    (b.) Cholelithiasis
    (c.) Cancer metatastic to the liver
    (d.) Cirrhosis of the liver
    (e.) Acute pancreatitis

 (f.) Cancer of the bile duct
 (g.) Congestive heart failure
 (h.) Alcoholism
 (i.) Barbiturate use
 (j.) Lipoid nephrosis
2. In myocardial infarction, YGT is usually normal. However, if there is an increase, it occurs about the fourth day after an MI and probably implies liver damage secondary to cardiac insufficiency.

LIPASE

Normal Values

0–1 unit/ml.

Explanation of Test

Lipase functions in the body to change fats to fatty acid and glycerol. The major source of this enzyme is the pancreas. Therefore, lipase appears in the bloodstream following damage to the pancreas.

 The test is used to diagnose pancreatitis and to differentiate pancreatitis from an acute surgical abdominal emergency. When secretions of the pancreas are blocked, the blood serum lipase levels rise.

Procedure

A venous blood sample of 10 to 20 ml. is obtained.

Clinical Implications

A. *In Pancreatic Disorders*
 1. Elevation of lipase may not occur until 24 to 36 hours after onset of illness.
 2. Elevation persists longer than changes in blood amylase, which is also related to pancreatic disorders (up to 14 days).

3. May be high when amylase levels are normal.
4. Thus the lipase test is useful in late diagnosis of acute pancreatitis.

B. *Increased lipase values* are associated with:
1. Pancreatitis
2. Obstruction of the pancreatic duct
3. Pancreatic carcinoma
4. Acute cholecystitis
5. Cirrhosis
6. Severe renal disease

C. Usually normal in mumps.

Interfering Factors

Drugs
1. Morphine
2. Codeine
3. Methylcholine
4. Bentanechol
5. Meperidine (Demerol)

PLASMA LIPIDS (TOTAL); LIPOPROTEINS: CHOLESTEROL, TRIGLYCERIDES, PHOSPHOLIPIDS

Normal Values

Total: 400–100 mg./dl. (published estimated ranges vary widely)

Cholesterol: 150–250 mg./dl.

Triglycerides: 40–150 mg./dl.

Phospholipids: 150–380 mg./dl. (The importance of phospholipids has not been generally agreed upon)

Explanation of Test. The blood lipids consist mainly of cholesterol, triglycerides and phospholipids. These three substances are also referred to as lipoproteins since they are bound to protein, and are therefore found in combination with the serum proteins. Chemically, the lipids resemble fatty acids and are related to fat metabolism.

Body lipids provide energy for metabolism and serve as precursors of steroid hormones (adrenals, ovaries, and testes) and bile acids. They also play an important role in the make-up of cell membranes.

Procedure
A venous blood sample of 20 ml. is obtained for total lipids.

Clinical Implications
1. Increased total lipids are most commonly associated with hyperlipidemia.
2. Decreased total lipids may be associated with fat malabsorption syndrome.

Hyperlipidemia
A. *General Considerations*

In certain diseases, the particular lipid fraction or the lipid level is elevated as a whole.
1. Hypothyroidism: Cholesterol is elevated.
2. Nephrotic syndrome: Total lipids are elevated.
3. Glycogen storage disease: Total lipids are elevated.
4. Ketosis: Total lipids are elevated.
5. Diabetes: Cholesterol is elevated.
6. Pancreatitis: Triglycerides elevated.
7. Obstructive liver disease: Cholesterol and phospholipids are elevated.
8. Myocardial infarction: Triglycerides are elevated.

B. *Congenital Forms*
1. There are five different types of congenital hyperlipidemia that are classified as I, II, III, IV, V.
2. In coronary heart disease, types II and IV are most noted:

Type II: cholesterol elevated; triglycerides slightly elevated

Type IV: cholesterol normal; triglycerides elevated

Interfering Factors
1. The total lipids will be increased after a fatty meal.
2. Oral contraceptives may cause increased total lipid levels.
3. Drugs which may cause decreased total lipid levels include:
   (a.) Cholestyramine resin
   (b.) Estrogens
   (c.) Fenfluramine

TABLE 5–2. PHENOTYPING OF HYPERLIPIDEMIA INTO 5 MAJOR TYPES*

Type	Cholesterol	Triglyceride
I (rare; familial; fat-induced)	++	+++
II (common; familial)	++++	+
III (uncommon; familial)	++	++
IV (common, carbohydrate-induced)	+	++++
V (uncommon; familial)	++	++++

*Blood lipids are elevated in hyperlipidemia. Two types of hyperlipidemia (Types II and IV) are important in cardiovascular disease.

Patient Preparation
1. Instruct patient to fast for 12 to 14 hours before the test.
2. Water is permitted.
3. Patient should be on a normal diet seven days prior to testing.

CLINICAL ALERT
If the patient breaks the fast, notify the laboratory.

Cholesterol

Normal Values. Normal values vary with age, diet, and from country to country.

Age (years)	Cholesterol (mg./dl.)
0–19	120–230
20–29	120–240
30–39	140–270
40–49	150–310
50–59	160–330

Background
Cholesterol is the most often measured blood lipid. Existing in muscles, red blood cells, and cell membranes, it is used by the

body to form steroid hormones, bile acids, and more cell membranes. Chemically, cholesterol exists in both a free and esterized form (60–75%) in the body. Much of the cholesterol ingested is esterized in the intestines, but since it is also esterized in the liver, cholesterol levels are frequently used as an indication of liver function.

In the public mind, however, cholesterol is associated with atherosclerosis and coronary artery disease. There is some evidence that populations consuming a smaller amount of fats in their total caloric intake (by eating vegetables rather than animal fats) have a lower cholesterol level and a lower incidence of atherosclerosis and coronary artery disease. Nevertheless, cholesterol levels are important detectors of disorders other than those directly related to coronary artery disease. Cholesterol levels are used to evaluate cellular damage to the liver, to aid in the prognosis in cases of jaundice, and to monitor the course of hyper or hypothyroidism.

Explanation of Test
The main use of this test is to diagnose a disorder of blood lipids. It is also used as a secondary aid in the study of thyroid and liver function.

Procedure.   A venous blood sample of seven ml. is obtained.

Clinical Implications
A. *Increased Levels*
  1. Levels above 250 mg. per dl. are considered elevated and call for a triglyceride test.
  2. Conditions related to elevated cholesterol:
      (a.) Cardiovascular disease and atherosclerosis
      (b.) Familial hypercholesterolemia
      (c.) Obstructive jaundice (also an increase in bilirubin)
      (d.) Hypothyroidism (decreased in hyperthyroidism)
      (e.) Nephrosis
      (f.) Xanthomatosis
      (g.) Uncontrolled diabetes

3. Free vs. esterized cholesterol
   There is a markedly abnormal ratio of free to
   esterified cholesterol in disease of the liver biliary
   tract, infectious diseases, and extreme cholesterol-
   emia.
B. *Decreased Levels*
   1. Instances when cholesterol is not absorbed from the
      GI tract:

   (a.) Malabsorption   (e.) Sepsis
   (b.) Liver disease   (f.) Stress
   (c.) Hyperthyroidism   (g.) Drug therapy
   (d.) Anemia

   2. General conditions related to decreased cholesterol
      levels
      (a.) Pernicious anemia
      (b.) Hemolytic jaundice
      (c.) Hyperthyroidism
      (d.) Severe infections
      (e.) Terminal stages of debilitating diseases such as
           cancer
   3. Esterol fraction decreases in liver diseases, liver cell
      injury, malabsorption syndrome, and malnutrition.

Interfering Factors
1. Cholesterol is normally slightly elevated in pregnancy.
2. Estrogen decreases plasma cholesterol, and oophorectomy
   increases it.
3. Many drugs may cause a change in the blood cholesterol.
   See appendix for a complete listing.

Triglycerides

Normal Values. 40–150 mg./100 ml.
   Values in the first two decades of life are slightly lower than
those in subsequent years. Values in women are about ten
milligrams lower than in men.

Background. Triglycerides, produced in the liver from
glycerol and fatty acids, are triesters of these two components.

Triglycerides which are absorbed from the intestines are called chlyomicrons, tiny fat droplets covered with a thin layer of protein. Meals rich in fats result in a heavy absorption of chlyomicrons which then give the serum a milky or creamy appearance (turbidity). A turbid serum or plasma calls for further analysis via electrophoresis to determine the fractioned breadkown of the lipids. A definite abnormal finding would signify the presence of triglycerides (chylomicrons) is a specimen taken while the patient had been fasting.

Explanation of Test. This test is used to evaluate patients with suspected atherosclerosis and as an indication of the body's ability to metabolize fat.

Procedure. A venous blood sample of at least three ml. is obtained.

Clinical Implications. Increased triglyceride levels are considered more important than increased cholesterol in the development of arterial disease.

A. *Increased Levels* occur in:
  1. Familial hyperlipidemia
  2. Liver disease
  3. Nephrotic syndrome
  4. Hypothyroidism
  5. Poorly controlled diabetes
  6. Pancreatitis
  7. Glycogen storage
  8. Myocardial infarction (increase may last a year)
B. *Decreased Level*
  Occurs in malnutrition and congenital alpha-beta lipoproteinemia.

Patient Preparation
1. Instruct patient about fasting overnight for 12 hours before the test.
2. Water is permitted.
3. Prior to fasting, the patient should be on a normal diet.

CEPHALIN FLOCCULATION; THYMOL TURBIDITY

Normal Values

Cephalin Flocculation: 24 or less negative units
Thymol Turbidity: 0–4 units

Background

In the laboratory, thymol is mixed with the patient's blood. Turbidity is usually increased in the presence of liver damage and related diseases. Moreover, the blood of patients with liver damage will flocculate (clump) a colloidal suspension of cephalin and cholesterol; the blood of healthy persons will not flocculate the suspension. The results of the test parallel one another.

Explanation of Test

These tests are used to diagnose liver damage, to differentiate liver disease from biliary obstruction, and to follow the course of cirrhosis. With these tests, it is often possible to detect cell damage before jaundice appears.

Procedure

A venous blood sample of ten ml. is obtained.

Clinical Implications

1. *Increased levels* are associated with:
    (a.) Acute hepatitis
    (b.) Cirrhosis (but can be normal)
    (c.) Multiple myeloma
    (d.) Sarcoidosis
    (e.) Hodgkin's disease
    (f.) Coccidioidosis
    (g.) Subacute endocarditis
    (h.) Rheumatoid arthritis

    (i.) Lupus erythematosus
    (j.) Tuberculosis (hematogenous)
    (k.) Histoplasmosis
    (l.) Malaria
    (m.) Lymphogranuloma venereum
2. Liver abscess and neoplasms will give a negative result.
3. In acute hepatitis, thymol turbidity becomes positive later than transaminase elevation and may remain positive after cephalin flocculation.

Interfering Factors

1. False positive results occur with blood samples that have a high fat content.
2. Refer to appendix for listing of drugs that cause falsely increased or decreased levels in this test.

FOLIC ACID (FOLATE)

Normal Values

5.9 to 21.0 μg/ml.

    Folic acid is needed for the normal function of red and white blood cells, and is required for the production of cellular genes. Folic acid is a more potent growth promoter than Vitamin B_{12}. Although fulfilling a different requirement, folic acid, like B_{12}, is required for DNA production. Folic acid is formed by bacteria in the intestines, is stored in the liver, and is present in foods such as eggs, milk, leafy vegetables, yeast, liver, fruits, and other elements of a well-balanced diet.

Explanation of Test

This test is indicated in the differential diagnosis of a hemolytic disorder and in the investigation of folic acid deficiency in altered utilization. When folic acid absorption is blocked, the liver and body stores of folic acid are depleted, and blood cell production and maturation are affected. If folic acid is deficient, large red cells are produced with shortened life span and impaired oxygen carrying capacity. Deficiency of folic acid also causes white abnormalities related to altered DNA or RNA synthesis. It takes several weeks for folate deficiency to develop. The folic acid level must remain at a decreased level for 20 weeks or more before anemia develops.

Procedure

A venous sample of 10 ml. is obtained.

Clinical Implications

1. The *major* causes of *decreased* folic acid (four μg./ml.) are:
   - (a.) Inadequate intake
   - (b.) Malabsorption of folic acid
   - (c.) Excessive utilization of folic acid by the body
   - (d.) Drugs which are folic acid antagonists (interfere with nuclei acid synthesis) such as:
     - (1.) Anticonvulsant drugs
     - (2.) Aminopterin and methotrexate used in leukemia treatment
     - (3.) Antimalaria drugs
     - (4.) Alcohol
2. *Decreased* folic acid levels are associated with:
   - (a.) Megaloblastic anemia
   - (b.) Hemolytic anemia
   - (c.) Liver disease associated with:
     - (1.) Alcoholism
     - (2.) Malabsorption syndrome
   - (d.) Sprue
   - (e.) Celiac disease
   - (f.) Ediopathic steatorrhea
   - (g.) Malignancies
   - (h.) Malnutrition
   - (i.) Drugs mentioned above
   - (j.) Elderly persons with inadequate diets
   - (k.) Hyperthyroidism
   - (l.) Vitamin C deficiency
   - (m.) Fibrile states
   - (n.) Chronic dialyses
3. The anemias due to folic acid deficiency include:

(a.) Megaloblastic anemia of pregnancy because of fetal requirements for folate.
(b.) Nutritional megaloblastic anemia by occurring in:
(1.) Infancy
(2.) Early childhood
(3.) Infections
(4.) Old age
(It occurs more commonly when infections or diarrhea increase folate requirements)
(c.) Macrocytic hemolytic anemia
(d.) Macrocytic anemia due to liver disease associated with alcoholism

CLINICAL ALERT
Elderly persons or those having inadequate diets in this country (U.S.A.) are known to develop folate deficient megaloblastic anemia.

SODIUM (NA+)

Normal Values

136–142 mEq./l. in adults under 65 years of age
132–140 mEq./l. in adults older than 65 years

Sodium, a blood electrolyte, is the most abundant cation (90% of the electrolyte fluid) and the chief base of the blood. Its primary functions in the body are to chenically maintain osmotic pressure and acid base balance, and to transmit nerve impulses. The body has a strong tendency to maintain a total base content and only slight changes are found even under pathologic conditions.

Sodium concentration is under the control of the kidneys and the central nervous system acting through the endocrine system. In health, the level of sodium is kept constant within narrow limits despite wide fluctuations in dietary intake. An average dietary intake of 90 to 250 mEq. per day is enough to maintain sodium balance in adults. The minimum daily need is approximately 15 mEq.

Explanation of Test

Determinations of plasma sodium levels are useful in detecting gross changes in water and salt balance but are of little help in detecting early or subtle changes. Urinary sodium is a more sensitive indicator of altered sodium balance. Numerous factors, as listed below, determine the content and volume of urine excreted. These, in turn, determine the content and flow rate in the renal vein returning processed blood.

Mechanisms for maintaining a constant sodium level in the plasma and extracellular fluid include:

1. *Renal blood flow*
   - (a.) Increased renal blood flow to the glomeruli will result in increased sodium and chloride excretions.
   - (b.) Decreased renal blood flow to the glomeruli will result in sodium and chloride retention and edema. This recurs in patients with reduced cardiac output.
2. *Carbonic anhydrase enzyme activity*
   - (a.) The level of activity of this system is an important factor in control of the rate of sodium excretion.
   - (b.) Inhibition of carbonic anhydrase enzyme activity results in increased sodium reabsorption in the tubules.
3. *Aldosterone*
   - (a.) Aldosterone acts on the distal tubules and also affects sodium reabsorption.
   - (b.) Regulation of aldosterone secretion is:
     - (1.) Primarily regulated by the renin-angiotensin system
     - (2.) Secondarily by ACTH, sodium, and potassium concentration
   - (c.) In primary hyperaldosteronism, Sodium will be retained and hypertension will result. In exchange for sodium, potassium will often be excreted and decreased potassium may be found in this condition.
4. *Action of other steroids* whose plasma level is controlled by the anterior pituitary gland.
   - (a.) These steroids can cause salt and water retention. During the menstrual cycle, estrogen and progesterone cause salt and water retention before menstruation, and diureses if fertilization has not taken place.
5. *Renin enzyme secretion*

   (a.) Renin is a potent stimulus to aldosterone secretion. It regulates renal blood flow, the glomerular filtration rate, and salt and water excretion. In renal diseases excessive amounts of renin secreted into the plasma result in salt and water retention and hypertension.
6. *ADH, antidiuretic hormone, vasopressin secretion*
   (a.) ADH controls the reabsorption of water at the distal tubules of the kidney.
   (b.) Secretion of this hormone is responsive to changes in extracellular fluid volume.

Procedure

A venous blood sample of seven ml. is obtained.

Clinical Implications

A. *Hyponatremia* (decreased levels)
   1. Hyponatremia usually reflects a relative excess of body water rather than a low total body sodium.
   2. *Reduced* sodium levels (hyponatremia) are associated with:
      (a.) Severe burns
      (b.) Severe diarrhea
      (c.) Vomiting
      (d.) Excessive IV's of nonelectrolyte fluids
      (e.) Addison's diseases (lack of adrenal steroids impairs sodium reabsorption)
      (f.) Severe nephritis
      (g.) Pyloric obstruction
      (h.) Malabsorption syndrome
      (i.) Diabetic acidosis
      (j.) Drugs
         (1.) Mercurial diuretics
         (2.) Chlorothiazide diuretics
      (k.) Edema
      (l.) Excessive sweating accompanied by large amounts of water by mouth
      (m.) Stomach suction accompanied by water or ice chips *by mouth*

B. *Hypernatremia* (increased levels)

Increased sodium levels are uncommon, but when they do occur they are associated with:

(a.) Dehydration and insufficient water intake
(b.) Conn's syndrome
(c.) Primary aldosteronism
(d.) Coma .
(e.) Cushing's disease
(f.) Diabetes insipidus
(g.) Tracheobronchitis

CLINICAL ALERT

1. IV therapy consideration
   a. Sodium balance is maintained in adults in an average dietary intake of 90 to 250 mEq. per day. The maximum daily tolerance to an acute load is 400 mEq. per day. If a patient is given three liters of isotonic saline in 24 hours, he will receive 465 mEq. of sodium. This amount exceeds the average, healthy adult's tolerance level. It will take a *healthy* person 24 to 48 hours to excrete the excess sodium.
   b. After surgery, trauma, or shock there is a decrease of extracellular fluid volume. Replacement of extracellular fluid is essential if water and electrolyte balance is to be maintained. The ideal replacement IV solution should have a sodium concentration of 140 mEq. per l.
2. Check patients for signs of edema, hypertension.

Interfering Factors

There are many drugs which may cause falsely increased or decreased levels of blood sodium. Refer to appendix for complete listing.

POTASSIUM (K+)

Normal Values

3.5–5.0 mEq./l.
4–4.7 mEq./l. (average)

Background

Potassium is the principal electrolyte (cation) of intracellular fluid, and primary buffer within the cell itself. 90 per cent of $K+$ is concentrated within the cell, only small amounts are contained in the bone and blood. A kilogram of tissue such as RBC or muscle contains about 90 mEq. of $K+$. Damaged cells release $K+$ into the blood.

The body is adapted to efficient potassium excretion. Normally, 80 to 90 per cent of the cells' potassium is excreted in the urine via the glomeruli of the kidneys. The remainder is excreted in sweat and in the stool. Even when no potassium is taken into the body (as in a fasting state), 40 to 50 mEq. are still excreted daily in the urine. The kidneys do not conserve potassium, and when an adequate amount of potassium is not ingested a severe deficiency will occur. The normal intake, minimal needs, and maximum tolerance for potassium is almost the same as that for sodium.

Potassium plays an important role in nerve conduction and muscle function. Moreover, it helps maintain acid-base balance and osmotic pressure. Along with calcium and magnesium, potassium controls the rate and force of contraction of the heart and thus, the cardiac output. Evidence of a potassium deficit can be noted on an ECG by the presence of a U wave.

Potassium and sodium ions are particularly important in the renal regulation of acid-base balance on account of hydrogen ions being substituted for sodium and potassium ions in the renal tubule. Potassium is more important than sodium since potassium bicarbonate is the primary intracellular inorganic buffer. In potassium deficiency there is a relative deficiency of intracellular potassium bicarbonate and the pH is relatively acid. The respiratory center responds to the intracellular acidosis by lower PCO_2, through the mechanism of hyperventilation.

Concentration of potassium is greatly affected by the adrenal hormones. A potassium deficiency will cause a marked reduction in protein synthesis.

Evaluation of Test

This test is used to evaluate changes in body potassium and is helpful in diagnosing disorders of acid base and water balance in the body. It is not an absolute value and varies with the circulatory volume and other factors. Thus it is important to check this value in severe cases of Addison's disease, uremic coma, intestinal obstruction, acute renal failure, gastrointestinal loss in the administration of diuretics, steroid therapy, and cardiac patients on digitalis.

Procedure

1. A venous blood sample of ten ml. is obtained.
2. Hemolysis in obtaining the sample should be avoided; it will give false to high results.

Clinical Implications

A. *Hypokalemia*
　　1. Values of 3.5 mEq. per l. are more commonly associated with deficiency, rather than normality.
　　2. A falling trend (0.1 to 0.2 mEq. per day) is indicative of a developing potassium deficiency.
　　　　(a.) Most frequent cause of K+ deficiency is gastrointestinal loss.
　　　　(b.) Most frequent cause of K+ depletion is diuretic administration without adequate K+ supplements.
　　3. Decreased levels, hypokalemia, are associated with:
　　　　(a.) Diarrhea
　　　　(b.) Pyloric obstruction
　　　　(c.) Starvation
　　　　(d.) Malabsorption
　　　　(e.) Severe vomiting
　　　　(f.) Severe burns
　　　　(g.) Primary aldosteronism
　　　　(h.) Excessive ingestion of licorice
　　　　(i.) Renal tubular acidosis
　　　　(j.) Diuretic administration
　　　　　　(1.) Mercurials
　　　　　　(2.) Ammonium chloride
　　　　　　(3.) Chlorothiazides
　　　　　　(4.) Deamox
　　　　(k.) Other drugs

(1.) Steroids
(2.) Estrogen
(l.) Familial periodic paralysis
(m.) Liver disease with oscites
(n.) Chronic stress
(o.) Crash dieting without K+
(p.) Chronic fever

B. *Hyperkalemia* (Increased levels)
1. The most frequent causes of increased levels are:
   (a) Inadequate excretion (renal failure)
   (b) Cell damage as in burns, accidents, surgery (damaged cells will release potassium into the blood)
   (c) Acidosis (drives potassium out of the cells)
2. Increased levels are associated with:
   (a) Addison's disease   (d) Internal hemorrhage
   (b) Acute renal failure   (e) Uncontrolled diabetes
      1. Oliguria   (f) Acidosis
      2. Anuria
   (c) Selective hypoaldo-steronism

Interfering Factors

1. Forearm exercise
Opening and closing the fist ten times with a tourniquet in place results in an increase of the K+ level by 10 to 20 per cent.
For this reason it is recommended that the blood sample be obtained without a tourniquet, or that the tourniquet should be released after the needle has entered the vein and two minutes allowed to elapse before the sample is withdrawn.

2. Drug usage:
   (a.) The IV use of *potassium penicillin* may cause hyperkalemia; *penicillin sodium* may cause an increased excretion of K+.
   (b.) Glucose tolerance testing or the ingestion/administration of large amounts of glucose in patients

with heart disease may cause a decrease of 0.4 mEq. per l. in K+ blood levels.

(c.) See appendix for complete listing of drugs that interfere with blood potassium levels.

CLINICAL ALERT

1. Notify the physician when K+ is three mEq./per l. or less or 6.5 mEq. per l. or greater. These levels may cause heart problems leading to death.

2. The most common cause of hypokalemia in patients receiving IV fluids is water and sodium chloride administration without adequate replacement for K+ lost in urine and drainage fluids. A patient receiving IV fluids needs potassium every day. The minimum daily dose should be 40 mEq., but the optimum daily dose ranges between 60 and 120 mEq. Potassium needs are greater in tissue injury, wound infection, gastric intestinal or biliary drainage. If adequate amounts of potassium are not given in IV solution (40 mEq./day) hypokalemia will develop eventually.

   A 40 mEq. dose of IV potassium should be given in one or more hours, not one or more minutes. 20 mEq. should be administered per hour. A burning sensation felt at the site of needle insertion may indicate that the concentration is toxic and the IV should be discontinued.

3. Patients taking digitalis and diuretics should be watched closely for hypokalemia since cardiac arrythmias can occur. Hypokalemia enhances the effect of digitalis preparations, creating the possibility of digitalis intoxication from even an average maintenance dose. Digitalis, diuretics and hypokalemia are a potentially lethal combination

4. The K+ blood level rises 0.6 mEq. per l. for every 0.1 decrease in blood pH.

5. Hyperkalemia can be altered by the use of hypertonic ion exchange resins orally, or orally by an enema (Kayexalate) to remove excess potassium.

6. If there is a massive loss of extracellular potassium, the potassium within the cells may have to support K+ concentration in the blood. This process cannot be measured directly and can only be inferred from an understanding of clinical signs. Recognizing signs and symptoms of hypokalemia and hyperkalemia is very important, since many of them originate in the nervous and muscular systems and are usually non-specific and similar.

7. *Evaluating changes in body Ka*

How to recognize excess K$^+$ even when the blood level is normal

How to recognize a K$^+$ deficiency or depletion even when the blood level is normal.

Hyperkalemic	Hypokalemic

Hyperkalemic

1. Record intake and output.
2. Check blood volume and venous pressure, which will give a clue to dehydrative or circulatory overload.
3. Identify electrocardiogram (ECG) changes:
   (a.) Elevated T wave heart block
   (b.) Flattened P wave
   (c.) Cardiac arrest may occur without any warning other than ECG changes.
4. Observe for slow pulse and oliguria.
5. Observe for neuromuscular changes:
   (a.) Muscle weakness and impaired muscle function
   (b.) Flaccid paralysis
   (c.) Tremors, twitching proceeding actual paralysis

Hypokalemic

1. Record intake and output.
2. Check blood volume and venous pressure which will give a clue to circulatory overload or dehydration.
3. Identify ECG changes:
   (a.) Depressed T waves
   (b.) Peaking of P waves
4. Observe for dehydration caused by severe vomiting, hyperventilation, sweating, diuresis, NG tube with gastric suction. Accurately record state of hydration or dehydration.
5. Observe for neuromuscular changes:
   (a.) Fatigue
   (b.) Muscle weakness, muscle pain, flabby muscles
   (c.) Parasthesia
   (d.) Hypotension and rapid pulse
   (e.) Respiratory muscle weakness leading to paralysis, cyanosis, and respiratory arrest
   (f.) Anorexia, nausea, vomiting, paralytic ileus
   (g.) Apathy, drowsiness, irritability, tetany, coma

CLINICAL ALERT

Be on the alert for these arrhythmias, which may occur with hyper-kalemia:

1. Sinus bradycardia
2. Sinus arrest
3. First degree AV block
4. Nodal rhythm

5. Idioventricular rhythm
6. Ventricular tachycardia
7. Ventricular fibrillation
8. Ventricular arrest

Be on the alert for these arrhythmias which may occur with hypo-kalemia:

1. Ventricular premature beats
2. Atriol tachycardia
3. Nodal tachycardia

4. Ventricular tachycardia
5. Ventricular fibrillation

CHLORIDE (CL⁻)

Normal Values

95–105 mEq./l.

Chloride, a blood electrolyte, is an anion that exists predominantly in the extracellular spaces, and in a lesser preponderancy in the intravascular spaces, and in the cell itself. Chemically, it exists primarily in combinations as sodium chloride or hydrochloric acid.

Chloride maintains cellular integrity through its influence on osmotic pressure. It is also significant in monitoring acid-base balance and water balance.

Chloride has the reciprocal power of increasing or decreasing in concentration whenever changes occur in the concentration of other anions. In metabolic acidosis, there is a reciprocal rise in chloride concentration when the bicarbonate concentration drops. Similarly, when aldosterone directly causes an increase in the reabsorption of sodium (which is a positive ion), the indirect effect is an increase in the absorption of chloride (the negative ion).

Chlorides are excreted with cations (positive ions) during massive diuresis from any cause and are lost from the gastrointestinal tract as a result of vomiting, diarrhea, or intestinal fistulas.

Explanation of Test

Alteration of serum chloride is seldom a primary problem. Thus, the measurement of chlorides is usually done for its inferential value and is helpful in diagnosing disorders of acid-base and water balance. Because of the relatively high concentration of chloride in the gastric juices, prolonged vomiting may lead to considerable chloride loss and lowered serum level.

Chloride is the least important electrolyte to measure in an emergency, but it is especially important to measure in the correction of hypokalemic alkalosis. If potassium is supplied without chloride, hypokalemic alkalosis may persist.

Procedure

A venous blood sample of ten ml. is obtained.

Clinical Implications

1. Whenever the serum level is much lower than 100 mEq. per l., the urinary excretion of chloride falls to a very low level.
2. The reason why decreased chloride levels often occur in acute infections is not clear.
3. Chloride measurements are of limited value in renal disease for the reason that plasma chloride can be maintained near normal limits even when a considerable degree of renal failure is present.
4. *Decreased* chloride levels occur in:
    - (a.) Severe vomiting
    - (b.) Severe diarrhea
    - (c.) Ulcerative colitis
    - (d.) Pyloric obstruction
    - (e.) Severe burns
    - (f.) Heat exhaustion
    - (g.) Diabetic acidosis
    - (h.) Addison's disease
    - (i.) Fever
    - (j.) Acute infections such as pneumonia
    - (k.) Use of drugs such as mercurial and chlorothiazide diuretics

5. *Increased* chloride levels occur in:
    (a.) Dehydration   (e.) Anemia
    (b.) Cushing's syndrome   (f.) Cardiac decompensation
    (c.) Hyperventilation   (g.) Some kidney disorders
    (d.) Eclampsia

Interfering Factors

1. The plasma chloride concentration of infants is usually higher than that of children and adults.
2. Many drugs may cause a change in chloride levels. See appendix for complete listing of drugs.

CLINICAL ALERT
1. In I.V. therapy, if the solution contains 100 mEq. per I. there is ample chloride present for the correction of urine metabolic acidosis.
2. If an electrolyte disorder is suspected, daily weight and accurate intake and output should be recorded.

TOXICOLOGY

ALCOHOL

Normal Values

Negative

Explanation of Test

Blood levels of *ethyl* alcohol are measured in cases of coma of unknown etiology or when the amount of alcohol must be determined, usually for legal purposes (traffic accidents or arrest). Most laws consider levels of 0.15 grams per 100 ml. (150 mg./dl.) as prima facie evidence of being under the influence of alcohol.

Procedure

A venous blood sample of four ml. is obtained.

Clinical implications

A. *Methyl Alcohol*

Methyl alcohol is a poisonous substance that can result in convulsions, blindness, and possible death if ingested in large enough quantities.
1. 25 mg./dl. or greater: toxic
2. 80 mg./dl. or greater: lethal

B. *Ethyl Alcohol*
1. 0.03–0.15 gm. per dl. or 30–150 mg. per dl.: "under the influence"
2. Levels between 50 to 150 mg. per dl. or .05 to 0.15 gm. per 100 ml. exert unmistakable effects on behavior and functioning, especially driving.

BARBITURATE (ASSAY)

Normal Values

Should be close to 0 (negative)

Explanation of Test

This test is indicated when accidental or intentional overdosage of barbiturates is suspected. Since patients with barbiturate intoxication are often unconscious, detection of the barbiturates and the possible identification of the type of compound ingested facilitates treatment.

Short-acting barbiturates are more potent and are eliminated from the body more slowly than long-acting barbiturates which are eliminated from the body at a faster rate.

The sample preferred is blood, but urine or aspirated stomach contents may be used.

Procedure

A venous blood sample, urine sample, or aspirated or vomited stomach contents can be examined.

Clinical Implications

1. Toxic level of short-acting barbiturates such as Seconal is three mg. per dl.
2. Toxic level of long acting barbiturates such as phenobarbitol is nine mg. per dl. Coma with shock is associated with these levels.
3. Other drugs such as tranquilizers and alcohol can have a compound effect on a moderate dose of barbiturates.

Interfering Factors

1. Drugs which may cause falsely increased levels are
     (a.) Antipyrine
     (b.) Theophylline in large doses

SALICYLATE

Normal Values

Negative

Background

Ingestion of aspirin is responsible for more cases of accidental poisonings in children that any other substance. Adults often use aspirin in suicide attempts, and often, large doses of salicylates are administered by enthusiastic self-healers. Toxic doses of salicylates initially produce a stimulation of the central nervous system as may be reflected in hyperventilation, flushes, fever, and ringing in the ears. This central nervous system stimulation is followed by depression.

A complex disturbance of acid-base balance results from severe hyperventilation. Initially, a respiratory alkalosis occurs, but this may be followed, especially in infants, by a metabolic acidosis. The net effect may be a decrease in the blood pH. Additionally, in the presence of salicylates, the liver fails to synthesize prothrombin from Vitamin K.

Explanation of Test

This test measures the level of salicylates in the blood and determines toxicity and therapeutic level.

Patients on aspirin for rheumatoid arthritis and related diseases should have their blood-salicylate level checked from time to time. Both blood and urine may be examined for salicylate levels.

Procedure

A venous blood sample of at least one ml. or urine sample is obtained.

Clinical Implications

1. Therapeutic level is 20 to 25 mg. per dl.
2. Toxic level is more than 30 mg. per dl.
3. A lethal level is more than 60 mg. per dl.

THEOPHYLLINE

Normal Values

None should be present

Therapeutic Values

5–20 ug/l.

Background

Theophylline (aminophylline), not a substance normally present in the blood, is a synthetic drug used in the treatment of restrictive airway diseases such as bronchial asthma, asthmatic bronchitis, and bronchospastic disorders.

Explanation of Test

This test measures the concentration of theophylline in the blood and indicates either a therapeutic or a toxic level. An important property of all medications is the relationship between therapeutic effect and toxicity.

Procedure

A venous blood sample is obtained.

Clinical Implications

1. Concentration of less than 20 μg. per l. is a toxic level and may cause nausea, vomiting, or other toxic symptoms.
2. A therapeutic level is 10 to 20 μg per l. depending on time and dosage.

Patient Preparation

1. Explain the purpose of the test.
2. Instruct the patient that no coffee, tea, cola, cocoa, or chocolate are permitted 12 hours prior to obtaining the blood sample, since these substances interfere with the laboratory results.

Interfering Factors

1. Drugs which may cause altered results include phenylbutazone, sulfonamides, theobromine, and xanthine.
2. Foods which may cause altered results include coffee, tea, cola, cocoa, and chocolate.

TESTOSTERONE

Normal Values

Males: 406 to 954 mg./dl.
Females: 40 to 120 mg./dl.

Background

Testosterone is a hormone responsible for the development of male secondary sexual characteristics. This substance is synthesized mainly in the Leydig cells of the testes. It is secreted by the adrenal glands and testes in men, and by the adrenal glands and ovaries in women.

Explanation of Test

Routine testosterone measurements in men have been found useful in the assessment of hypogonadism, pituitary gonadotropin function, impotency, and cryptorchidism; these measurements are also useful in the detection of ovarian and adrenal tumors in women.

Procedure

1. Three venous blood samples of ten ml. may be obtained from males.
2. Five venous blood samples of ten ml. may be obtained from females. (The quantity will vary according to laboratory procedure.)

Clinical Implications

1. Decreased testosterone levels are associated with:
   a. Male hypogonadism
   b. Klinfelter's syndrome in men
2. Increased testosterone levels are associated with:
   a. Adrenogenital-syndrome in women
   b. Stein-Leventhal syndrome in women when virilization is present

c. Adrenal neoplasms
d. Ovarian tumors, benign or malignant

PROTEIN-BOUND IODINE (PBI);
BUTANOL-EXTRACTABLE IODINE (BEI)

Normal Values

4.0–8.0 μg/dl. PBI
3.5–6.5 μg/dl. BEI

Explanation of Test

This measurement of organic iodine bound to protein is one of the most widely used tests of thyroid function. The thyroid is the only gland that actively metabolizes iodine. Circulating iodine is in the form of thyroid derived compounds, thyroxine (T_4) being the principle hormone. The level of PBI in the blood correlates with the thyroid status by accurately reflecting bound thyroxine. However, it has limited value since it is subject to interference by iodine drugs; the T_3 and T_4 must be normal, and the TBG and TBPA must be normal.

BEI is similar functionally to the PBI, but it is a more accurate and more specific method, since it is less subject to interference by drugs containing iodine.

Procedure

1. A venous blood sample of at least three ml. is obtained.
2. The sample should be obtained shortly after a meal, when lipids are usually not present in large amounts.

Clinical Implications

1. *Increased* PBI and BEI levels are found in:
    (a.) Hyperthyroidism
    (b.) Acute thyroiditis
        In hyperthyroidism, PBI levels of 8 to 25 μg. per dl. are found.

2. *Decreased* PBI and BEI levels are found in:
   (a.) Hypothyroidism
   (b.) Chronic thyroiditis
   (c.) Myxedema
   (d.) Nephrosis
3. In hypothyroidism, PBI levels of 0 to 4.0 μg per dl. are found.

Interfering Factors

1. A diet high in iodine (iodized salt) will interfere with the true picture of PBI and BEI.
2. A mild elevation of the PBI level may normally occur in pregnancy.
3. False elevations are caused by the use of:
   (a.) Iodine contrast substance in an IVP, gall bladder x-rays, myelograms, bronchograms, and CAT scans
   (b.) Thyroid hormones
   (c.) Estrogens
   (d.) Vaginal suppositories
   (e.) Amebicides
4. Refer to appendix for complete listing of drugs that cause falsely elevated or decreased levels of PBI.

Patient Preparation

1. Explain the purpose of the test, special diet, and drug restrictions to the patient. Check with laboratory for regulations.
2. An iodine-free diet is necessary for three days before the test. No iodized salt can be used for this period of time.
3. Drugs containing inorganic iodine such as Lugol's solution must be discontinued for one week before test.
4. Patient should wait at least one week after IVP x-ray and at least four weeks after gallbladder x-ray before having PBI.

CLINICAL ALERT
This test should be scheduled before an IVP, gallbladder X ray myelogram, or CAT scan, for the iodine contrast material used in these studies will cause false elevations. Check with individual testing department

for regulations. Since the contrast media is absorbed so slowly in the serum proteins, it may take up to five years to completely clear the body of this iodine.

BROMSULPHALEIN (BSP)

Normal Values

5% BSP retention 45 min. after injection of dye

Explanation of Test

This test of hepatic function is valuable in detecting early liver disease and in following the progress of known liver disease. It is most useful in liver cell damage without jaundice, in cirrhosis, and acute hepatitis. The BSP test is based on the ability of the liver to remove the injected dye. A definite amount of the dye (0.1 cc. of 5% BSP dye per kg. of body weight) is injected and the amount remaining in the blood after a definite time, usually 45 minutes, is measured. The removal rate is more rapid after meals because of increased blood flow. For this reason, the test must be done on fasting patients.

Procedure

1. Fasting is necessary for eight to 12 hours before and during testing
2. Record patient's weight.
3. An intravenous dose of bromsulphalein is injected slowly (5 mg. of dye per kg. of body weight), and exactly 45 minutes later, a venous blood sample of at least three ml. is obtained from a vein in the opposite arm. Avoid hemolysis of blood sample.

Clinical Implications

1. Increased abnormal retention of the dye is generally due to:
   (a.) bile duct obstruction
   (b.) liver cell damage

2. Increased retention is associated with:

(a.) Acute hepatitis

(b.) Hepatic necrosis

(c.) Chronic hepatitis

(d.) Cirrhosis

(e.) Cancer of liver

(f.) Heart failure

(g.) Shock

(h.) Acute hemorrhage

Interfering Factors

1. Drugs which cause false abnormal retentions (positives) of the dye:
   (a.) Phenolsulfonphthalein
   (b.) Pyridium
   (c.) Contrast dyes used in GB and IVP x-rays
   (d.) Hemolysis of blood sample
   (e.) See appendix for complete listing of the many drugs that interfere with testing.
2. Falsely low values are associated with:
   (a.) Low serum albumin
   (b.) Injection of the dye in a non-fasting state
   (c.) Drugs such as kanamycin and placebos

Patient Preparation

1. Explain purpose and procedure of test.
2. Fasting from food is necessary for eight to 12 hours the day of test and until a blood sample is obtained. Patient may drink water, coffee, or tea without sugar or cream.

Patient Aftercare

Eating and drinking can be resumed after the blood sample is obtained.

CLINICAL ALERT
Observe patient closely for allergic reaction to dye, and anaphylactic shock.

REFERENCES

Benson, McDermott: TEXTBOOK OF MEDICINE. 14th Ed., Philadelphia, W. B. Saunders, 1975.

French, Ruth M.: GUIDE TO DIAGNOSTIC PROCEDURES. 4th Ed., New York, McGraw-Hill Book Company, 1975.

Garb, Solomon: LABORATORY TESTS IN COMMON USE. 6th Ed., New York, Springer Publishing Company, 1976.

McGehee, Harvey, *et al.:* PRINCIPLES AND PRACTICE OF MEDICINE. 19th Ed., New York, Appleton-Century Crofts, 1976.

Preston, Joseph, and Troxel, David: BIOCHEMICAL PROFILING IN DIAGNOSTIC MEDICINE. Tarrytown, N.Y. Technicon Instruments Corporation, 1971.

Stroot, Violet R., Lee, Carla A., and Shaper, C. Ann: FLUIDS AND ELECTROLYES. 2nd Ed., Philadelphia, F. A. Davis Company, 1977.

Thorn, George W, *et al.:* Harrison's PRINCIPLES OF INTERNAL MEDICINE. 8th Ed., New York, McGraw-Hill Book Company, 1977.

Tilkian, S. M., Conover, M. H., and Tilkian, A. G.: CLINICAL IMPLICATIONS OF LABORATORY TESTS. 2nd Ed., St. Louis, The C. V. Mosby Company, 1979.

Wallach, Jacques: INTERPRETATION OF DIAGNOSTIC TEXTS—A HANDBOOK SYNOPSIS OF LABORATORY MEDICINE. 3rd Ed., Boston, Little, Brown and Company, 1978.

White, Abraham, *et al.:* PRINCIPLES OF BIOCHEMISTRY. 5th Ed., New York, McGraw-Hill Book Company, 1973.

6 □ MICROBIOLOGICAL STUDIES

INTRODUCTION

Diagnostic Testing and Microbial Flora

Microorganisms of interest in diagnostic testing are known as *pathogens*. The word pathogenic is usually defined as "causing infectious disease"; however, organisms which are pathogenic at certain times may reside in or on the human body at other times without causing disease. When these organisms are indeed present without causing harm to the host, they are considered *commensals*. But once they begin to multiply excessively and cause tissue damage, they are regarded as pathogens, for they will then have the potential for increasing pathogenicity.

Host Factors

Certain important factors influence the development of an infectious disease:

General health of the patient
Patient's defense mechanisms
Previous contact with the particular organism
Development of immune substances, or antibodies
Past clinical history
Type of tissue involved in the infection
Stress to the body, not necessarily of microbial origin
Age of patient
Exposure to antibiotics

COLLECTION OF SPECIMENS

General Principles

The health care professional responsible for collecting specimens used for diagnostic examinations must know the correct method for:

Obtaining the specimen
Delivering the specimen to the laboratory
Preserving it, when necessary
Reporting the results

The professional must also have an understanding of:

The indications for the diagnostic test
The nature of the test procedure
The implications of the results

Precautions

Certain routine precautions must be taken in the collection and handling of specimens. Without these precautions the patient's condition may be incorrectly diagnosed, much laboratory time wasted, and the pathogenic organisms transmitted to health care workers and to other patients.

Source of Specimens

Microbiological specimens may be collected from many

sources: blood, pus or wound exudates, urine, sputum, feces, the genital tract, cerebrospinal fluid, an eye, or an ear. During collection the following general procedures should be followed:

1. Labeling Specimens

    Specimens should be labeled with

    (a.) Patient's name, age, sex, address (or hospital number or physician's name and address)

    (b.) Site of specimen (*e.g.*, throat, conjunctiva)

    (c.) Time of collection

    (d.) Nature of studies desired

    (e.) Clinical diagnosis; microorganisms suspected

    (f.) Duration of illness

    (g.) Patient's immune state

    (h.) Previous infection

    (i.) Nature of any antibiotic therapy

2. Avoiding Contamination

    Collection should be as aseptic as possible. Observe the following:

    (a.) Use only sterile specimen containers.

    (b.) Do not spill any material on the outside of the container.

    (c.) Use only standard plugs to stopper tubes and bottles.

    (d.) Discard plugs and caps that have come in contact with nonsterile surfaces.

3. Preserving Specimens

    Prompt delivery to the laboratory is desirable, however, many specimens may be refrigerated (not frozen) for a few hours without any adverse effects. Note the following:

    (a.) Urine cultures must be *refrigerated* if results of diagnostic tests are to be of value.

    (b.) Cerebrospinal fluid specimens should be quickly transported to the laboratory. If this is impossible, the culture should be *incubated*, for the suspected meningococcus will not withstand refrigeration.

4. Transporting Specimens

    Care and speed of transport of specimens to the laboratory is urged. The material should be transported quickly to prevent drying out of the specimen and consequent death of the microorganisms.

TABLE 6–1. PATHOGENS DETECTABLE IN BODY TISSUE AND FLUID BY DIAGNOSTIC METHODS

Nasopharynx	Sputum	Feces
Beta hemolytic streptococci	Blastomyces dermatitidis	Candida albicans
Bordetella pertussis	Bordetella pertussis	Clostridium botulinum
Candida albicans	Candida albicans	Entamoeba histolytica
Corynebacterium diphtheriae	Coccidioides immitis	Escherichia coli (in infants)
Hemophilus influenzae (large counts)	Hemolytic streptococci	Mycobacterium tuberculosis
Meningococci	Hemophilus influenzae	Proteus
Pneumococci (large counts)	Histoplasma capsulatum	Pseudomonas (large counts)
Staphylococcus aureus	Klebsiella species	Salmonella
	Mycobacterium tuberculosis	Shigella
	Pasteurella pestis	Staphylococci
	Pasteurella tularensis	Vibrio cholerae
	Pneumococci	Vibrio comma
	Staphylococcus aureus	Other parasites

Urine	Skin	Ear
Beta hemolytic streptococci, group B & D	Bacteroides species	Aspergillus fumigatus
Coliform bacilli (100,000 count or more), including Escherichia coli, Klebsiella, Enterobacter-Serratiae	Clostridium	Candida albicans and other fungi
	Coliform bacilli	Coliform bacilli
	Fungi	Hemolytic streptococci
	Proteus	Proteus series
Enterococci (Streptococcus faecalis)	Pseudomonas	Pneumococci (Streptococcus pneumoniae)
Gonococci-(Neisseria gonorrhoeae)	Staphylococcus aureus	Pseudomonas aeruginosa
Klebsiella, positive and negative coagulase	Streptococcus pyogenes	Staphylococcus aureus
Mycobacterium tuberculosis		
Proteus species		
Pseudomonas aeruginosa		
Staphylococci		
Salmonella and Shigella species		
Trichomonas vaginalis		

TABLE 6-1. PATHOGENS DETECTABLE IN BODY TISSUE AND FLUID BY DIAGNOSTIC METHODS *(Continued)*

Cerebrospinal Fluid	Vaginal Discharge	Urethral Discharge
Actinebacter calcoaceticus	Candida albicans	Hemophilus ducreyi
Bacteroides species	Enterococci	Mima polymorpha
Coliform bacilli	Hemophilus ducreyi	Neisseria gonorrhoeae
Cryptococcus neoformans	Hemophilus vaginalis	Treponema pallidum
Edwardsiella tarda	Listeria monocytogenes	Trichomonas vaginalis
Hemophilus influenzae	Neisseria gonorrhoeae	
Leptospira species	Treponema pallidum	
Mycobacterium tuberculosis		
Neisseria meningitidis		
Pneumococci, streptococcus pneumonia		
Pseudomonas		
Staphylococci		
Streptococci		
Viruses and fungi		

(a.) With anaerobic cultures, no more than ten minutes should elapse between collection and culture.

(b.) Urine should be *refrigerated* during transport to the laboratory.

(c.) Specimens suspected of containing anaerobic bacteria should be injected into a butyl rubber-stoppered gassed-out glass tube.

(d.) Feces suspected of having *Salmonella* or *Shigella* organisms should be placed in a special transport medium such as buffered glycerol-saline if culturing will be delayed.

5. Quantity of Specimens

(a.) The quantity of specimens should be as large as possible. When only a small quantity is available, swabs should be moistened with sterile saline. This procedure is especially important in nasopharyngeal cultures.

6. Scheduling the Collection of Specimens

(a.) Whenever possible, specimens should be collected before an antibiotic regimen is instituted.

(b.) Collection must be geared to the rise in symptoms. (The practitioner should be familiar with the clinical course of the suspected disease.)

DIAGNOSIS OF BACTERIAL DISEASE:
GENERAL OBSERVATIONS

Bacteriological studies are done to try to determine the specific organism that is causing an infection. This organism may be specific for one disease such as Mycobacterium tuberculosis, the causative agent of tuberculosis, or it may be organisms such as the staphylococci species that can cause a variety of infections. Antibiotic susceptibility or sensitivity tests to antibiotics are also done to determine the reactions of a specific organism to antibiotics.

The questions asked in searching for bacteria as the cause of a disease process are: (1) Are bacteria responsible for this disease? and (2) Is antimicrobial therapy indicated? Most bacterial diseases follow a febrile course. From a practical standpoint, relatively soon in the evaluation of a patient with fever a diagnosis must be reached and a decision made concerning antimicrobial therapy.

At this time there is no practical and rapid method of distinguishing patients with febrile illness of bacterial origin from patients with febrile illness of nonbacterial origin. (It would be very helpful to distinguish between the two classes of disease so that antimicrobial therapy could be initiated.) The nitroblue tetrazolium (NBT) test may be such an aid, but it is not possible at this time to determine its overall accuracy and it is not in current use at this time. Along with the total and differential of the WBC and sedimentation rate, the NBT does seem to be an important test.

Disease due to anaerobic bacteria is commonly associated with localized, necrotic abscesses, each of which may yield 2 to 13 different strains of bacteria. Because of the multiple species that can be isolated, the term "polymicrobic disease" is sometimes used to refer to anaerobic bacterial diseases. Diseases caused by anaerobic bacteria are in sharp contrast to the "one organism - one disease" concept that characterizes infections such as typhoid fever, cholera, and diphtheria. The isolation and identification of different strains of anaerobic bacteria are desirable so that appropriate therapy is given. For instance, it is important when planning therapy for patients with anaerobic disease to know that certain drugs are not an effective or appropriate treatment.

TABLE 6–2. BACTERIAL DISEASES AND THEIR LABORATORY DIAGNOSIS*

Disease	Causative Organism	Source of Specimen	Diagnostic Tests
Anthrax	*Bacillus anthracis*	Blood, sputum, sore	Blood, sputum, and skin smear and culture; specific serologic test; biopsy
Brucellosis (Undulant Fever)	*Brucella melitensis, Br. abortus, Br. suis*	Blood, bone marrow	Blood and bone marrow culture; skin test; specific serologic test
Bubonic plague	*Pasteurella pestis, Yersinia pestis*	Buboes (enlarged and inflamed lymph nodes), Blood, sputum	Skin, blood, and sputum smear; culture; agglutination test
Chancre	*Hemophilus ducreyi*	Penis	Penis smear culture; biopsy; serologic test
Cholera	*Vibrio cholerae*	Feces	Stool smear and culture; skin biopsy
Diphtheria	*Corynebacterium diphtheriae*	Pharynx	Pharyngeal smear and culture; Schick test
Dysentery	*Shigella dysenteriae*	Feces	Stool culture; serologic test
Endocarditis	*Staphylococcus aureus*	Petechiae	Petechial smear
Glander's Disease	*Actinobacillus mallei*	Skin sore	Skin smear and culture; serologic test
Gonorrhea	*Neisseria gonorrhoeae*	Vagina, urethra, CSF, blood, joint fluid	Smear, culture, and serologic tests
Granuloma inguinale	*Donovania granulomatis*	Penis, groin	Smears and culture from penis and groin
Leprosy (Hansen's disease)	*Mycobacterium leprae*	Skin scrapings	Skin smear, biopsy, histamine lepromin, serologic test
Listeriosis	*Listeria monocytogenes*	Pharynx, blood, CSF	Pharyngeal, blood, and CSF smears and culture; serologic test
Meningitis	*Neisseria meningitidis*		Pharyngeal, CSF, and blood smears and cultures
	Angiostrongylus cantonensis	Pharynx, CSF, Blood	
Pertussis (Whooping Cough)	*Bordetella pertussis*	Trachea, bronchi, nasopharynx	Cultures of swabs of trachea and nasopharynx and bronchi; serologic test
Pharyngitis	*Streptococcus pyogenes*	Pharyngeal swab, sputum	Smear of sputum and pharyngeal swab culture; Antistreptolysis O (ASO) test; C-reactive protein (CRP) test; serologic test

Table continued on the following page

TABLE 6–2. BACTERIAL DISEASES AND THEIR LABORATORY DIAGNOSIS
(Continued)

Disease	Causative Organism	Source of Specimen	Diagnostic Tests
Pneumonia	Hemophilus influenzae, Klebsiella pneumoniae, Staphylococcus aureus, Diplococcus pneumoniae	Pharyngeal swab CSF, sputum blood, exudates, effusions	Smear and culture of sputum, blood, CSF, nasopharyngeal specimens, and exudates and effusions
Tetanus	Clostridium tetani	Wound	Wound smear and culture
Tuberculosis	Mycobacterium tuberculosis	Sputum, gastric washings, urine, CSF	Smears and culture of sputum; gastric washings, urine and CSF; skin biopsy; skin test
Tularemia	Pasteurella tularensis	Skin, lymph node, pharynx	Foshay skin test, serologic test
Typhoid	Salmonella typhosa	Blood (after first week of infection) Feces (after second week of infection)	Culture and serologic test

*Modified from Collins, R. D.: ILLUSTRATED MANUAL OF LABORATORY DIAGNOSIS. 2nd Ed., Philadelphia, J. B. Lippincott Company, 1975.

SENSITIVITY/SUSCEPTIBILITY OF BACTERIA TO ANTIMICROBIAL AGENTS

A sensitivity (susceptibility) test detects the amount of antibiotic or chemotherapeutic agent required to inhibit the growth of bacteria. Often a sensitivity test is ordered with a culture procedure.

With the increasing number of drugs and the changing patterns of resistance and susceptibility among bacteria (particularly the gram-negative colon bacteria), sensitivity testing is relied upon for the selection of appropriate drugs or for the alteration of an already imposed regimen of treatment.

The most common and most useful test for antibiotic sensitivity is the disc method (Fig. 6–1). A basic set of antibiotic-impregnated discs for routine testing against the commonly isolated microorganisms is available. The basis of the sensitivity testing is that specific amounts of an antibiotic are inoculated with a culture of the specific bacteria to be tested. After a suitable period of incubation, sensitivity of the organisms is determined by microscopic observation of the presence, or absence of growth in the antimicrobial agent.

Clinical Implications

1. The term *sensitive* implies that an infection caused by the strain tested, such as streptococcus, may be expected to respond favorably to the indicated antimicrobial, such as penicillin, for that type of infection and pathogen.
2. The term *resistant* means that the strain tested is not inhibited completely by therapeutic concentrations of a specific drug.
3. Many doctors rely more upon published reports of the antibiotics usually effective against the organism isolated than upon the sensitivity report, for sensitivity is an *in vitro* (in glass) test, and the antibiotic will be working *in vivo* (in the body).

DIAGNOSIS OF RICKETTSIAL DISEASE: GENERAL OBSERVATIONS

Overview

Rickettsiae are small rod-shaped to coccoid-shaped organisms that structurally resemble bacteria, but on the average are only one-tenth to one-half as large.

Rickettsiosis is the general name given to any disease caused by Rickettsiae. The organisms are considered to be *obligate intracellular parasites*; that is, they cannot exist anywhere except inside the bodies of living organisms. Diseases caused by rickettsiae are transmitted by *arthropod vectors*: lice, fleas,

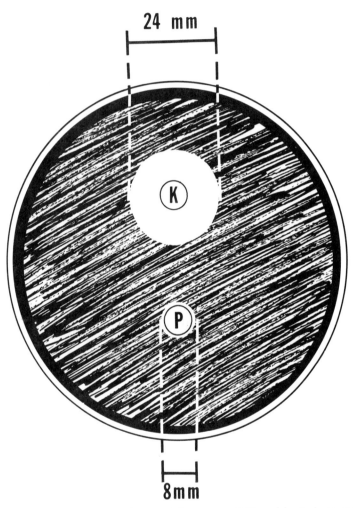

Fig. 6-1. Disc method of determining susceptibility of bacteria to antibiotics. The disc marked "K" is saturated with kanamycin; the disc marked "P" is saturated with penicillin. Escherichia coli, the bacterial organism growing on the plate, is resistant to penicillin and susceptible to kanamycin. (From Moffet, Hugh L.: PEDIATRIC INFECTIOUS DISEASES—A PROBLEM-ORIENTED APPROACH. Philadelphia, J. B. Lippincott Company, 1975.)

TABLE 6–3. RICKETTSIAL DISEASES AND THEIR LABORATORY DIAGNOSIS*

Disease	Causative Organism	Source of Specimen	Diagnostic Tests
Q Fever	Coxiella burnetii	Skin, blood	Skin smear and negative Weil-Felix test; complement fixation
Rocky Mountain Spotted Fever	Rickettsia rickettsii	Skin exudate, blood	Skin smear, blood culture, Weil-Felix test, complement fixation
Scrub Typhus	Rickettsia tsutsugamushi	Skin exudate, blood	Serodiagnostic test
Typhus Fever	Rickettsia prowazekii	Skin exudate, blood	Skin smear, blood culture, Weil-Felix test

*Modified from Collins, R. D.: ILLUSTRATED MANUAL OF LABORATORY DIAGNOSIS. 2nd Ed., Philadelphia, J. B. Lippincott Company, 1975.

ticks, or mites. Generally, these disease entities are divided into the following groups:

1. Typhus-like fevers
2. Spotted fever
3. Scrub typhus
4. Q fever
5. Other miscellaneous groups

Signs and Symptoms of Rickettsial Diseases

1. Fever
2. Skin rashes
3. Parasitism of blood vessels
4. Prostration
5. Stupor and coma
6. Headache
7. Ringing in the ears
8. Dizziness

Note: Rickettsial diseases are often characterized by an incubation period of 10 to 14 days, with an abrupt onset of the above signs and symptoms following a history of arthropod bites.

DIAGNOSIS OF PARASITIC DISEASE: GENERAL OBSERVATIONS

Many parasitic infections are asymptomatic, producing only mild symptoms. Routine blood and stool examinations will uncover many unsuspected infections.

TABLE 6–4. PARASITIC DISEASES AND THEIR LABORATORY DIAGNOSIS*

Disease	Causative Organism	Source of Specimen	Diagnostic Tests
Amebiasis	Entamoeba histolytica	Stool	Stool smear, rectal biopsy, and serologic test
Ascariasis	Ascaris lumbricoides	Stool, sputum	Stool and sputum smear
Cestodiasis of intestine (Tapeworm disease)	Taenia saginata Taenia solium Diphyllobothrium latum	Stool	Stool smear and Scotch tape test
Chagas' disease	Trypanosoma cruzi	Blood Spinal fluid	Blood and spinal fluid smear; animal inoculation
Cysticercosis	Taenia solium larvae		Muscle and brain cyst biopsy
Echinococcosis	Echinococcus granulosus	Sputum Urine	Sputum and urine smear; serologic test; Casoni skin test; liver and bone biopsy
Enterobiasis (Pinworm disease)	Enterobius vermicularis	Stool	Scotch tape smear
Filariasis	Wuchereria bancrofti	Blood	Blood smear; lymph node biopsy
Hookworm disease	Ancylostoma duodenale Necator americanus	Stool	Stool smear
Kala-azar	Leishman's anemia	Liver Bone marrow Blood	Liver, bone marrow, and blood smear and culture; animal inoculation; lymph node and spleen biopsy
Malaria	Plasmodium falciparum Plasmodium malariae Plasmodium vivax Plasmodium ovale	Blood Bone marrow	Blood and bone marrow smear; serologic test; Wassermann test
Onchocerciasis	Onchocerca volvulus		Skin biopsy
Paragonimiasis	Paragonimus westermani	Sputum Stool	Sputum and stool smear; serologic test; skin test
Scabies	Sarcoptes scabiei	Skin	Skin smear; serologic test; skin test

TABLE 6-4. PARASITIC DISEASES AND THEIR LABORATORY DIAGNOSIS
(Continued)

Disease	Causative Organism	Source of Specimen	Diagnostic Tests
Schistoso-miasis of intestine and bladder	Schistosoma mansoni Schistosoma japonicum Schistosoma haematobium	Stool Urine	Urine and stool smear; serologic test; skin test; rectal, bladder, and liver biopsy
Strongyloi-diasis	Strongyloides stercoralis	Stool Duodenal aspirate	Stool and gastric smear
Toxoplas-mosis	Toxoplasma gondii		Animal inoculation; serologic test; skin test
Trichinosis	Trichinella spiralis		Serologic test; skin test; muscle biopsy
Trichomoni-asis	Trichomonas vaginalis	Vagina Bladder Urethra	Vaginal and urethral smear and culture
Trichuriasis	Trichuris trichiura	Stool	Stool smear
Trypanoso-miasis	Trypanosoma rhodesiense Trypanosoma gambiense	Blood Spinal fluid Lymph node	Blood, spinal fluid, and lymph node smear; animal inoculation; serologic test
Visceral larva migrans	Toxocara canis Toxocara cati		Serologic test; skin test; liver biopsy

*Modified from Collins, R. D.: ILLUSTRATED MANUAL OF LABORATORY DIAGNOSIS. 2nd Ed., Philadelphia, J. B. Lippincott Company, 1975.

Parasites and their products act as antigens that stimulate the production of antibodies when introduced into the body of the host. The parasites invading the tissues produce the most pronounced immunologic response. Approximately 70 species of animal parasites commonly infect the body. More than half can be detected by examination of stool specimens, for the parasites inhabit the gastrointestinal tract and its environs. Of the parasites that can be diagnosed by stool examinations, one third are single-celled protozoa and two thirds are multicellular worms. Only six or seven of the intestinal protozoa are clinically important, but almost all of the worms are potentially pathogenic.

Collection of Specimens: General Principles

1. In general, it is not possible to accurately identify a parasite from one submitted specimen.

2. Most parasites in humans are identified from blood or feces, but organisms may also be obtained from urine, sputum, tissue fluid, and biopsies.

CLINICAL ALERT
The number of worms harbored is the most important factor in the diagnosis of parasitic worms.

Clinical Findings

A. General
   1. *Eosinophilia* is regarded as a definite indication of a parasitic infection. Infections with parasitic worms and protozoa may have associated eosinophilia, which varies considerably depending on the reaction of the patient.
   2. Protozoa and helminths, particularly larvae, may be found in various organs and tissues of the body, as well as in the blood.
B. According to Specimen
   1. *Hepatic puncture* is useful in the diagnosis of visceral leishmaniasis. Liver biopsy may reveal toxocara larvae and schistosomal worms and eggs.
   2. *Bone marrow* may be examined in trypanosomiasis and malaria when the blood is negative. Specimens are obtained by puncturing the sternum, crest of the ilium, vertebral processes, trochanter, or tibia.
   3. *Lymph nodes* may be examined for the diagnoses of trypanosomiasis, leishmaniasis, toxoplasmosis, and filariasis either by puncture or biopsy.
   4. Material from *mucous membranes* and *skin* may be obtained for examination by scraping, aspirating, or biopsy. Material may be obtained from the ulcer or nodule of the sore by puncturing the indurated margin of the lesion with a sterile hypodermic needle and aspirating gently.
   5. The *cerebrospinal fluid* may be examined for trypanosomes and toxoplasma.

6. *Sputum* may be examined for presence of eggs of *Paragonimus westermani* (the lung fluke). Occasionally, the larvae and the hookworm of *Strongyloides stercoralis* and *Ascaris lumbricoides* may be coughed up during their pulmonary migration. In pulmonary echinococcosis (hydatid disease), the contents of the hydatid cyst may be evacuated in the sputum.

DIAGNOSIS OF FUNGAL DISEASE: GENERAL OBSERVATIONS

The isolation and identification of the causative agents of fungal diseases have been developed only in comparatively recent years. Fungal diseases, the mycoses, are now believed to be more common than in the past because of the widespread rise of the use of antibacterial agents and immunosuppressive drugs.

Of more than 50,000 species of fungi, approximately 50 are generally recognized as being pathogenic for man. Fungi are organisms that live in a soil enriched by decaying nitrogenous matter and are capable of maintaining a separate existence via a parasitic cycle in humans or animals. The systemic mycoses are not communicable in the usual sense of man-to-man or animal-to-man transfer. Man becomes an accidental host by the inhalation of spores or by their introduction into his tissues through trauma. Altered susceptibility may result in fungus lesions, as in patients having debilitating disease, diabetes, or impaired immunological mechanisms resulting from steroid or antimetabolite therapy. Prolonged administration of antibiotics can result in a superinfection by a fungus.

Fungal diseases can be classified according to the type of tissues involved:

1. *Dermatophytoses* includes the superficial and cutaneous mycoses such as athlete's foot, ringworm, and "jock itch." Species of microsporum, epidermophyton, and trichophyton are the causative organisms of the dermatophytoses.
2. *Subcutaneous mycoses* involve the subcutaneous tissues and muscles.
3. *Systemic mycoses* involve the deep tissues and organs, and are the most serious of all three groups.

TABLE 6–5. FUNGAL DISEASES AND THEIR LABORATORY DIAGNOSIS.*

Disease	Causative Organism	Source of Specimen	Diagnostic Tests
Actinomy-cosis	Actinomyces israelii	skin, subcutaneous tissue, sputum	skin, subcutaneous tissue, and sputum culture and smear; biopsy
Blastomyco-sis	Blastomyces dermatitidis	skin, sputum	skin and sputum smear and culture; serologic test; skin test
Candidiasis	Candida albicans	Mucous membrane, sputum	mucous membrane and sputum smear and culture
Coccidioido-mycosis	Coccidioides immitis	sputum	sputum smear, culture, animal inoculation, serologic test, skin test, biopsy
Histoplas-mosis	Histoplasma capsulatum	sputum urine blood bone marrow	smear, culture, animal inoculation, serologic test, skin test, and biopsy
Mucormy-cosis	members of the order Muco-rales (Absidia, Rhizopus, and Mucor)	nose pharynx stool CSF	nose, pharynx, stool and CSF culture; biopsy
Nocardiosis	Nocardia aster-oides Nocardia brasi-liensis	sputum spinal fluid	sputum and spinal fluid culture and smear; biopsy
Sporotri-chosis	Sporothrix schen-ckii	skin	skin culture and biopsy
Torulosis	Cryptococcus neoformans	sputum spinal fluid	sputum and spinal fluid smear and culture
Tinea pedis (Athlete's foot)	Epidermophytons and Candida albicans	skin	hair, skin, and nail scrapings for culture
Tinea capitis (Ringworm of scalp)	(Microsporum (any species) and Trichophy-ton (all except T. concentri-cum)	skin	hair, skin, and nail scrapings for culture
Tinea barbae (Ringworm of the beard, Bar-ber's itch)	Trichophytons and Microspo-rums	skin	hair, skin, and nail scrapings for culture
Tinea cruris (Jock itch)	Epidermophytons and Candida albicans	skin	hair, skin, and nail scrapings for culture

*(Modified from Collins, R. D.: ILLUSTRATED MANUAL OF LABORATORY DIAGNOSIS. 2nd Ed., Philadelphia, J. B. Lippincott Company, 1975.)

Collection of Hair and Skin Specimens

1. Cleanse area of suspected infection with 70 per cent alcohol to remove bacteria.
2. Scrape area with a sterile scalpel or wooden spatula, and place specimen in a small sterile container with a lid.
3. Hair of the infected scalp or beard should be clipped and placed in a covered sterile container.
4. Hair stubs should be plucked out with a tweezer since the fungus is usually found at the base of the hair shaft. Using a Wood's light in a darkened room will help to identify the infected hairs.

The Most Common Methods Used in the Diagnosis of Fungal Infections Include:

1. Direct microscopic examination of material on a slide to determine whether a fungus is actually present.
2. Wood's light to determine presence of a fungus. A Wood's light is a lamp using 3,660 Angstrom units of ultraviolet rays. When used in a darkened room, infected hairs will fluoresce a bright yellow-green color.
3. KOH (Potassium hydroxide) test to determine the presence of fungus involves the use of a special low pH agar plate that is incompatible with bacterial growth. The test is positive for fungus if hyphae are present.
4. Culture is done to identify the specific type of fungus.

Types of Specimens Collected Include:

1. Skin
2. Nails
3. Hair
4. Ulcer scrapings
5. Pus
6. Cerebrospinal fluid
7. Urine
8. Sputum
9. Blood
10. Bone marrow
11. Stool
12. Bronchial washings
13. Biopsies

DIAGNOSIS OF SPIROCHETAL DISEASES: GENERAL OBSERVATIONS

Spirochetes are spiral and curved bacteria. There are four genera of spiral and curved bacteria, which include a number of human pathogens. The genera are *Borrelia, Treponema, Leptospira,* and *Spirillum.*

Clinical Considerations

1. *Borrelia*
    - (a.) *Borrelia* appears in the blood at the onset of various forms of relapsing fever. This genus is responsible for European and American relapsing fever.
    - (b.) *Borrelia vincentii* is the species responsible for ulcerative gingivitis (trench mouth).
2. *Treponema*
    - (a.) *Treponema pallidum* is the species responsible for venereal and nonvenereal syphilis in humans.
    - (b.) *Treponema pertenue* is the causative agent of yaws.
    - (c.) *Treponema carateum* causes pinta (carate).
3. *Leptospira*
    - (a.) *Leptospira* is the genus of microorganism responsible for Weil's disease (infectious jaundice), swamp fever, swineherd's disease, and canicola fever.
    - (b.) The organism is widely distributed in the infected individual and appears in the blood early in the disease.
    - (c.) After 10 to 14 days the organisms are present in considerable numbers in the urine.
    - (d.) Patients with Weil's disease show striking antibody responses, and serologic testing is useful in diagnoses.
4. *Spirillum*
    - (a.) *Spirillum minus* (as well as *Streptobacillus moniliformis*) is the species responsible for rat-bite fever; the condition occurs in Japan and the United States.

TABLE 6–6. SPIROCHETAL DISEASES AND THEIR LABORATORY DIAGNOSIS*

Disease	Causative Organism	Source of Specimen	Diagnostic Tests
Pinta	*Treponema carateum*	Skin	Skin smear, serologic test
Rat-bite fever	*Spirillum minus* *Streptobacillus moniliformis*	Blood Joint fluid	Skin, blood, and joint fluid culture and serologic test
Relapsing Fever	*Borrelia recurrentis*	Blood	Blood smear and culture and serologic test
Syphilis	*Treponema palidum*	Skin	Skin smear; TPI and FTA-Ab test
Weil's disease (leptospiral jaundice)	*Leptospira icterohaemorrhagiae*	Urine, blood	Urine and blood smear; culture-muscle biopsy; serologic test
Yaws	*Treponema pertenue*	Skin	Skin smear and serologic test

*Modified from Collins, R. D.: ILLUSTRATED MANUAL OF LABORATORY DIAGNOSIS, 2nd Ed., Philadelphia, J. B. Lippincott Company, 1975.

DIAGNOSIS OF VIRAL AND MYCOPLASMAL DISEASE: GENERAL OBSERVATIONS

Viruses are submicroscopic, filterable, infectious organisms that exist as intracellular parasites. They are divided into two groups according to the type of nucleic acid they contain: ribonucleic acid (RNA) or deoxyribonucleic acid (DNA).

Mycoplasmas are scotobacteria without cell walls and are surrounded by a single triple-layered membrane. They are also known as pleuropneumonia-like organisms (PPLO).

Viruses and mycoplasmas are both small, infectious agents that are capable of passing through bacteria-retaining filters. Although smallness is the only property they have in common, viruses and mycoplasma cause illnesses that are often indistinguishable from each other in clinical signs and symptoms, and both are found together frequently as a double infection. Thus, the serologic (antigen-antibody) procedures that are used commonly in the diagnosis of viral disease are also used for diagnosing cases of mycoplasmal infection.

Physiologically, mycoplasms are considered generally as an intermediate disease stage between bacteria and rickettsiae.

TABLE 6–7. VIRAL DISEASES AND THEIR LABORATORY DIAGNOSIS*

Diseases	Causative Organism	Source of Specimen	Diagnostic Tests
Cat-scratch fever	not isolated	Skin scraping	Skin test; lymph node biopsy
Colorado tick fever	Arborvirus	Blood, serum	Blood serologic test
Cytomegalic inclusion disease	Cytomegalovirus	Urine Sputum	Urine and sputum culture and serologic test
Dengue	Arborvirus	Blood	Blood serologic test
Herpes Zoster (Varicella)	Herpesviruses	Skin scrapings	Blood serologic test, culture, and smear
Encephalitis	Arborvirus	Blood	Blood serologic test
Lympho-granuloma venereum	Chlamydia strain	Blood	VDRL serologic test; Frei test
Measles (Rubeola)	Pseudomyxovirus	Sputum, blood	Throat sputum, blood culture, serologic test
Mumps	Pseudomyxovirus	Saliva, CSF	Saliva and CSF culture; serologic test
Poliomyelitis	Poliovirus	Stool	Stool culture and serologic test
Psittacosis (Parrot fever)	*Chlamydia psittaci*	Blood, sputum, lung tissue	Blood, sputum, and lung tissue culture
Rabies	RNA virus	Saliva	Saliva culture and animal inoculation
Rubella (German Measles)	Rubella virus	Nasopharynx	Nasopharyngeal culture
Smallpox	Poxvirus	Skin lesions	Skin smear culture and serologic tests
Trachoma	TRIC agents	Conjunctiva, urethra, or cervix	Conjunctival (urethral or cervical) smear and culture; serologic test
West Nile Fever	Arborvirus	Blood	Animal inoculation and serologic test
Yellow fever	Arborvirus	Blood	Animal inoculation and serologic test

*(Modified from Collins, R. D.: ILLUSTRATED MANUAL OF LABORATORY DIAGNOSIS. 2nd ed., Philadelphia, J. B. Lippincott Company, 1975.)

One species, *Mycoplasma pneumoniae,* is recognized as the causative agent of primary atypical pneumonia and bronchitis. Other species are suspected as possible agents in urethritis, infertility, early abortion, rheumatoid arthritis, myringitis, and erythema multiforme.

Approach to Diagnosis

The general approach to diagnosis of viral and mycoplasmal infections is based upon:

1. Microscopic examination of infected tissues for presence of viral material or pathologic changes.
2. Isolation and identification of a viral agent.
3. Demonstration of a significant increase in antibody titer to a given virus during the course of disease.

Collection of Specimens for Diagnosis of Viral and Mycoplasmal Diseases

1. Acute-phase blood specimens and materials should be collected within the first few days of illness (no later than 5–7 days).
2. The convalescent-phase specimen should be collected 14 to 21 days or longer after onset.
3. Blood specimens for serologic testing are examined to determine whether antibodies have appeared or increased in titer during the course of illness.
4. It is preferred that the first specimen sent for viral and mycoplasmal examination be identified with the following information:
    (a.) Date of onset of symptoms
    (b.) Type of suspected disease
    (c.) Major clinical signs and symptoms

DIAGNOSTIC PROCEDURES

Six classes of laboratory tests are used in the diagnosis of infectious diseases: smears, cultures, animal innoculation, tissue biopsy, serologic testing, and skin testing. Cultures and skin testing are described in detail in this chapter. A brief description of each of these procedures follows.

Smears and Stains

A. The Smear. A smear is a specimen for microscopic study that is prepared by spreading a small quantity of material across a glass slide. If the material is to be stained, it is generally fixed to the slide by passing the slide quickly through the flame of a Bunsen burner.

B. The Stain.   Smears are most often observed after they have been stained. Stains are salts composed of a positive and negative ion, one of which is colored. Structures in the specimen pick up the stain, thereby making the organism visible under the light microscope. One staining procedure, called the *negative stain,* colors the background and leaves the organisms uncolored. The gross structure of the organisms can then be seen.

Types of Stains.   Bacterial stains are of two major types: *simple* and *differential.* A simple stain consists of a coloring agent such as gentian violet, crystal violet, carbol fuscin, methylene blue, or safranin. A thin smear of organisms is stained and then observed under the oil-immersion lens. A *differential stain* is one in which two chemically different stains are applied to the same smear. Organisms that are physiologically different will pick up different stains.

The Gram Stain.   The Gram stain, which is the most important of all bacteriologic differential stains, divides bacteria into two physiologic groups: gram-positive and gram-negative.

The staining procedure has four major steps: (1) staining the smear with gentian or crystal violet, (2) washing off the violet stain and flooding the smear with an iodine solution, (3) washing off the iodine solution and flooding the smear with 95 per cent alcohol, and (4) counterstaining the smear with safranin, a red dye.

In addition to allowing for morphologic study of the bacteria under question, the Gram stain divides all bacteria into two physiological groups according to their ability or inability to pick up one or both of the two stains. The two categories of bacteria (gram-positive and gram-negative) exhibit different properties, which thereby help in their identification.

Other stains besides the Gram stain are used in examinations of bacteriologic smears. Some, such as the acid-fast stain, are used in identifying organisms of the genus *Mycobacterium.* Others are employed in the differentiation of certain structures, such as capsules, endospores, and flagella.

Cultures

A *culture* is the growth of microorganisms or living tissue cells on special media conducive to the growth of this material. Cultures may be maintained in test tubes, petri dishes, dilution bottles, or any other suitable container. The container holds a food (called the *culture medium*) that is either solid, semisolid, or liquid. Each organism has its own special requirements for growth (proper combination of nutritive ingredients, temperature, and presence or absence of oxygen). The culture is prepared in accordance with the food needs. Later, it is either refrigerated or incubated according to the temperature requirements for growth.

Animal Inoculation

Animal inoculation is the means for isolating bacteria when other means have failed. For example, when tuberculosis is suspected, but smears have failed to confirm the disease, guinea pig inoculation is used. The organisms responsible for plague *(Pasteurella pestis)* and tularemia *(Pasteurella tularensis)* may be isolated by animal inoculation. When viruses, certain spirochetes, certain fungi, and some parasites must be identified, animal inoculation is often used.

Tissue Biopsy

At times, microorganisms are isolated from small quantities of body tissue which have been surgically removed in the operating room or in the physician's office. Such tissue is removed using full aseptic technique, and is transferred to a sterile container to be transported rapidly to the laboratory for analysis. Generally, the specimens are ground finely in a sterile homogenizer and plated out.

Serologic Testing

Serologic testing, which will be discussed in detail in Chapter 7, Serologic Studies, is a method for analysis of blood specimens for antigen-antibody reactions. This form of testing is generally valuable in diagnosis only late in the course of the infection. Specimens should be collected immediately after the patient has been admitted to the hospital, and again, three to four weeks after the onset of the disease.

Skin Testing

Skin testing, which will be described later in this chapter, is used to determine hypersensitivity of an individual to the toxic products formed in the body by pathogens. Three types of skin tests are generally employed: scratch tests, patch tests, and intradermal tests.

BLOOD CULTURES

Background

Blood for culture is probably the single most important specimen submitted to the microbiological laboratory for examination. Blood cultures are collected whenever there is reason to suspect bacteremia or septicemia. Although a mild transitory bacteremia is a frequent finding in many infectious diseases, the persistent, continuous, or recurrent type of bacteremia is indicative of a more serious condition.

Indications for Blood Culture

1. Bacteremia
2. Septicemia
3. Unexplained postoperative shock
4. Postoperative shock following genitourinary tract manipulation
5. Unexplained fever of more than several days duration
6. Chills and fever in patients with
    (a.) Infected burns
    (b.) Urinary tract infections
    (c.) Rapidly progressing tissue infections
    (d.) Postoperative wound sepsis
    (e.) Indwelling venous or arterial catheters

7. Debilitated patients undergoing therapy with
   (a.) Antibiotics
   (b.) Corticosteroids
   (c.) Immunosuppressives
   (d.) Antimetabolites
   (e.) Parenteral hyperalimentation

Note: In typhoid fever and certain other diseases such as tularemia and plague, blood cultures are positive only in certain stages of the disease. Therefore, the clinician should be familiar with the clinical course of the disease, so that the most advantageous time for taking a blood sample may be known.

Procedure for Obtaining Blood Culture

CLINICAL ALERT

In venipuncture the potential for infecting the patient as a result of the diagnostic procedure is very high. Therefore, aseptic technique must be rigorously followed.

1. The proposed puncture site should be scrubbed with soap or pHisohex and with an antiseptic such as Betadine (povidone-iodine)
2. The tops of culture bottles should be cleansed with iodine and allowed to air dry. They should then be cleansed with 70 per cent alcohol.
3. The venipuncture area should be draped.
4. Venipuncture should be performed with a sterile syringe and needle.
5. Approximately 8 ml. quantities of blood should be taken in 20 ml. syringes.
6. After the specimen is obtained, the needle should be passed over a flame before the sample is injected into the culture bottle.
7. The neck of the culture bottle must not be touched during or after transfer of the specimen.
8. With cultures drawn for anaerobic bacteria, culture bottle should not be shaken, so as not to disturb the interface on the broth.

9. Specimens should be properly labeled with patient's name, age, date, time, and number of culture, and any other information the laboratory requires.

CLINICAL ALERT
(a.) Handle all blood specimens as if they are capable of transmitting disease.
(b.) After disinfection, do not probe the venipuncture site with your finger unless sterile gloves are worn or the finger has been disinfected.
(c.) Attending physician should be notified immediately about positive cultures so that appropriate treatment may be started at once.

Equipment

Culture bottles: one for aerobic bacteria
                 one for anaerobic bacteria
                 one for agar slant

Sterile towel	Disinfectant
Drape	Gown
Tourniquet	Mask
20 ml. syringe (disposable)	Gloves
Labels	

Clinical Implications

A. Negative Cultures
   If all cultures, subcultures, and gram-stained smears are negative, the blood culture may be reported as: NO GROWTH, AEROBIC OR ANAEROBIC, AFTER THREE DAYS INCUBATION. FURTHER REPORT TO FOLLOW. FINAL REPORT: NO GROWTH AFTER 7 to 14 DAYS' INCUBATION.

B. Positive Cultures
   Pathogens most commonly found in blood cultures include the following:

Bacteroides species	Filariae*
Brucella species	*Francisella tularensis*
Coliform bacilli	*Hemophilus influenzae*

Leptospira species	*Staphylococcus aureus,*
Listeria monocytogenes	*S. epidechidis* and
Malaria*	*S. saphrolyticus*
Neisseria meningitidis	*Streptococcus pyogenes*
Pneumococci	*Salmonella* species
Rickettsiae*	Trypanosomes*

*Note: Culture is not the ideal method for isolating parasites. Peripheral blood smears are the usual method for detection of parasites.

Interfering Factors

Blood cultures are subject to contamination, especially by skin bacteria. These organisms should therefore be identified in the laboratory.

Special Situation

With patients who have already received antibacterial therapy, certain enzymes may be incorporated into the growth medium to eliminate the activity of the antibacterial agent in the blood.

URINE CULTURES

Normal Values

Negative: less than 10,000 organisms/ml.
  Any bacteria found are either contaminants from the skin or invading pathogens.

CLINICAL ALERT
Urine cultures of *E. coli* are not definitely significant unless they contain more than 100,000 organisms per ml.

Background

Urine cultures are most commonly used to diagnose a bacterial infection of the urinary tract (kidneys, ureter, bladder, and urethra). Urine is an excellent culture medium for most organisms that infect the urinary tract, growing within the urine in the body, and resulting in high counts in established untreated infection.

1. Infection of the urinary tract is one of the most common bacterial diseases. Bacterial infections of the urinary tract affect patients of all ages and both sexes, varying in severity from an unsuspected infection to a condition of severe systemic disease.
2. Most urinary tract infections result from ascending infection by organisms introduced through the urethra.
3. Acute infections are more common in females than in males because of a shorter urethra and the greater likelihood of its becoming contaminated.
4. Infections are usually associated with bacterial counts of 100,000 (10^5) or more organisms per ml. of urine. (This level indicates significant bacteriuria.)
5. The combination of pyuria (pus in the urine) and significant bacteriuria strongly suggests the diagnosis of urinary tract infection.
6. A bacterial count of less than 10,000 bacteria per ml. is not indicative of infection and may possibly be contamination. A count of 100,000 or more bacteria per ml. indicates infection.

Collection of Specimens for Culture: General Principles

1. Early morning specimens should be obtained whenever possible because of bacterial counts being highest at that time.
2. A clean voided urine specimen should be collected in a sterile container. Specimens may also be collected by catheterization, suprapubic aspiration, or directly from an indwelling catheter. Urine must not be obtained from a urine-collecting bag.

CLINICAL ALERT
Catheterization heightens the risk of introducing infection. Whenever possible, avoid collecting urine by this method. DO NOT catheterize when merely a bacteriological specimen is needed.

3. Urine should be examined immediately. When this is not possible the urine can be refrigerated overnight until cultured, if necessary.
4. Two successive clean voided midstream specimens should be collected in order to be 95 per cent certain that true bacteriuria is present.
5. Whenever possible, specimens should be obtained before antibiotics or other antimicrobial agents have been administered.
6. The instruction for collection of all specimens should be the responsibility of professional health personnel (nurse, physician, medical technologist). Failure to isolate a causative organism is frequently the result of faulty collection techniques that can come from misinformation about the collection procedure.
7. Proper supplies and privacy for cleansing and collection should be provided. (Sterile specimen container and antiseptic sponges should be available.)
8. Properly instructed patients will usually cleanse their pelvis or vulva and perineum at least as well as the health attendant. However, when the patient is unable to follow the procedure, a trained individual can cleanse the patient and collect the specimen.
9. The specimen should be covered and labeled with:
   - (a.) Patient's name
   - (b.) Suspected clinical diagnosis
   - (c.) Method of collection
   - (d.) Precise time obtained
   - (e.) Whether forced fluids or IV's have been administered
   - (f.) Any specific chemotherapeutic agents being administered

Equipment

Sterile, wide-mouthed, screw-capped bottles
Urine collection bag (for infants and children)
Antiseptic sponges
Labels

Procedure for Collection of Midstream or Clean-Catch Urine Specimen

CLINICAL ALERT

Urine is an excellent culture medium, which at room temperature allows the growth of many organisms. Collection of specimens, therefore, should be as aseptic as possible. Samples should be taken immediately to the laboratory, where they can be examined while still warm. If prompt analysis is not possible, the specimen must be refrigerated.

1. Females
   (a.) Lower undergarments are to be removed.
   (b.) Patient should thoroughly wash hands with soap and water and then dry them with a disposable towel.
   (c.) The cap from a sterile container should be removed and placed with outer surface down in a clean area.
   (d.) The area around the urinary meatus must be cleaned from front to back with an antiseptic sponge.
   (e.) With one hand, the patient should spread the labia, keeping them apart until the specimen is collected.
   (f.) After cleansing, the patient voids. After the first 25 ml. has been passed into the toilet bowl, the urine is caught directly into the sterile container without stopping the stream. The patient voids until the container is almost full. The collection cup should be held in such a way that contact with the legs, vulva, or clothing is avoided. Fingers should be kept away from the rim and inner surface of the container.
2. Males
   (a.) Patient washes as above in (b.).
   (b.) The foreskin is completely retracted to expose the glans.
   (c.) The area around the meatus is cleansed with antiseptic sponges.
   (d.) Patient is to pass the first portion of urine (25 ml.) directly into the toilet bowl and then pass a portion of the remaining urine into the sterile specimen con-

tainer. Patient voids until the container is almost full. The last few drops of urine should not be collected.
3. Infants and Children

In infants and young children, urine may be collected in a plastic collection apparatus. Since the collection bag touches skin surfaces and thereby picks up commensals, the specimen must be analyzed as soon as possible.

Clinical Implications

When present in significant titer, the following organisms, present in the urine, may be considered pathogenic:
1. Coliform bacilli
2. Enterococci
3. Gonococcus
4. *Klebsiella* (often)
5. *Mycobacterium tuberculosis*
6. *Proteus* species
7. *Pseudomonas aeruginosa*
8. Staphylococci, coagulase positive and coagulase negative
9. Streptococci, beta hemolytic, usually Groups B and D
10. *Trichomonas vaginalis*

Interfering Factors

1. The urine of patients who are receiving forced fluids may be sufficiently diluted to reduce the colony count below 10^5 per ml.
2. Bacterial contamination comes from sources such as:
    (a.) Hair from the perineum
    (b.) Bacteria from beneath the prepuce in males
    (c.) Bacteria from vaginal secretions from the vulva or from the distal urethra in females
    (d.) Bacteria from the hands, skin, or clothing

Patient Preparation

1. Explain purpose and procedure of test to patient.
2. The cleansing procedure must remove contaminating or-

ganisms from the vulva, urethral meatus, and perineal area so that bacteria found in the urine can be assumed to have come from the bladder and urethra only.

CLINICAL ALERT

The urine studied for culture should *not* be a sample taken from a urinal or bedpan and should *not* be brought from home. The urine is to be collected directly into a sterile container that will be used for culture.

Special Situation

With suspected urinary tuberculosis, the specimen should consist of three consecutive early-morning samples that are pooled in the laboratory. Special care should be taken in washing the external genitalia to reduce contamination with commensal acid-fast *M. smegmatis*.

RESPIRATORY TRACT CULTURES

Four major types of cultures may be used to diagnose infectious diseases of the respiratory tract: (1) sputum, (2) throat swabs, (3) nasal swabs, and (4) nasopharyngeal swabs. At times the purposes for which certain tests are ordered will overlap. Each of these cultures will be described below.

Normal Values. The following organisms may be present in the nasopharynx of apparently healthy individuals:
1. *Candida albicans*
2. Diphtheroid bacilli
3. *Hemophilus hemolyticus*
4. *Hemophilus influenzae*
5. *Neisseria catarrhalis*
6. *Staphylococcus aureus* (occasionally)
7. Staphylococci (coagulase-negative)
8. Streptococci (alpha-hemolytic)
9. Streptococci (nonhemolytic)

SPUTUM

Background. Sputum is *not* material from the postnasal region and is *not* spittle or saliva. A specimen of sputum must be coughed up from deep within the bronchi.

Indications for Collection. Sputum cultures are important in the diagnosis of the following conditions:
1. Bacterial pneumonia
2. Pulmonary tuberculosis
3. Chronic bronchitis
4. Bronchiectasis
5. Suspected pulmonary mycotic infections
6. Mycoplasma pneumonia infection
7. Suspected viral pneumonia

Procedure for Collection of Specimen
1. Sputum must be coughed up from the bronchi.
2. The specimen must be collected in a clear, sterile container, and the container must be capped.
3. The volume of the expectorate need not exceed one to three ml. of purulent or mucopurulent material. This quantity is sufficienct for most examinations except tuberculosis testing.
4. The specimen should be examined prior to delivery to the laboratory to determine whether the specimen is truly sputum and not saliva. Too often the culturing of unsuitable material (saliva) results in misleading information because of the true infecting agent not having been observed.

Maintenance and Delivery of Specimen
1. Specimens should not be refrigerated.
2. Specimens should be delivered to the laboratory rapidly, so that organisms are still viable.

3. All specimens should be labeled with the name of the patient, date, room number, and suspected disease.

Patient Preparation
1. Patient should be instructed that this test requires tracheobronchial sputum, a substance from the lungs which is brought up by a deep cough.
2. The use of superheated hypertonic saline aerosols for sputum induction is recommended when the cough is not productive. Proper decontamination of the equipment must be carried out.

CLINICAL ALERT
In children or adults who cannot produce sputum, a laryngeal swab may be taken.

THROAT CULTURE (SWAB)

Indications for Collection
1. Throat cultures are important in the diagnosis of the following conditions:
    (a.) Streptococcal sore throat
    (b.) Diphtheria
    (c.) Thrush (Candidal infection of the mouth)
    (d.) Tonsillar infection
2. Throat cultures are useful in establishing the focus of infection in:
    (a.) Scarlet fever
    (b.) Rheumatic fever
    (c.) Acute hemorrhagic glomerulonephritis
3. Throat cultures can be used in detecting the carrier state of such organisms as:
    (a.) Beta hemolytic streptococcus
    (b.) *Neisseria meningitidis*
    (c.) *Corynebacterium diphtheriae*
    (d.) *Staphylococcus aureus*

Procedure for Collection of Throat Culture
1. Patient must be placed in a good light.
2. A sterile throat culture kit with a polyester-tipped applicator, or swab, is used.
3. A sterile container or tube of culture medium must be available.
4. With the patient's tongue depressed via a tongue blade and the throat well exposed and illuminated, the swab must be rotated firmly and gently over the back of the throat, both tonsils or fossae, and areas of inflammation, exudation, or ulceration.
   (a.) Care should be taken to avoid touching the tongue or lips with the swab.
   (b.) Since most patients will gag or cough, the collector should preferably wear a mask or should stand to the side of the patient.
5. The swab is replaced in the inner tube and the ampule is crushed. The swab is then forced into the released medium. The medium is covered and the specimen is sent immediately to the lab.
6. If throat culture cannot be examined within one hour, it can be refrigerated.

Pediatric Cases: Procedure for Collection of Throat Culture
1. The child is seated on the collector's lap; the collector encircles the child's arms and chest with his or her left arm.
2. The child's head is held firmly against the collector's chest.
3. Swab is taken as described above in the general procedure.

NASAL CULTURE (SWAB)

Indications for Collection
1. Acute leukemia patients
2. Transplant recipients
3. Intermittent dialysis patients
4. In tracing epidemics

Equipment. Swabs

Procedure.   Swab both external nares and deeper, moister, recesses of the nose.

NASOPHARYNGEAL CULTURE (SWAB)

Background.   Nasopharyngeal specimens can be obtained by inserting a special tube through the nose and then into the nasopharynx. The tube contains a cotton swab wrapped on the end of a flexible wire.

Indications for Collection of Specimen
1. Isolation of pneumococci, meningococci, or *Hemophilus influenzae*
2. Isolation of *Bordetella pertussis* (causative agent of whooping cough)
3. Identification of carriers of *Neisseria meningitides* (causative agent of meningitis)

Procedure for Collection of Specimen
1. Patient's head must be held firmly.
2. A special thin swab is passed quickly and gently through the nose into the nasopharyngeal area.
3. The swab is gently rotated and removed. Care must be taken to avoid mouth and throat contamination of the swab.
4. Inoculated swab is placed into the inner tube of the sterile container holding the medium and cover.
5. Specimen must be taken immediately to the laboratory.

Clinical Implications.   When present in significant titer, the following organisms may be considered pathogenic in the nasopharynx:

Bordetella pertussis
Candida albicans
Corynebacterium diphtheriae
Hemophilus influenzae, in large numbers
Meningococcus
Pneumococci, in large numbers
Staphylococcus aureus (coagulase positive)
Streptococci (beta hemolytic; Group A, and possibly, Groups B, C, and G)

WOUND CULTURES

Normal Values

Clinical specimens taken from wounds may be expected to have any of the following microorganisms. The pathogenicity of the organisms is dependent on the quantity present.
1. *Actinomyces* species
2. *Bacteroides* species
3. *Clostridium perfringens* and other species
4. *Escherichia coli*
5. Other Gram-negative enteric bacilli
6. *Mycobacterium* species
7. *Nocardia* species
8. *Pseudomonas* species
9. *Staphylococcus* species
10. *Staphylococcus epidermidis*
11. *Streptococcus faecalis*
12. *Streptococcus pyogenes*

Background

Material from infected wounds will reveal a variety of aerobic and anaerobic microorganisms. Because anaerobic microorganisms are the predominant microflora in humans and are constantly present in the upper respiratory tract, gastrointestinal tract, and genitourinary tract, they are also likely to invade other parts of the body, causing severe and often fatal infections.

Clinically significant pathogens are likely to be found in the following specimens:
1. Pus from any deep wound or aspirated abscess, especially if associated with a foul odor.
2. Necrotic tissue or debrided material from suspected gas gangrene tissue.
3. Material from infections bordering mucous membranes.
4. Drainage from postoperative wounds.
5. Ascitic fluid

Equipment

Blood agar plate
Half-antitoxin plate
Several tubes of cooked, meat broth
Serum-dipped swabs
Wide-mouthed, sterile, screw-capped containers (for dressings)

Culture Maintenance

All media must be incubated under strictly anaerobic conditions.

Procedure for Collection of Specimens for Wound Culture

1. Open collection container; remove swab. Take sample by applying sterile swab directly to source of culture.
2. Insert swab into container. Break swab and discard top portion.
3. Seal container.
4. Do not touch swab tip or inner surface of collection container.
5. Label specimen with
   (a.) patient's name
   (b.) date of sample
   (c.) source of specimen
   (d.) clinical diagnosis
   (e.) any other pertinent information required by laboratory
6. Take culture in such a way that exposure to oxygen is minimized or excluded.
7. If infection from mycobacteria or fungi is suspected, exudate or tissue should be collected in place of a swab.
8. With cultures of dry wounds, swab should be moistened in sterile saline prior to use.

CLINICAL ALERT

A microscopic examination of pus and wound exudates can be very helpful in diagnosis of the pathogenic organism. Consider the following:

(a.) Pus from streptococcal lesions is thin and serous.
(b.) Pus from staphylococcal infections is gelatinous.
(c.) Pus from Ps. pyocyanea infections is blue-green.
(d.) Actinomycosis infections show "sulfur" granules.

CLINICAL ALERT

The most useful specimens for analysis are pus or excised tissue. Dressings from discharging wounds are also acceptable. If swabs must be used, at least three swabs from one site must be submitted, and these swabs should be serum-coated. Swabs with a light smearing of pus dry out very quickly and are virtually useless.

SKIN CULTURES

Normal Values

The following organisms may be present on the skin of a healthy individual. When present in low numbers, certain of these organisms may be considered normal commensals; but at other times, when they multiply to excessive quantities, these same organisms may be pathogens.

1. *Clostridium* species
2. Coliform bacilli
3. Diphtheroids
4. Enterococci
5. Mycobacteria
6. *Proteus* species
7. Staphylococci
8. Streptococci
9. Yeasts and fungi

Background

The most common bacteria involved in skin infections are staphylococci, streptococci (Group A), and *Corynebacterium diphtheriae*.
The common abnormal, skin conditions include:
1. Pyoderma
    (a.) Staphylococcal impetigo characterized by bullous lesions with thin, amber, varnish-like crusts
    (b.) Streptococcal impetigo characterized by thick crusts
2. Erysipelas
3. Folliculitis
4. Furuncles
5. Carbuncles
6. Secondary invasion of burns, scabies, and other skin lesions
7. Dermatophytes, especially athlete's foot, scalp and body ringworm, and "jock itch."

CLINICAL ALERT
The most useful and common specimens for analysis are skin scrapings, nail scrapings, and hairs (See fungal diseases).

Clinical Implications

When present in significant quantities on the skin, the following organisms may be considered pathogenic, and therefore indicative of an abnormal condition:
1. *Bacteroides* species
2. *Clostridium* species
3. Coliform bacilli
4. Fungi (sporotrichum, *actinomyces, Nocardia, Candida albicans, Trichophyton, Microsporum, Epidermophyton*)
6. *Staphylococcus aureus* (coagulase positive)
7. *Streptococcus pyogenes*

SKIN TESTS

Background.   Skin testing is done for three major reasons: (1) to detect a person's sensitivity to allergens such as dust and pollen, (2) to determine a person's sensitivity to microorganisms believed to cause disease, and (3) to determine whether a person's cellmediated, immune function is normal. The test which detects sensitivity to allergens will be mentioned only briefly in this chapter. Most of the discussion will center on tests used in the determination of sensitivity to pathogens.

In general, three types of skin tests are used:

1. SCRATCH TESTS

Scratches approximately 1.0 cm. long and 2.5 cm. apart are made in rows on a patient's back or forearm. Extremely small quantities of allergens are introduced into these scratches. Positive reaction: swelling or redness at the site within 30 minutes.

2. PATCH TESTS

A small square of gauze is impregnated with the substance in question and is applied to the skin of the forearm. Positive reaction: swollen or reddened skin at the site of the patch after a given period of time.

3. INTRADERMAL TESTS

The substance which is being tested is introduced within the layers of skin via a tuberculin syringe fitted with a short-bevel, 26- or 27- gauge needle. Positive reaction: red and inflamed area at the site of the injection within a given period of time (*e.g.*, 72 hours in the Mantoux test for tuberculosis).

Skin tests revealing a hypersensitivity to a toxic product from a disease-producing agent may also indicate an immunity to the disease. Positive reactions may additionally indicate the presence of an active or inactive case of the disease under study. The following is a categorization of skin tests according to their nature and purpose:

1. Tests to determine possible susceptibility (or resistance) to infection.

Examples: Schick test (positive reaction = lack of immunity to diphtheria)

Dick test (positive reaction = lack of immunity to scarlet fever)

2. Tests to indicate a present or past exposure with the infectious agent.

Example: Tuberculin test (positive reaction = presence of active or inactive tuberculosis)

3. Tests to show sensitivity to various types of materials to which a person may react in an exaggerated manner.

Example: Allergenic extracts such as house dust and pollen (positive reaction to sensitivity to allergen extracts)

4. Tests to Detect Impaired Cellular Immunity

Intradermal skin testing with several common antigenic, microbial substances is one way of determining whether immune function is normal. This would be important in treating leukemias and cancer patients with chemotherapy.

Example: PPD tuberculin skin tests; mumps virus; *candida albicans;* skin fungi; and streptokinase-streptodornase. (Negative reaction to any intradermal antigen is indicative of impaired, immunity due to abnormal cell mediated immune function)

Indications for Tests.   Diagnostic skin tests may be used to determine the presence of the following disease entities:

1. Blastomycosis
2. Brucellosis
3. Echinococcosis
4. Histoplasmosis
5. Lymphogranuloma venereum
6. Mumps
7. Toxoplasmosis
8. Tuberculosis
9. Tularemia

Procedure for Taking Skin Test

1. Most diagnostic skin tests come in an unopened, sterile kit. Follow manufacturer's instructions carefully.
2. Generally, 0.1 ml. of the substance under question is injected intradermally in the volar aspect of the forearm.
3. Positive reaction: Redness or swelling of more than one cm. in diameter. A central area of necrosis is an even more significant finding.

CLINICAL ALERT
Material for diagnostic skin tests may be inadvertently injected subcutaneously rather than intradermally. A subcutaneous injection will yield a false negative result.

Procedure for Taking Patch Test
1. Skin is cleansed and allowed to dry.
2. Remove protective cover from a specially prepared adhesive patch or gauze square impregnated with testing substance and firmly apply to the forearm or the interscapular region of the back.

Procedure for Taking Scratch Test
The scratch method is especially recommended in patients who give a history of extreme sensitivity.
1. Skin is cleansed with either alcohol or ether and allowed to dry. Sites to be used are the forearm or the interscapular region of the back. The elbow and wrist areas are less reactive and should be avoided.
2. The skin is stretched taut, using the thumb and index finger.
3. Using a sterile lancet to puncture the epidermis, a scratch approximately 1 to 4 mm. long is made. The purpose is to raise the skin. The skin should be abraided without drawing blood. In the event that blood is drawn, the site should not be used.
4. One drop of substance used for testing is applied to the scarification, taking care not to touch the skin with the dropper.
5. A control test should be performed for comparison purposes.

TUBERCULIN SKIN TEST (FOR DETECTION OF TUBERCULOSIS)

Normal Values. See "Reading the Test Results."

Explanation of Test. Although the tuberculin skin test is an intradermal test used to detect tuberculin infection, it does not distinguish active from dormant infections. *Tuberculin* is a protein fraction of tubercle bacilli, and when it is introduced into the skin of a person with active or dormant tuberculosis infection, it causes a localized thickening of the skin because of an accumulation of small, sensitized lymphocytes. There are several methods of testing with tuberculin for the evidence of infection.

Methods of Testing for Tuberculosis

1. PPD-t Test. (Purified Protein Derivative tuberculin antigen test). PPD-t stabilized with Tween 80 is the material used in an intermediate-strength tuberculin skin test. Tests are read 48 to 72 hours after injection, since the response develops over a period of 24 to 72 hours.
2. Mantoux Test. A 0.1 ml. quantity of a solution containing 0.5 tuberculin unit of PPD-t is injected via a small needle into the skin of the volar aspect of the forearm. This test is used in exacting clinical situations and is preferred over the Tine Test, which is often used in mass surveys.
3. Tine Test. A stainless steel disc with four tines impregnated with PPD-t is pressed to the skin. This instrument is available in individual sterile units and is disposable, so it offers certain practical advantages for use in mass surveys.

Procedure for Tuberculin Skin Test
A. Intradermal Skin Test
    1. PPD-t is drawn up into a tuberculin syringe. (Follow manufacturer's directions carefully.)
    2. The skin on the volar or dorsal aspect of the forearm is cleansed with alcohol and allowed to dry.
    3. Skin is stretched taut.
    4. The tuberculin syringe is held close to the skin so that the hub of the needle touches it as the needle is introduced.
    5. The PPD-t is injected into the superficial layers of the skin. If the injection is too deep, no wheal (zone of raised skin) will appear, and the test may therefore yield a false negative result.
B. Vollmer's Patch Test
    Two pieces of filter paper that have been impregnated

with concentrated Old Tuberculin and attached to adhesive tape are applied to the skin.

1. Skin is cleansed and allowed to dry.
2. Patch is warmed and firmly applied to either the forearm or the interscapular region of the back.
3. Patch is removed after 48 hours, and the reaction is noted after another 48 hours.
4. A positive reaction is characterized by a reddened raised area or by an area of several distinct papules.

Reading the Test Results

1. The test should be read within 48 to 72 hours.
2. The patient should be examined in a good light.
3. Have the patient flex his forearm at the elbow.
4. The skin should be inspected for induration (hardening of the skin).
5. The examiner's finger should be rubbed lightly from the area of normal skin to the indurated zone.
6. The zone of induration should be circled with a pencil, and the diameter measured in millimeters.

Interpreting the Test Results.

The interpretation of the test is based on the size of the zone of induration (thickening).

Negative: zone less than 5 mm. in diameter
Doubtful or Probable: zone 5 to 10 mm. in diameter
Positive: zone 10 mm. or more in diameter

Note: Positive reactions are recorded also using the criteria of the National Lung Association:

1. Doubtful (+1−): Slight erythema and a trace of edema that measures 5 mm. or less in diameter.
2. One Plus (+): Erythema and edema that measures 5 to 10 mm. in diameter.
3. Two Plus's (+ +): Erythema and edema that measures 10 to 20 mm. in diameter.
4. Three Plus's (+++): Marked erythema and edema that exceeds 20 mm. in diameter.
5. Four Plus's (++++): Erythema, edema, and central necrosis.

Clinical Implications

1. Since a positive reaction to intermediate PPD-T indicates the presence of a tuberculosis infection without distinguishing between an active and a dormant infection, the stage of infection can be diagnosed from the results of clinical bacteriologic tests of the sputum and from x-rays.
2. A positive reaction in a patient who is clinically ill means that active tuberculosis cannot be dismissed as a diagnostic possibility.
3. A positive reaction in healthy persons usually signifies healed tuberculosis or an infection caused by a different mycobacteria.

CLINICAL ALERT
1. The frequency of repeated tuberculin tests depends upon the risk of exposure and on the prevalence of tuberculosis in the population groups.
2. BCG vaccine is an attenuated tuberculosis vaccine, which is indicated for persons in geographical areas (South America) or specific social circumstances (crowded living conditions) where the risk of infection is high. However, a positive tuberculin test renders BCG ineffective and potentially dangerous.

Interfering Factors

1. False negative results may occur even in the presence of active tuberculosis and whenever sensitized T lymphocytes are temporarily depleted in the body, as in patients who have the following conditions:
   - (a.) Clinical illness
   - (b.) Fever
   - (c.) Pleural effusion
   - (d.) Miliary tuberculosis
2. In persons ill enough to be admitted to a hospital, as stated above, false negative results may be as high as 10 to 30 per cent.

SCHICK TEST (FOR SUSCEPTIBILITY TO DIPHTHERIA)

Normal Values.   See "Clinical Implications."

Background

1. Diphtheria is a respiratory disease by the bacterium *Corynebacterium diphtheriae.*
2. A person who is immune to diphtheria will produce anti-toxins that will circulate in his blood in significant quantities.
3. A person who is susceptible to diphtheria will lack (or have very low levels of) antitoxins, and therefore will not be able to neutralize the diphtheria toxin injected intradermally in the test.

Explanation of Test

1. The Schick test is a means for determining the presence or absence of a significant quantity of diphtheria antitoxins in the blood. The presence of these antitoxins indicates immunity to the disease.
2. If the skin test causes erythema and flaking of the skin at the site of the injection, the person tested is susceptible to diphtheria. This is a positive reaction.
3. A negative reaction, indicated by no flaking or erythema, means that under normal conditions of exposure, the person will not contract diphtheria.
4. The test gives a rough estimate of the quantity of antitoxins circulating in the blood.

Procedure

1. A 0.1 ml. quantity of purified diphtheria *toxin* (.02 of the amount necessary to kill a guinea pig) dissolved in human serum albumin is injected intradermally on the volar surface of the forearm. A 0.1 ml. quantity of inactivated diphtheria *toxoid* is injected into the other arm as a control to rule out sensitivity to culture proteins.
2. These areas are examined at 24 and 48 hours and between the third and fourth days.

Interpreting Test Results

1. Positive Test: Site of toxin injection begins to redden in 24 hours, increases and reaches a maximum size in about one week, when it will be swollen and tender, and as large as three cm. in diameter. There is usually a small, dark-red

central zone that gradually turns brown and leaves a pigmented area. The area of *toxoid* injection shows no reaction.
2. Negative Test: No reaction at either site.

Clinical Implications

1. If a reaction occurs (*i.e.*, a positive test), the person does not have enough antibodies to neutralize the toxin and is therefore susceptible to diphtheria. The person has no immunity to diphtheria.
2. Persons who have been well immunized with four injections of diphtheria toxoid show uniformly negative reactions to the Schick test.
3. If the test is positive in a well-immunized person, this is strong evidence of the individual's inability to produce antibodies.
4. A negative test means that the person has immunity to exposure to diphtheria.

CLINICAL ALERT
1. The major significant reservoirs of diphtheria are immunized persons, particularly the elderly whose immunity has waned, and children who have not been immunized.
2. The recommended schedule for active immunization against diphtheria in normal infants and children is:

2 months	18 months
4 months	4 to 6 years
6 months	

These are the ages in which a child should receive DTP, a diphtheria and tetanus toxoid combined with pertussis vaccine.
3. An adult (any person older than 16 years of age) requiring immunization against diphtheria would receive TD combined with tetanus and diphtheria toxoids.

DICK TEST (FOR SUSCEPTIBILITY TO SCARLET FEVER)

Normal Values. See "Clinical Implications"

Background
1. The Dick test is a diagnostic skin test that measures an individual's susceptibility to scarlet fever. It also indicates immunity to the disease.
2. Scarlet fever, also called Scarlatina, is a communicable, hemolytic streptococcal infection caused by *Streptococcus pyogenes*. The condition causes generalized toxemia, a typical rash and scaling of skin, during the recovery period.
3. Occurrence of scarlet fever has been decreasing in recent years.
4. Scarlatinal or erythrogenic toxin is responsible for the rash of scarlet fever.

Explanation of Test. A solution of dilute scarlatinal toxin is injected intradermally to detect antibody and to determine immunity to scarlet fever.

Procedure
1. A 0.1 ml of dilute solution of scarlet fever (Dick) toxin is injected intradermally on the volvar surface of the forearm.
2. The test area is examined within a 24-hour period.

Interpreting Test Results
1. The test should be read within 18 to 24 hours.
2. Positive reaction: Site of injection is very red and markedly swollen (3 to 5 cm. in diameter). Swollen area has sharply raised edges. A positive test indicates damage done by the injected toxin that has not been neutralized by antibodies present in the body.
3. Negative reaction: No more than a faint pink streak along the course of the needle.
4. Slightly positive reaction: Faint red area measuring less than 1 cm. in diameter; no swelling.

Clinical Implications
1. A positive reaction signifies that the individual has insufficient circulating antitoxins to the Dick toxin and is susceptible to scarlet fever. A positive test reverts to a negative reaction following infection.
2. A negative reaction signifies that an individual is relatively immune to the disease.

CLINICAL ALERT
There are three immunologically rare but distinct toxins, which may account for second attacks of scarlet fever.

SKIN TESTS FOR ASSORTED BACTERIAL DISEASES

BRUCELLOSIS (UNDULANT FEVER) TEST

Causative Agent.   Brucellosis is caused by *Brucella melitensis, Brucella abortus,* and *Brucella suis.*

Explanation of Test.   Antigen (0.1 ml.) is injected intradermally. Two types of antigen are used:
1. A killed suspension of *Brucella* organisms
                 or
2. A protein solution, Brucellergan, derived from the organism.

Interpreting Test Results
1. The test is read in 48 hours.
2. Positive reaction: Characterized by edema, redness, and induration.
      In infected persons, exacerbation of symptoms may accompany a local reaction. The hypersensitive patient may have both a systemic and a local reaction.

SOFT CHANCRE TEST

Causative Agent.   Soft chancre is caused by *Hemophilus ducreyi.*

Explanation of Test.   An antigen prepared from cultures of *Hemophilus ducreyi* or Bubo pus is injected intradermally.

Interpreting Test Results
1. The test is read in 72 hours.

2. Positive reaction: Characterized by an area of erythema of 14 mm. or more in diameter and an area of induration of 8 mm. or more in diameter. A positive reaction may persist for weeks, and it indicates that the patient has had an active chancroid infection or has been injected in the past. (The skin hypersensitivity may last for many years.)

TULAREMIA TEST

Causative Agent. Tularemia is caused by *Pasteurella tularensis.*

Explanation of Test. The Foshay antigen, which is prepared from a culture of the causative organism, is injected intradermally.

Interpreting Test Results
1. The test is read in 48 hours.
2. Positive reaction: Characterized by an area of erythema and induration. Positive reactions are known to occur during the first week of the disease.

CLINICAL ALERT
Blood for agglutination tests should be drawn before the antigen is injected, since the skin-test antigen may cause false positive agglutinins.

PARASITIC DISEASE SKIN TESTS

ECHINOCOCCOSIS (HYDATID DISEASE) TEST

Causative Agent. Hydatid disease is an infection of the liver caused by hydatid cysts (larval forms) of tapeworms belonging to the genus *Echinococcus.*

Explanation of Test. An antigen made from infected hydatid cysts in human or dog tapeworms is injected intradermally. Usually a control material from uninfected animals is also infected.

Interpreting Test Results
1. The test is read in 15 to 20 minutes.
2. Positive reaction: Immediate erythema and swelling.

Clinical Implications
1. A positive reaction is usually indicative of echinococcosis
2. More reliable diagnostic results are obtained by complement fixation, hemagglutination, and precipitation tests.

Interfering Factors. False positive reactions may be due to:
1. Other cestode infections
2. Hypersensitivity to foreign protein in the antigen

TOXOPLASMOSIS TEST

Causative Agent. Toxoplasmosis, caused by *Toxoplasma gondii*, is a protozoan disease affecting humans. Toxoplasmosis is characterized by CNS lesions, and the condition may lead to blindness, brain damage, and ultimate death.

Explanation of Test. An antigen from infected mice is injected intradermally, as is a control from noninfected mice.

Interpreting Test Results
1. The test is read in 24 to 48 hours.
2. Positive reaction: Area of erythema and induration more than ten mm. in diameter.

Clinical Implications
1. A positive test indicates the presence of antibodies to *Toxoplasma gondii*.

2. A positive test gives diagnostic results similar to the Sabin-Feldman dye test, a serologic test for the diagnosis of toxoplasmosis. (The Sabin-Feldman dye test is based on the failure of living toxoplasmas, in the presence of specific antibody and accessory factor, to take up methylene blue dye.)

TRICHINOSIS TEST

Causative Agent. Trichinosis is a disease caused by eating undercooked meat containing the parasitic nematode, *Trichinella spiralis.* The condition is characterized by fever, colic, nausea, diarrhea, pain, stiffness, muscle swelling, eosinophilia, sweating, and insomnia.

Explanation of Test. An antigen made from material drawn from animals infected with trichinosis is injected intradermally. A control material from uninfected animals is also injected intradermally. This test is a valuable aid in the diagnosis of trichinosis, especially when only mild symptoms occur.

Interpreting Test Results
1. The test is read in 15 to 20 minutes.
2. Positive reaction: Immediate; characterized by a blanched wheal surrounded by an area of erythema.

Clinical Implications
1. A positive test is usually indicative of trichinosis.
2. The skin test is not positive until about the second week of infection.

CLINICAL ALERT
Blood for precipitins, agglutination, or complement fixation tests should be obtained before skin testing.

Interfering Factors. Up to ten per cent of positive reactions may be false.

VIRAL DISEASE SKIN TESTS

FREI TEST (FOR CONFIRMATION OF LYMPHOGRANULOMA VENEREUM)

Causative Agent.   Lymphogranuloma venereum (LGV) is an infectious venereal disease caused by a member of the genus *Chlamydia*. The condition begins with a small, ulcerative lesion of the genitals and later progresses to a systemic infection with enlargement of the regional lymph nodes. LGV may lead to chronic infection resulting in elephantiasis of genital tissues.

Explanation of Test.   An antigen made from the yolk sac of infected chick embryos is injected intradermally. A control material made from normal yolk sac is also injected intradermally.

Interpreting Test Results
1. The test should be read in 48 to 72 hours.
2. Positive reaction: A raised papule six by six mm. in diameter; a reaction to the control material of five mm. or less.
3. Negative reaction: Even in cases of apparently "negative" reactions, the test area should be examined for several days because of the frequency of delayed reactions.

Clinical Implications.   The test becomes positive one to six weeks after infection begins and remains positive for the life of the patient.

CLINICAL ALERT
Persons who are known to be allergic to eggs or chicken may react unfavorably.

MUMPS TEST

Causative Agent.   Mumps, the common disease causing swelling and tenderness of the parotid glands, is caused by a myxovirus.

Explanation of Test.   An antigen made from injected monkeys or chickens is injected intradermally, and a control material made from noninfected monkeys or chickens is also injected intradermally.

Interpreting Test Results
1. The test should be read in 48 hours.
2. Positive reaction: Erythema and a lesion larger than 10 mm. in diameter.
3. Negative reaction: No erythema and a lesion less than 10 mm. in diameter.

Clinical Implications
1. A positive reaction indicates resistance to the mumps virus.
2. A negative reaction indicates susceptibility to the mumps virus.

MYCOTIC INFECTION SKIN TESTS

BLASTOMYCOSIS (GILCHRIST'S DISEASE) TEST

Causative Agent.   Blastomycosis, a condition characterized by cutaneous, pulmonary, and systemic lesions, is caused by organisms of the genus *Blastomyces*.

Explanation of Test.   Blastomycin, an antigen, is injected intradermally. The test is reasonably specific for blastomycosis, but in practice this skin-test antigen is usually injected simultaneously with histoplasmin, coccidioiden and tuberculin.

Blastomycosis is also diagnosed by the recovery of the organism from pus, sputum, or tissue specimens.

Interpreting Test Results
1. The test should be read in 48 hours.
2. Positive reaction: Area of erythema and induration five by five mm. or greater.
3. Doubtful reaction: Area of induration less than five mm. in diameter or erythema only.
4. Negative reaction: No induration or erythema less than five mm. in diameter.

Clinical Implications
1. A positive reaction may be indicative of:
   - (a.) Past infection
   - (b.) Mild, chronic, or subacute infection
   - (c.) Improvement in cases of serious symptomatic blastomycosis that previously had been blastomycin-negative

COCCIDIOIDOMYCOSIS TEST

Causative Agent. Coccidioidomycosis, an infectious fungus disease occurring in both an acute form and a progressive form, is caused by *Coccidioides immitis*.

Explanation of Test. Coccidioidin, an antigen prepared from culture, is injected intradermally. A skin reaction will appear 10 to 21 days after infection, and a sensitivity continues throughout life. Coccidioidomycosis can also be diagnosed by recovery of the causative organism from pus, sputum, or tissue specimens.

Interpreting Test Results
1. The test must be read in 24 to 72 hours. If an immediate reaction occurs, it is nonspecific for coccidioidomycosis and is ignored.
2. Positive reaction: Area of erythema and induration of five mm. or more in diameter. Reaction disappears within 24 to 72 hours.

Clinical Implications
1. The skin test becomes positive in 87 per cent of the cases of coccidioidomycosis during the first week of clinical symptoms and in almost 100 per cent of patients after the first week.
2. A positive reaction persists for many years, but this does not imply that active infection is present. However, when there is a positive reaction during the course of infection in which an earlier test was negative, it can indicate active infection.

HISTOPLASMOSIS TEST

Causative Agent.   Histoplasmosis, a systemic fungus infection of the reticuloendothelial system, is caused by the organism *Histoplasma capsulatum.*

Explanation of Test.   Histoplasmin, an antigen prepared from culture, is injected intradermally. Skin reactions to histoplasmin are of relatively little diagnostic value, since energy may provide false negative results. Histoplasmosis is also diagnosed by identification of the causative agent in pus, sputum, or tissue specimens.

Interpreting Test Results
1. The test should be read in 24 to 48 hours. If an immediate reaction occurs, it is nonspecific for histoplasmosis and is ignored.
2. Positive reaction: Area of erythema and induration of five mm. or more in diameter.
3. Negative reaction: No induration; erythema less than five mm. in diameter.

Clinical Implications
1. A positive test indicates past or present infection.
2. Acutely ill patients may not have a positive reaction.

CEREBROSPINAL FLUID (CSF) CULTURES AND SMEARS

Normal Values

No flora are normally present.

In healthy individuals the specimen may be contaminated by normal skin flora.

Pathogens Found in CSF:

1. *Bacteroides* species
2. Coliform bacilli
3. *Cryptococcus* and other fungi
4. *Haemophilus influenzae* (especially in infants and children)
5. *Leptospira* species
6. *Listeria monocytogenes*
7. *Mycobacterium tuberculosis*
8. *Neisseria meningitidis*
9. Pneumococci
10. Staphylococci
11. Streptococci

Indications for Collection of CSF

1. Viral meningitis
2. Pyogenic meningitis
3. Tuberculosis meningitis
4. Chronic meningitis (due to *Cryptococcus neoformans*)

Explanation of Test

Culture of bacteriological examination of cerebrospinal fluid is an essential step in the diagnosis of any case of suspected meningitis. Acute bacterial meningitis is an infection of the meninges, or membrane covering the brain and spinal cord, and is a rapidly fatal disease if untreated or if given inadequate treatment. Prompt identification of the causative agent is necessary for appropriate antibiotic therapy. Meningitis is caused by a variety of gram-positive and gram-negative micro-organisms. Bacterial meningitis can also be secondary to infections in other parts of the body.

It is recommended that a smear and culture be carried out in all CSF specimens from persons with suspected meningitis, whether the fluid is clear or cloudy. (Normal cerebrospinal fluid is clear.)

In bacterial meningitis, which is caused by a variety of bacteria, the CSF shows the following characteristics:
1. Purulent (usually)
2. Increased WBC
3. Predominance of polymorphonuclear cells
4. Decreased CSF glucose

In meningitis, which is caused by tubercule bacillus, viruses, fungi, or protozoa, the CSF shows the following characteristics:
1. Nonpurulent (usually)
2. Decreased count of mononuclear white cells
3. Normal or decreased CSF glucose

In persons with suspected meningitis the fluid is generally submitted for chemical and cytological examinations, as well as for culture.

Procedure for Collection of Specimens

1. The specimen must be collected under sterile conditions, sealed immediately to prevent leakage or contamination, and sent to the laboratory without delay.

> **CLINICAL ALERT**
> It is very important that a diagnosis be made as quickly as possible. Since some organisms cannot tolerate temperature changes, it is very important that the culture be done as quickly as possible.
> If a viral etiology is suspected, a portion of the fluid must be immediately frozen for subsequent attempts at isolation of the virus.

2. Specimen should be labeled with patient's name, age, date, room number, and suspected disease. Laboratory staff

should be alerted so that they can prepare to examine specimen immediately.

CLINICAL ALERT
The laboratory should be given adequate warning that a CSF sample will be delivered. Time is a critical factor; the cells disintegrate if the sample is kept at room temperature for more than one hour.

---

3. The attending physician should be notified as soon as results are obtained so that appropriate treatment can be started.
4. CSF specimens can be incubated after collection but can never be refrigerated.

Maintenance of Culture

1. If specimen cannot be delivered at once to the laboratory for analysis, the container should be kept at 37° C.
2. No more than four hours should elapse before laboratory analysis, because of the low survival rate of the organisms causing meningitis, especially *H. influenzae* and the meningococcus.

Special Situation

In cases of suspected tuberculous meningitis, the specimen may be left standing at 37° C (98.6° F) for an hour to form the characteristic "spider web" clot. This technique is best left for later in the course of the disease, for the clot is often not found early, or it is used as a sign of the progress of chemotherapy.

Clinical Implications

1. Positive cultures occur in:
   (a.) Meningitis
   (b.) Trauma
   (c.) Abscess of brain or ependyma of spine
   (d.) Septic thrombophlebitis of venous sinuses

VAGINAL, URETHRAL, AND ANAL CULTURES AND SMEARS FOR GONORRHEA

Background

The laboratory diagnosis of gonorrhea depends upon the demonstration of intracellular diplococci in smears and upon identification of the causative agent *Neisseria gonorrhoeae* by culture procedure. Usually, gonococci can be found in the smears of pus from acute infections, particularly in the male. In chronic infections, especially of females, the value of smears decreases and culture methods usually yield a higher percentage of positive results. (Direct smears are made by rolling the swab over the slide.)

Collection of Specimens: General Principles

1. In female patients the cervix is the best site to obtain a culture specimen. This specimen should be collected with care by a trained, experienced professional.
2. In male patients the urethra is the best site to obtain a culture specimen.
3. In male homosexuals oropharyngeal and anal specimens should be obtained.
4. A swab packaged in a container with culture medium should be used. Dry swabs are not acceptable for gonorrhea culture. All specimens should be sent immediately to the laboratory and incubated.

Procedure for Obtaining Cultures for Gonorrhea

For Female Patients
1. *Cervical Culture.* The cervix is the best site to obtain a culture specimen (Fig. 6–2).
   (a.) Moisten speculum with warm water; do NOT use lubricant.
   (b.) Remove cervical mucus, preferably with a cotton ball held in ring forceps.
   (c.) Insert sterile, cotton-tipped swab into endocervical

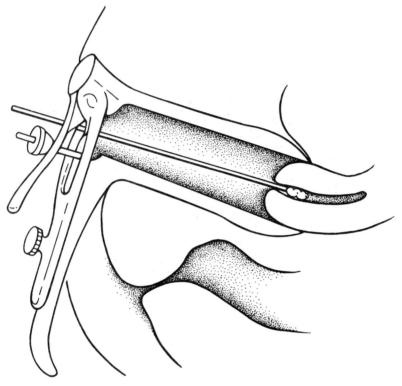

Fig. 6–2. *Method for obtaining the endocervical culture.*

canal; move swab from side to side; allow several seconds for absorption of organisms by the swab.

2. *Anal Canal Culture.* This is the most likely site to be positive when a cervical culture is negative.

Note: The anal canal specimen can be obtained after the cervical specimen without changing patient's position and without using the anoscope.

  (a.) Insert sterile, cotton-tipped swab approximately one inch into the anal canal. (If swab is inadvertently pushed into feces, use another swab to obtain specimen.)

  (b.) Move swab from side to side in the anal canal to

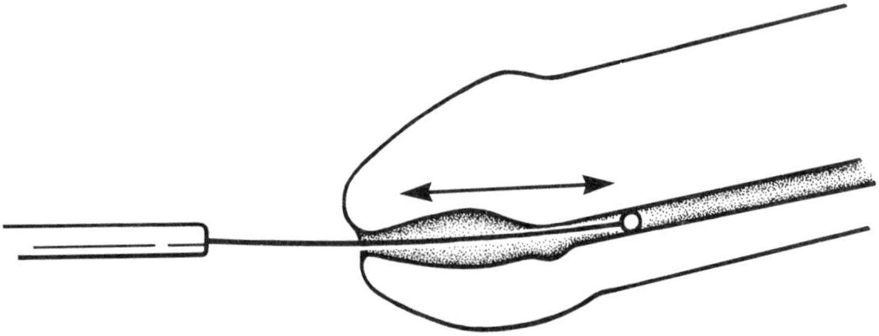

Fig. 6–3. *Method for obtaining the urethral culture.*

sample crypts; allow several seconds for absorption of organisms by the swab.

For Male Patients

1. *Urethral Culture*

   Use a sterile swab to obtain the specimen from the anterior urethra by gently scraping the mucosa (Fig. 6–3).

CLINICAL ALERT
If urethral culture in males is negative, but gonorrhea is still suspected, prostatic massage may increase the number of organisms in urethral discharge.

2. *Anal Canal Culture*

   Follow the same procedure as in female patients.

Both Male and Female Patients

1. *Oropharyngeal Culture*

   Culture specimens should also be obtained from the oropharynx in persons engaging in oral sex.

Procedure for Inoculating Culture Medium

1. Use culture bottles containing Modified Thayer-Martin Medium, a culture medium designed for the cultivation of *N. gonorrhoeae.*
2. Keep neck of bottle elevated to minimize loss of carbon dioxide.
3. Remove cap of bottle only when ready to inoculate medium.

4. Soak up excess moisture in bottle with specimen swab. Roll swab from side to side across medium, beginning at the bottom of the bottle.
5. Discard swab.
6. Label the bottle and send to the laboratory as soon as possible after collection.

> **CLINICAL ALERT**
> Repeated culturing for gonococci without detection does not exclude a diagnosis of gonorrhea.

Patient Preparation

1. Patient is to be placed in dorsal lithotomy position and appropriately draped.
2. Person collecting specimen should wear sterile, disposable gloves.

STOOL AND ANAL CULTURES AND SMEARS

Normal Values

The following organisms may be present in the stool of apparently healthy individuals:
1. *Candida albicans*
2. Clostridia
3. Enterococci
4. *Escherichia coli*
5. *Proteus* species
6. *Pseudomonas aeruginosa*
7. *Salmonella* species
8. Staphylococci

> **CLINICAL ALERT**
> *Candida albicans* in large numbers in the stool is considered pathogenic in the presence of previous antibiotic therapy. Alterations

of the normal flora by antibiotics often changes normally harmless organisms into pathogens.

Background

Stool cultures are commonly done to identify parasites, enteric disease organisms, and viruses in the intestinal tract. Of all specimens collected, feces are most likely to contain the greatest number and greatest variety of organisms. In a routine culture the stool is examined to rule out *Salmonella, Shigella,* enteropathogenic *E. coli* (in the newborn), and pure cultures of staphylococcus.

A single negative stool culture should not be regarded as confirmation of noninvolvement of infectious bacteria. At least three cultures are usually done if the clinical picture of the patient suggests a bacterial involvement and if the first two cultures are negative. Moreover, after a positive diagnosis has been made, personal contacts of the patient and the convalescent patient should also have three negative stool cultures to prevent spread of infection.

Procedure for Collection of Stool Specimen

1. Feces should be collected in a dry container free of urine.
2. A freshly passed stool is the specimen of choice. The entire stool should be collected.
3. Only a small amount of stool is needed. A stool the size of a walnut is usually adequate; however, the entire passed stool should be sent for examination.
4. A diarrheal stool usually gives good results.
5. Stool passed into the toilet bowl must not be used for culture.
6. No toilet paper should be placed in the bedpan or specimen container, for it may contain bismuth, which interferes with laboratory tests.
7. Stool should be transferred to a container via use of tongue blades. Specimen should be labeled and sent immediately to the laboratory.

Patient Preparation for Collection of Stool Specimen

1. Patient should be instructed to defecate into a clean bedpan or a large-mouthed container.
2. Patient should be told not to defecate into the toilet bowl or to urinate into the bedpan or collecting container, since urine has a harmful effect on protozoa.
3. Toilet paper should not be placed in bedpan or collection container.

Procedure for Taking a Rectal Swab

1. Swab is inserted gently into the rectum and rotated to obtain a visible amount of fecal material (Fig. 6–4).
2. Swab is placed in a clean container and the cover closed.
3. Specimen is properly labeled and sent immediately to the laboratory.

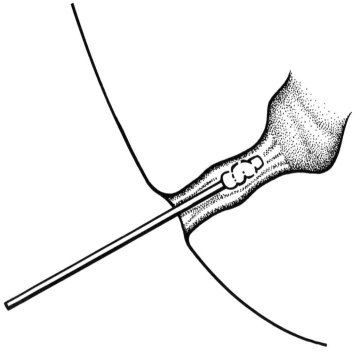

Fig. 6–4. *Method for obtaining the rectal culture.*

CLINICAL ALERT

Fecal specimens are far superior to rectal swabs. Often "rectal" swabs are merely "anal" and provide little material of diagnostic significance.

Culture Maintenance

1. Examination should be within a few hours of collection.
2. If delays of over 18 to 24 hours are suspected, specimen should be mixed with an equal volume of buffered glycerol-saline (Gillies, 1978).
3. Swabs must be examined immediately to prevent drying out of specimen.

Procedure for Taking Cellophane Tape Test

1. Tape test is indicated in cases of suspected enterobiasis (pinworms).
2. A strip of clear cellophane or Scotch tape (not micropore or adhesive) is applied to the perineal region. It is then removed and spread on a slide for microscopic examination.
3. A paraffin-coated swab can be used in place of the cellophane tape test. If it is used, it is placed in a covered test tube.
4. Repeated examinations on consecutive days may be necessary.
5. The test for eggs is made preferably in the morning before the patient has defecated or bathed.
6. Test in children: In about one third of infected children, eggs can also be obtained from beneath the fingernails. Follow the instructions on the kit provided.

Interfering Factors

Feces from patients receiving barium, bismuth, oil, or antibiotics are unsatisfactory for the identification of protozoa.

CLINICAL ALERT
1. In hospitalized patients, a preliminary report of *Salmonella* or *Shigella* will require the initiation of isolation with stool or enteric precaution.
2. Liquid or semiliquid stools should be examined immediately.
3. Feces should be examined before administration of barium or bismuth and not until one week after their use.

REFERENCES

Baily, Robert W., and Scott, Elvyn G.: *Diagnostic Microbiology.* 4th ed., St. Louis, C. V. Mosby Company, 1974.

Berkow, Robert (ed.): *The Merck Manual of Diagnosis and Therapy.* 13th ed., Rahway, N.J., Merck Sharp & Dohme Research Laboratories, 1977.

Collins, R. Douglas: *Illustrated Manual of Laboratory Diagnosis.* 2nd ed., Philadelphia, J. B. Lippincott Company, 1975.

Gillies, R. R.: *Lecture Notes on Medical Microbiology.* 2nd ed., Oxford, Blackwell Scientific Publications, 1978.

Lennette, Edwin H., Spaulding, Earl H., and Triant, Joseph P.: *Manual of Clinical Microbiology.* 2nd ed., Washington, D.C., American Society for Microbiology, 1974.

Moffet, Hugh L: *Pediatric Infectious Diseases—A Problem-Oriented Approach.* Philadelphia, J. B. Lippincott Company, 1975.

Stratford, Bryan C.: *An Atlas of Medical Microbiology: Common Human Pathogens.* Oxford, Blackwell Scientific Publications, 1977.

Tilkian, Sarko M., and Conover, Mary H: *Clinical Implications of Laboratory Tests.* St. Louis, The C. V. Mosby Company, 1975.

Washington, John A. II (ed.): *Laboratory Procedures in Clinical Microbiology.* Boston, Little, Brown and Company, 1974.

Widmann, Frances K.: *Clinical Interpretation of Laboratory Tests.* 8th ed., Philadelphia, F. A. Davis Co., 1979.

Wilson, Marion E., and Mizer, Helen Eckel: *Microbiology in Patient Care.* 2nd ed., New York, Macmillan Publishing Company, Inc., 1974.

Youmans, Guy, Paterson, Philip Y., and Sommers, Herbert M.: *The Biologic and Clinical Basis of Infectious Diseases.* Philadelphia, W. B. Saunders Company, 1975.

7 □ □ SEROLOGIC STUDIES

INTRODUCTION

Overview

Serology is the study of antigen-antibody reactions *in vitro.*

Diagnostic serology, or *serodiagnostic testing,* utilizes serologic tests to aid in the diagnosis of infectious disease and allergic reactions.

General Principles

1. Tests involve the study of serum proteins with immunologic action.
2. Immunologically active proteins are called *antibodies* or *immunoglobulins.*
3. Patient's blood serum is tested to determine whether it contains antibodies against a particular antigen.
4. Methods of serology are usually based on a rise in titer of a specific antibody between the *acute phase* (beginning) of an illness and the *convalescent phase* (2–4 weeks later).

Antigen-Antibody Reaction

The concepts of antigen and antibody are so interdependent that it is impossible to discuss one without the other.

1. *Antigen:* any substance that stimulates the formation of antibodies in the body and reacts with them specifically.
2. *Antibody:* a substance usually appearing in the body as a result of the introduction of an antigen and which reacts specifically with that antigen.

The body's antigen-antibody response is the method of natural defense against invading organisms.

Purpose of Antigen-Antibody Diagnostic Tests

1. To demonstrate a change in antibody titer between the acute and the convalescent phases of an illness.

    Titer: Reciprocal of the highest dilution of the patient's serum that will cause agglutination of the presence of a specific antigen.

2. To diagnose a condition when microbiologic testing has proved ineffective because:
    (a.) Antimicrobial therapy has suppressed the growth of invading organisms.
    (b.) Culture methods are not effective enough to substantiate growth.
3. To confirm a diagnosis when the etiologic agent has already been isolated.

Types of Serologic Tests

Serologic methods demonstrate that antigen-antibody reactions have taken place. There are five or six major laboratory techniques for demonstrating this reaction. The tests described in this chapter generally fall into one of these categories.

1. *Immunofluorescence Tests.*
    (a.) Antibody molecules can be treated with fluorescent dyes such as fluorescein without interfering with the molecule's function.
    (b.) When an antigen-antibody reaction occurs, the fluorescent material can be shown under the microscope.
    (c.) This immunofluorescence is the basis of the fluorescent-antibody group of tests.
    (d.) The following are examples of tests commonly used to diagnose syphilis, malaria, tularemia and to detect typhoid carriers:
        (1.) FTA (Fluorescent treponemal antibody test for syphilis)
        (2.) FTA-ABS (Fluorescent treponemal antibody test for syphilis)
        (3.) FA (Fluorescent antibody test for malaria)
2. *Precipitation Tests*
    (a.) The reaction between a soluble antigen and its antiserum leads to a visible result in the form of precipitation.
    (b.) Antigen and antibody must be mixed in a favorable ratio for a precipitate to form.
    (c.) The following are examples of tests commonly used to diagnose:

(1.) CM fungal antibody test for coccidioido-mycosis

(2.) Circumoral precipitin test for Schistoso-miasis—best done on cerebrospinal fluid

(3.) C-reactive protein is the test most often used to evaluate the severity and cause of many in-flammatory diseases and necrotic lesions

3. *Agglutination Tests*

(a.) When a particulate antigen, such as a saline suspen-sion of red blood cells, mixes with a homologous antiserum, cells clump together and settle to the bot-tom of the fluid.

(b.) This type of test is relatively easy to do and is the most popular form of serologic test.

(c.) Examples:

(1.) Thyroid hemagglutination test

(2.) HI or HIA test for determination of immunity for rubella

(3.) Cold agglutinins test

4. *Complement Tests*

Complement is a substance in blood serum that causes lysis when it combines with complexes of antigen and antibody.

There are several types of serologic tests involving complement:

(a.) Complement-fixation test: A patient's serum is incu-bated with complement and the antigen being tested. Complement will "fix" or attach to the antigen-antibody complex if it forms. The test is commonly used to diagnosis:

(1.) Histoplasmosis

(2.) Rickettsial disease

(3.) Blastomycosis

(4.) Trichinosis

(5.) Schistosomiasis

(b.) Cytolysis: Cellular antigens and their antibodies in the presence of complement lead to the dissolving of the antigen.

(c.) Immune Adherence: Certain microorganisms adhere

to nonphagocytic cells in the presence of homologous antimicrobial serum and complement.
5. *Neutralization of Toxins Tests*
When exotoxins are formed, they may be neutralized by small quantities of homologous antibodies, also called antitoxins. This neutralization is tested by inoculation of laboratory animals.

Collection of Serum for Serologic Tests

1. *Take two samples.* One sample should be taken at the beginning of the illness (the acute phase), and the other should be taken three to four weeks later (the convalescent phase). In general, the usefulness of the serologic tests depends on an increase in titer between the acute and convalescent phase.

   Note: In a few serologic tests, one serum sample may be adequate since (a) presence of antibody indicates an abnormal condition, or (b) the antibody titer is unusually high. One sample may be used in the following tests:
   (a.) Antinuclear antibody
   (b.) Heterophilic antibody titer
   (c.) Histoplasmosis CF
   (d.) TPM test
   (e.) Rubella HI titer
   (f.) VDRL test
2. *Take serologic test before skin testing.* Skin testing often induces antibody production and therefore may interfere with the results of the serologic test.
3. *Identify sample plainly and provide appropriate clinical data.* The sample should have information on the patient's name, age, suspected diagnosis, vaccinations, therapy, and previous infections.
4. *Send samples to laboratory before hemolysis occurs.* Hemolysis can interfere with the interpretation of the results. The presence of hemoglobin in serum can destroy complement and can interfere with the determination of complement-fixing antibodies.

Factors of Diagnostic Significance

More important than the mere detection of antibodies is the demonstration of a *titer change* between acute and convalescent stages of a disease.

When interpreting the results of a serologic test, keep the following in mind:

1. A single test has little or no significance unless the titer is unusually high or the presence of *any* antibody is abnormal.
2. Blood should be tested during the acute phase of the disease and then a short time later (2–4 weeks).
3. Testing of serum later in the course of a disease has no significance, since there is no baseline with which it can be compared.

Interpreting Results of Serologic Tests

Certain factors will affect the interpretation of test results:

1. History of previous infection by the same organism.
2. Previous vaccination (Determine how recent it has been).
3. Anamnestic reactions caused by heterologous antigens.
    (An *anamnestic reaction* is the appearance in the blood of antibody after administration of an antigen to which the patient had developed a primary immune response.)
4. Cross-reactivity
    Antibodies produced by one species of an organism frequently react with an entirely different species.
    Examples:
    (a.) Tularemia antibodies may agglutinate *Brucella* and vice versa.
    (b.) Rickettsial infections may produce antibodies that react with *Brucella*.
    (c.) Typhoid patients may produce antibodies to Proteus OX-19.
5. Presence of other serious conditions.
    No immunologic response can be demonstrated in some individuals having either agammaglobulinemia, leukemia, or advanced carcinoma.

Serologic vs. Microbiologic Methods

Chapter six provided descriptions of many microbiologic tests for diagnosing a disease entity. The best means of establishing the etiology of an infectious disease is by isolation and confirmation of the pathogen involved.

Serologic methods can aid or confirm microbiologic analysis when:

1. The patient is observed late in the course of the disease.
2. Antimicrobial therapy has suppressed growth of the invading organism.
3. Culture methods were ineffective in substantiating growth of the suspected causative agent.

BLOOD GROUPS; ABO RED CELL GROUPS

Normal Values

Antigen Present on Red Blood Cell	Antibodies Present in Serum	Major Blood Group Designation	Distribution in U.S.	
None	anti-A, anti-B	O (universal donor)*	O	46%
A	anti-B	A	A	41%
B	anti-A	B	B	9%
AB	None	AB (universal recipient)†	AB	4%

*Named "universal donor" on account of the individual having no antigens on red blood cells, and, therefore, being able to donate to all blood groups.

†Named "universal recipient" on account of the individual having no antibodies in serum and, therefore, being able to receive blood from all blood groups.

Explanation of Test

Blood typing is a test required of all blood donors and all potential blood recipients. The main purpose of this test is to prevent the transfusion of incompatible blood.

Human blood is grouped according to the presence or absence of specific chemical structures called *blood group antigens*. These antigens, which are found on the surface of the red blood cells, are substances capable of inducing the body to produce antibodies. Since 1900, more than 100 distinct antigens have been recognized on the red cell surface. However, there are only two major antigens, A and B, forming the basis of the ABO blood group system. Group A contains RBC's with the A antigen, group B with B antigen, AB with both A and B antigens, and O cells contain neither A nor B antigens.

In general, patients are given blood of their own ABO group, for antibodies against the other blood antigens may be found in the blood serum. These antibodies are designated anti-A or anti-B, according to the antigen they act against. Under normal conditions a person's blood serum will *not* contain the antibody that is able to destroy its antigen. For example, an individual with antigen A will *not* have anti-A in his serum. But he may or will have anti-B antibodies. Therefore, in addition to detecting antigens on red cells, it is necessary to test the patient's blood for the presence of specific antibodies to confirm ABO grouping.

CLINICAL ALERT

To prevent antigen-antibody reactions in the blood, a situation which could be extremely dangerous and potentially fatal, a patient's blood group must be determined *in vitro* prior to any transfusions.

Before a blood transfusion is begun, two professional persons must check the recipient's identified blood group with the donor type to be used in the transfusions.

Procedure

A venous blood sample of ten ml. is obtained.

Rh FACTORS; Rh TYPING

Normal Values

Whites: 85% Rh-positive (*i.e.*, has the Rh antigen)
           15% Rh-negative (*i.e.*, lacks the Rh antigen)

Blacks: 90% Rh-positive
         10% Rh-negative

Background

Human blood may be classified as Rh-positive or Rh-negative, depending on the presence or absence of Rh antigen on the red cell membrane. The Rh antigen, first discovered in 1939, has been extensively studied since 1943. Different systems of naming these antigens have been developed and each system has its particular merits. The two nomenclatures used most frequently are given below.

COMPARISON OF TERMS USED IN Rh SYSTEM*

Wiener	Fisher-Race
Rh_o	D
rh'	C
rh''	E
hr'	c
hr''	e
hr	f (ce)
rh^G	G

*The term "Rh factor," without qualification, means Rh_o (D = Rh:1). "Rh-positive" means RH_o (D) positive.

Explanation of Test

The Rh system is composed of antigens tested for in conjunction with the ABO group. D (Rh_o) factor is often the only factor tested for. When this factor is not present, further typing is done to identify any of the less common Rh factors before the individual is identified as Rh-negative. Rh-negative blood differs from Rh-positive in that the anti-Rh antibodies are not usually present in significant quantities until the patient is exposed to the Rh-positive factor by transfusion or during pregnancy.

To determine the presence or absence of Rh antigen, the red blood cells are tested with anti-D. Agglutination of the cells indicates presence of antigen D. Absence of agglutination indicates absence of the antigen.

Three major techniques are used in the typing of blood for the Rh factor:

1. Saline tube test
2. Slide test
3. Modified tube test
    - (a.) Serum-suspended cells
    - (b.) Saline-suspended cells

Need for Rh Typing

Rh typing must be conducted for:
1. The administration of Rh-positive blood to an Rh-negative person may sensitize the person to form anti-D.
2. The administration of D-positive blood to a recipient having anti-D in the serum could be fatal.
3. To identify Rho GAM (Rh immunoglobins) candidates:
    - (a.) Rh-negative, pregnant women with Rh-positive partners may carry Rh-positive fetuses. Cells from the fetus may pass through the placenta to the mother and cause production of antibodies in the maternal blood. The maternal antibody, in turn, may pass through the placenta into the fetal circulation and cause destruction of fetal blood cells. This condition, called hemolytic disease of the newborn (formerly called erythroblastosis fetalis), may cause reactions ranging from anemia (slight or severe) to death *in utero*. This condition can be prevented if an Rh-negative woman who gives birth to an Rh-positive child is given an injection of Rh immunoglobulins (Rho GAM).
    - (b.) Rh typing must also be done in abortion patients.

Clinical Implications

1. The significance of Rh factors is based on their capacity to immunize in transfusions or pregnancies. The Rh_0 (D) factor is by far the most antigenic, and the other Rh factors are much less likely to produce isoimmunization. The following general conditions must be met in immunization to Rh factors:
    - (a.) The blood factor must be absent in the immunized person.

    (b.) The blood factor must be present in the immunizing blood.

    (c.) The blood factor must be of sufficient antigenic strength.

2. Antibodies for Rh' (C) are frequently found together with anti-Rh_0 (D) antibodies in the Rh-negative, pregnant woman whose fetus or child was type Rh and thus possessed both factors.

3. Factors other than Rh_0 (D) may induce formation of antibodies in Rh-positive persons.

4. With exceedingly rare exceptions, Rh antibodies do not occur without preceding antigenic stimulation as in :

    (a.) Pregnancy and abortions

    (b.) Blood transfusions

    (c.) Deliberate immunization consistency, most commonly of repeated IV injections of blood

Rh ANTIBODY TITER TEST

Normal Values

Normal is zero, no antibody

Explanation of Test

This antibody study is performed on a blood specimen to obtain the Rh-antibody level in a pregnant woman who is Rh-negative but whose partner is Rh-positive. If the Rh-negative woman is carrying an Rh-positive fetus, the antigen from the blood cells of the fetus causes antibody production in the serum of the mother. The firstborn child usually shows no ill effects, but with subsequent pregnancies the antibodies in the mother's serum increase and are sufficient to cause destruction of the red cells of the fetus (hemolytic disease of the newborn).

Procedure

A venous blood sample of ten ml. is obtained.

Clinical Implications

If the Rh-antibody titer in the pregnant woman is greater than 1:64, an exchange transfusion is considered.

CROSSMATCH (COMPATIBILITY TEST)

Normal Values

Compatibility is shown by the absence of clumping or hemolysis when serum and cells are appropriately mixed and incubated in the laboratory. (The major crossmatch is that between recipient serum and donor cells; the minor crossmatch is that between recipient cells and donor serum.)

Background

The primary purpose of the crossmatch, or compatibility test, is to prevent a transfusion reaction. The compatibility test includes the *major crossmatch* and the *minor crossmatch*. (The minor crossmatch is not usually done anymore.)

1. Major crossmatch is done to detect antibodies in the recipient's serum that may damage or destroy the cells of the proposed donor. Of the two tests, the major crossmatch is the more important.
2. Minor crossmatch is done to detect antibodies in the donor's serum capable of affecting the red blood cells of the recipient. Since donor antibodies will be greatly diluted *in vivo* by the recipient's plasma, these antibodies are considered to be of minor importance.

Explanation of Test

Crossmatching in the laboratory must be done to detect the following:
1. Different types of antibodies
2. High protein medium-acting antibodies
3. Saline-acting antibodies
4. Antibodies recognizable only with the antiglobulin technique.

CLINICAL ALERT

Even the most carefully performed crossmatch will not detect all possible sources of incompatibility.

Procedure

A venous blood sample of ten ml. is obtained.

Clinical Implications

1. A *transfusion reaction* will occur when incompatible blood is transfused, specifically if antibodies in the recipient's serum would cause rapid destruction of the red blood cells of the proposed donor.

   (a.) Certain antibodies, though not causing immediate red cell destrucion and transfusion reaction, may nevertheless reduce the normal lifespan of transfused incompatible cells, necessitating subsequent transfusions.

   (b.) Obviously, the patient will derive maximum benefit from red cells that survive longest in his circulation.

CLINICAL ALERT

The most common cause of hemolytic transfusion reaction is the administration of blood to the wrong recipient because of improper patient identification and labeling of donor blood. The error, then, is often one of negligence.

Symptoms of Transfusion Reaction

1. Feeling of heat along the vein into which blood is transfused.
2. Constricting pain in chest and lumbar region of back.
3. Flushing of face
4. Hemoglobinuria
5. Generalized oozing of blood
6. Bleeding from operative wounds

2. The probable benefits of each blood transfusion must be weighed against risks such as the following:

TABLE 7–1. ANTIBODIES FOUND IN CROSSMATCHING*

Antibody	Frequency of Occurence in Crossmatch	Description
Anti-B	Almost universal	Natural antibody-immune forms; may be hemolytic
Anti-A	Almost universal	Natural antibody-immune forms; may be hemolytic
Anti-Rh$_o$(D)	1 in 400	Most common immune antibody; enzyme enhanced
Anti-Rh$_o$' (D + C)	1 in 600	rh' (C) alone is rare-combination frequent; enzyme enhanced
Autoantibody	1 in 2000	Acquired hemolytic anemia, lupus; occasionally specific (anti-hr'' anti-hr', anti-c, anti-e)
Cold agglutinin	1 in 2000	Viral pneumonitis, reacts with all cells
Anti-hr' (c)	1 in 5000	Most common immunization in Rh-positive persons
Anti-rh'' (E)	1 in 6000	Common immunization in Rh-positive persons; enzyme enhanced
Anti-hr' + rh'' (c + E)	1 in 6000	Combination occurs in Rh$_1$Rh$_1$ (DCe/CDe); enzyme enhanced
Anti-A$_1$	1 in 10,000	Natural antibody occurs in A$_2$ and A$_2$B donor and recipient
Anti-K (Kell)	1 in 15,000	Potent antibody in erythroblastosis fetalis
Anti-(D + E)	1 in 15,000	Combination found in Rh-negative (rh) persons (cde/cde)
Anti-Le (Lewis)	1 in 20,000	Natural antibody-complex system; may be hemolytic; enzyme may enhance
Anti-Fy^a (Duffy)	1 in 20,000	Acquired by transfusion and pregnancy; enzyme may destroy
Anti-P	1 in 20,000	Natural-weak-often at refrigerator temperature
Anti-M	1 in 30,000	Natural-rarely immune; enzyme destroys
Anti-(C + D + E)	1 in 30,000	Acquired antibodies in the Rh-negative person
Anti-Jk^a (Kidd)	1 in 30,000	Acquired; enzyme enhanced
Anti-rh' (C)	1 in 50,000	Acquired-rare in Rh-negative person as single antibody
Anti-hr'' (e)	1 in 100,000	Acquired by transfusion and pregnancy in Rh$_2$Rh$_2$ (cDE/cDE)
Anti-S	1 in 100,000	Natural or acquired; MN system; reacts more often with M or MN cells
Anti-rh$^w_1$(C^w)	1 in 100,000	Acquired; "pure" anti-rh$^w_1$ (anti-C^w) in type Rh$_1$Rh$_1$ or type Rh$_1$rh
Anti-k (Cellano)	1 in 100,000	Acquired; factor allelic to K

TABLE 7-1. ANTIBODIES FOUND IN CROSSMATCHING *(Continued)*

Antibody	Frequency of Occurrence in Crossmatch	Description
Anti-Jk^b (Kidd)	1 in 100,000	Acquired-enzyme enhanced; factor allelic to Jk^a
Anti-Fy^b (Duffy)		Acquired-enzyme may destroy; factor allelic to Fy^a
Anti-N		Natural-enzyme destroys
Anti-Lu^a (Lutheran)		Acquired-enzyme may destroy
Anti-hr (f)		Acquired-positive with cells of individuals having gene r or gene R^o

(*Adapted from Bauer, John D., et al.: BRAY'S CLINICAL LABORATORY METHODS. St. Louis, The C. V. Mosby Co., 1974.)

(a.) Hemolytic transfusion reactions due to infusion of incompatible blood which can be fatal

(b.) Induction of febrile or allergic reactions

(c.) Transmission of infectious disease, especially hepatitis

(d.) Stimulation of antibody production which could complicate later transfusion or childbearing

COOMB'S ANTIGLOBULIN TEST

Normal Values

Direct Coomb's Test negative, done on rbc
Indirect Coombs' Test negative, done on serum

Explanation of Test

The Coombs' Test is used to show certain antigen-antibody reactions. It differentiates between types of hemolytic anemias, determines minor blood types (such as the Kell factor), and tests for suspected erythroblastosis fetalis. There are two types of tests: direct and indirect.

A. *Direct Coombs' Test*

    1. Detects the presence of antibody on red blood cells (done *in vivo*)

2. Diagnoses the following conditions:
  (a.) Erythroblastosis fetalis when the red cells of the infant are tested for sensitization
  (b.) Acquired hemolytic anemia when the patient may have produced an antibody that coats his own cells
  (c.) Transfusion reaction when the patient may have received incompatible blood that has sensitized his red cells

B. *Indirect Coombs' Test*
  1. Detects presence of antibody in blood serum (*e.g.,* a major crossmatch).
  2. Reveals presence of anti-Rh antibodies in mother's blood during pregnancy.
  3. Is valuable in detecting incompatibilities not found by other methods.

Procedure

A venous blood sample of 10 ml. is obtained.

Clinical Implications

A. *Direct Coombs' Test*
  1. Positive Test in:
    (a.) Erythroblastosis fetalis
    (b.) Autoimmune hemolytic anemia (most cases)
    (c.) Transfusion reaction
    (d.) Patients receiving cephalothin therapy (75% of cases) and some penicillin
    (e.) Also drugs like alpha methyl dopa-aldomet
  2. Negative Test in:
    (a.) Nonautoimmune hemolytic anemias

B. *Indirect Coombs' Test*
  1. Positive Test in:
    (a.) Presence of specific antibody, usually as a result of a previous transfusion or pregnancy
    (b.) Presence of a nonspecific antibody, as in cold agglutination disease and drug induced hemolytic anemia

Interfering Factors

The following drugs may cause a positive direct Coombs' test:

(a.) Cephalexin	(l.) Mephalan
(b.) Chlorpromazine	(m.) Methyldopa
(c.) Cephaloridine	(n.) Oxyphenisatin
(d.) Diphenylhydantoin	(o.) Penicillin
(e.) Cephalothin	(p.) Procainamide
(f.) Dipyrone	(q.) Quinidine
(g.) Ethosuximide	(r.) Rifampin
(h.) Hydralazine	(s.) Streptomycin
(i.) Isoniazid	(t.) Sulfonamides
(j.) Levodopa	(u.) Tetracyclines
(k.) Mefenamic acid	

COLD AGGLUTININS (ACUTE AND CONVALESCENT STUDIES)

Normal Values

Normal: 0 ÷ 8

Background

Cold agglutinins are complete antibodies that cause the agglutination of the patient's own red blood cells at temperatures in the range of 0 to 10°C. These antibodies, with maximum activity, at temperatures below 37°C are termed *cold* and are found in the blood of normal persons in small amounts. Cold agglutinins have been demonstrated in the blood of 55 per cent of patients suffering from primary atypical pneumonia. They have also been demonstrated in persons having tonsillitis, scarlatina, Raynaud's syndrome, gangrene, staphylococcemia, African trypanosomiasis, influenza, pulmonary embolism and viral pneumonia.

Diagnosis depends on the demonstration of a four-fold or higher increase in antibody titers between an acute blood serum sample taken as early as possible in the course of the infection and a blood serum sample taken in convalescence. The titer is high in convalescence.

Explanation of Test

The test is used most commonly to diagnose atypical pneumonia and in diagnosing the disease entity in patients with prolonged illness.

CLINICAL ALERT
In cases of suspected primary atypical pneumonia, there is a titer rise eight to ten days after onset, a peak in titer 12 to 25 days after onset, and a decrease in titer 30 days after onset.

Clinical Implications

An antibody titer > 16 is significant.
1. An antibody titer of 1:32 to 1:64 is positive.
2. High titers are commonly associated with the following conditions:
   - (a.) Atypical pneumonia
     - (1.) Mycoplasma pneumonia
     - (2.) Influenza A and B
   - (b.) Congenital syphilis
   - (c.) Severe hemolytic anemia of cold variety-paroxysmal cold hemoglobinurias
   - (d.) Cirrhosis
   - (e.) Lymphatic leukemia
   - (f.) Malaria
   - (g.) Peripheral vascular disease
3. In patients with a titer in the tens of thousands, agglutination of red blood cells may occur within their blood vessels after exposure to cold, causing such conditions as the following:
   - (a.) Frostbite
   - (b.) Focal gangrene
   - (c.) Raynaud's syndrome
   - (d.) Anemia
4. More important than any single high titer is the rise in titer

during the course of illness. The titer will usually decrease by the fourth to sixth week after onset of illness.

CLINICAL ALERT
Specimens should be collected at 37° C and then transported to the laboratory submerged in water at 37° C. When this procedure is not possible, the specimen should be warmed for 30 minutes to 37° C before the serum is separated from the cells.
    Since cold agglutinins will attach themselves to the bed blood cells and therefore will not be present in the serum for testing, these precautions are taken.

Interfering Factors

1. A high titer of cold agglutinins can interfere with typing and cross-matching.
2. High titers sometimes appear spontaneously in older persons. The high antibody titer may persist for years.
3. Antibiotic therapy may interfere with the development of cold agglutinins.

HEMAGGLUTINATION INHIBITION (HI OR HAI) TEST

Normal Values

No real normal.
Titer 1:10 indicates patient susceptible to rubella infection
Titer 1:20 indicates previous rubella infection and, therefore, protection from rubella

Background

Rubella is a paramyxovirus that is the causative agent of German measles, a mild systemic disease characterized by fever and transient rash.
    It is important to identify exposure to rubella infection and susceptibility status in pregnant women, since infection in the

first trimester of pregnancy is associated with congenital abnormalities, abortion, or stillbirth in about three per cent of infected women.

Explanation of Test

The hemagglutination inhibition test, which detects hemagglutinin-inhibition 19S-type antibodies of active infection, determines susceptibility or immunity to the rubella virus. It is used to identify those persons who are susceptible to rubella (those without antibodies), to diagnose infection, and to help monitor the levels of immunity in infected and vaccinated populations. A history of rubella illness in childhood is not reliable enough to exclude children from immunization.

All pregnant women should have an HAI antibody screening test during the first antepartum visit.

Indications

To identify persons who are potential carriers of rubella and who may infect women of childbearing age, the following groups of individuals should be administered the HAI test:
1. Hospital personnel responsible for maternal and child care.
2. Persons who may be frequently exposed to rubella infection (*e.g.* teachers, nurses, doctors, midwives)

Procedure

A venous blood sample of five ml. is obtained.

Clinical Implications

1. If the patient has a rash, diagnosis of rubella can be established if a first specimen is obtained three days after onset of rash and a second specimen three weeks later.
   A four-fold increase in titer from the first to the second specimen is an indication that the rash was caused by rubella.
2. When immunity to rubella is being established, a single specimen with a titer of 1:20 or greater indicates immunity.

When pregnant women are exposed to rubella, HI tests for susceptibility to rubella virus should be done (a) at time of exposure, (b) again six weeks later. A rise in antibody titer indicates that both mother and fetus have been infected. If the mother had been exposed in the first trimester, the fetus is at risk for congenital heart defects, cataract, mental retardation, and deafness. If the exposure was late in the pregnancy, the infant will be born with the disease in the same stage as the mother's.

3. A Rubacele test which detects only immune status can also be done. In a pregnant woman who has been exposed to rubella, if the test is positive, she has immunity and is protected from rubella. She can be instructed that she need not worry about risk to the fetus.

RHEUMATOID FACTOR (RA FACTOR); RHEUMATON

Normal Values

Negative (<1:20)

Background

The blood of many people with rheumatoid arthritis contain a macroglobulin type of antibody which has been called *rheumatoid factor* (RF). Rheumatoid factor(s) has the property of an antibody. There is some evidence indicating that rheumatoid factors are anti-gammaglobulin antibodies; however, until a specific antigen eliciting the production of RF is discovered, the exact nature of RF can only be speculated. Even more uncertain is the role which RF plays in rheumatoid arthritis. Although, RF may cause or perpetuate the destructive changes associated with rheumatoid arthritis, it may be incidental to these changes, or may even serve some beneficial purpose. Rheumatoid factor is not limited to blood from patients with rheumatoid arthritis but may sometimes be found in serum from patients with a variety of other diseases. However, the incidence and titers of rheumatoid factors are higher in patients with rheumatoid arthritis than in patients with other diseases. It has been proposed that the antiglobulins in rheumatoid arthritis result from chronic stimulation by an unknown antigen, perhaps microbial in origin.

Explanation of Test

This is a specific test for rheumatoid arthritis and is both a qualitative and quantitative determination of the rheumatoid factor in the blood serum. "Rheumatoid arthritis" is essentially a clinical diagnosis and many physicians have placed more reliance on the rheumatoid factor test than it deserves.

Procedure

A venous blood sample of ten ml. is obtained.

Clinical Implications

1. When a patient with a positive test improves, the test will remain positive, except in a small number of patients whose titers were initially low.
2. A positive RA factor test often supports a tentative diagnosis of early rheumatoid arthritis (*e.g.*, in a young adult in whom a distinction must be made between RA and rheumatic fever) and may lend credence to a diagnosis of inactive rheumatoid arthritis in a patient with a compatible history but only a mild deformity and no obvious synovitis at the time of examination.
3. High titers occur in a variety of diseases other than rheumatoid arthritis, including lupus erythematosus, endocarditis, tuberculosis, syphilis, sarcoid, cancer, viral infections, and diseases affecting the liver, lung, or kidney.

Interfering Factors

The titer is normally higher in older patients.

THYROID HEMAGGLUTINATION TESTS

Normal Values

1:20 or negative

Background

Autoantibodies are substances produced by the body against its own tissue antigens. The production of autoantibodies to thyroid constituents is associated with destructive inflammatory lesions of the thyroid gland. Antibodies to two of these constituents, thyroglobulin and microsomal antigen, are of particular importance for diagnostic purposes. It is important to note that the titer of antibodies to the antigens does not correlate with the symptoms of thyroiditis. Antibodies are detectable only about four weeks after symptoms appear.

Antibody Detection Tests

1. Complement Fixation Test (CFT) for detection of thyroglobulin (this test is rarely done today).
2. Tanned Red Cell Agglutination Test (TRC) for detection of microsomal antigen

Explanation of Tests

These tests are used to measure thyroid autoantibodies to human thyroglobulin and to detect primary hypothyroidism in adults. These methods are also used in familial studies and genetic surveys of thyroid disorders.

Indications for Test

1. Hashimoto's thyroiditis
2. Graves' disease
3. Pernicious anemia
4. Lupus erythematosus

5. Rheumatoid arthritis
6. Various connective tissue disorders

Procedure

A venous blood sample of two ml. is obtained.

Clinical Implications

1. In *Hashimoto's thyroiditis* and *Graves' disease,* high titers (up to 1:1000) occur.
2. In 50 per cent of patients with *pernicious anemia,* the incidence of thyroid antibodies is increased.
3. Antibodies are present in a high proportion of the *relatives* of patients having *Hashimoto's thyroiditis.* This phenomenon is due to the fact that the tendency to develop thyroid autoimmunity is familial.
4. In systemic lupus erythematosus, rheumatoid arthritis, and other connective tissue diseases, the tests are positive.

Interfering Factors

In normal individuals the hemagglutinating antibody (IgG) is occasionally detected in titers up to 1:20. This incidence increases with age in normal persons. The titer is greater in women than in men, especially women over 60 years of age.

TOXOPLASMOSIS (TPM) TEST

Normal Values

Negative or <1:64 titer

Background

Toxoplasmosis is a condition caused by the sporozoal parasite *Toxoplasma gondii.* It may be a severe generalized disease or a granulomatous disease of the CNS. The condition may be either congenital or postnatal.

Congenital toxoplasmosis may lead to fetal death. Symptoms of subacute infection may also appear shortly after birth or months and even years later. Complications of congenital toxoplasmosis include hydrocephaly, microcephaly, convulsions, and chronic retinitis.

Acquired toxoplasmosis may begin as pneumonitis, a condition which resembles atypical pneumonia. If the patient passes into the subacute phase, he may be incorrectly diagnosed as having infectious mononucleosis. Infection of the eye is often associated with acquired toxoplasmosis. Latent toxoplasmosis is the most common form of the disease. It is believed that one-quarter to one-half of the adult population is asymptomatically infected with toxoplasmosis. The Center for Disease Control therefore recommends that physicians consider serologic testing of their pregnant patients for detection of this disease.

Explanation of Test

The TPM test helps to differentiate toxoplasmosis from infectious mononucleosis.

It is also a valuable screening test for latent toxoplasmosis.

Procedure

1. A venous blood sample of five ml. is obtained.
2. In the laboratory infected cells will rupture in the preparation of slides, and the parasite will be freed.

Clinical Implications

The test may be considered positive under any of the following conditions:
1. The titer is 1:256 or higher.
2. The patient is over four months old.
3. The same or higher titer is obtained on a repeat test four months after the first test.

Interfering Factors

Newborn infants may have a high titer because of transfer of antibodies from the mother. It is therefore necessary to repeat the test after four months, when passively transferred antibodies will have disappeared.

ENTAMOEBA HISTOLYTICA (AMEBIASIS) DETECTION AND HK9 ANTIGENS

Normal Values

Negative

Explanation of Test

Entamoeba histolytica, the causative agent of amebiasis, is a pathogenic parasite found in the intestine. The *Entamoeba histolytica* test is used to detect the presence or absence of specific serum antibodies (HK9 antigens) to this parasite. The usual definitive method of diagnosis of amebiasis is stool examination. However, the absence of detectable organisms in the stool does not necessarily rule out the disease, on account of antibiotic therapy, oil enemas, and barium making a stool identification impossible.

Procedure

A venous blood sample of five ml. is obtained.

Clinical Implications

1. A positive test may reflect only past, not current infections.
2. Positive results occur in:
    (a.) Amebic liver abscess
    (b.) Amebic dysentery

ALPHA₁-ANTITRYPSIN TEST

Normal Values

Average Normal 159–400 mg./dl.

Background

Alpha₁-antitrypsin is a protein produced by the liver. It is believed that this protein inhibits protease released into body fluids by dying cells. Deficiency of this protein is associated with pulmonary emphysema and liver disease. Human blood serum is known to contain at least three inhibitors of protease, two of which are best known as alpha₁-antitrypsin and alpha₂-macroglobulin. Total antitrypsin levels in blood are composed of approximately 90 per cent alpha₁-antitrypsin and 10 per cent alpha₂-macroglobulins.

Explanation of Test

This test is a nonspecific method of diagnosing inflammation, severe infection, and necrosis. This measurement is becoming important clinically because of the direct relation this protein has been shown to have in pulmonary and other metabolic disorders. It appears that pulmonary problems such as emphysema may be brought about by the inability of antitrypsin-deficient individuals to ward off the action of endoproteases.

Procedure

1. A venous blood sample of five ml. is obtained.
2. Fasting is required if patient has elevated cholesterol or triglyceride levels.

Clinical Implications

1. The following should facilitate an adequate interpretation of levels of alpha₁-antitrypsin:

- (a.) High levels: generally found in normal individuals
- (b.) Intermediate levels: found in persons with a predisposition to pulmonary emphysema
- (c.) Low levels: found in patients with obstructive pulmonary disease and in children having cirrhosis of the liver

2. *Increased* levels indicate the following:
   - (a.) Acute and chronic inflammatory
   - (b.) After infections of typhoid vaccine
   - (c.) Cancer
   - (d.) Thyroid infections
   - (e.) Use of oral contraceptives
   - (f.) Stress syndrome
   - (g.) Hematologic abnormalities

3. *Decreased* levels are associated with two progressive diseases:
   - (a.) Early-onset, chronic pulmonary emphysema in adults
   - (b.) Liver cirrhosis in children
   - (c.) Pulmonary disease
   - (d.) Severe hepatic damage
   - (e.) Nephrotic syndrome
   - (f.) Malnutrition

Interfering Factors

Serum levels may increase normally by 100 per cent in pregnancy.

Patient Preparation

1. Instruct patient about fasting if necessary.
2. Water is permitted.

CLINICAL ALERT

Individuals with deficient antitrypsin levels should be counseled to avoid smoking and occupations where significant levels of air pollutants such as fumes and dust can lead to respiratory inflammation.

ANTI-STREPTOLYSIN O (ASO), STREPTOZYME, STREPTODORNASE-B, ASLO TEST

Normal Values

200 I.U. or less than 160 Todd units
Mean normal levels are age-dependent:

Preschool	1:60
School age	1:70
Adult	1:85

Background

Streptolysin "O" is a hemolytic factor produced by most strains of Group A beta-hemolytic streptococci. Antistreptolysin "O" (ASO) is the specific neutralizing antibody produced after infection with these organisms. Antistreptolysin O appears in the blood from one week to one month after the onset of a streptococcal infection.

Explanation of Test

This test is widely used to diagnose recent streptococcal infection. It is useful in the diagnosis of rheumatic fever and glomerulonephritis. This test detects antibodies to the exoenzymes of streptococcus Group A, which may develop in rheumatic fever, glomerulonephritis, bacterial endocarditis, scarlet fever, and other related conditions. Serial determinations with a rising titer over a period of weeks are more significant than a single determination.

Procedure

1. A venous blood sample of 45 ml. is obtained.
2. Subsequent testing is advisable two times a week for four to six weeks following a streptococcal infection.

Clinical Implications

1. The titer that is considered elevated varies, but in general a titer of 166 Todd units or higher is definitely elevated. A

repeated low titer is good evidence that there is no active rheumatic fever. However, a high titer does not necessarily mean rheumatic fever or glomerulonephritis, yet it does indicate a focus of streptococcal infection. The deciding factors in diagnosis are clinical symptoms and other laboratory tests.

2. The production of ASO is especially high in cases of rheumatic fever and glomerulonephritis. It is characteristic for each of these conditions to show a marked increase of the ASO titer during the symptomless period preceding an attack of the illness.

Interfering Factors

1. An increased titer is found in healthy carriers.
2. Antibiotic therapy will suppress the streptococcal antibody response.
3. Increased beta lipoprotein levels inhibit streptolysin O, thereby giving falsely high ASO titer.

CLINICAL ALERT
The ASO test is impractical in patients who have recently received antibiotics, or who are scheduled for antibiotic therapy, since the treatment suppresses the antibody response.

AGM TEST FOR IMMUNOGLOBULINS IgG, IgA, AND IgM

Normal Values

The following values refer to the serum concentrations of immunoglobulins:

IgG—700–1350 mg./dl.   IgD—very small amount
IgA—75–370 mg./dl.   IgE—small amount
IgM—35–200 mg./dl.

Background

"Immunoglobulin" is a general term for *antibody*. Five classes of immunoglobulins, IgG, IgA, IgM, IgD, and IgE, have been isolated in humans. Each of the immunoglobulins bears a structural similarity to the other antibody molecules. The basic functions of immunoglobulins are to neutralize toxic substances (antigens) entering the body, to allow for phagocytosis, and to kill microbial organisms.

Since the AGM test is useful for detection of only three immunoglobulins (IgG, IgA, and IgM), a brief description of their properties follows:

IgG
1. Major immunoglobulin of blood
2. Accounts for 85 per cent of total human immunoglobulin
3. Serum concentration of 800 to 1680 mg. per 100 ml.
4. Possesses antibody activity against viruses, some bacteria, and toxins
5. The only immunoglobulin that crosses the placenta

IgA
1. Main immunoglobulin in body secretions such as colostrum, saliva, tears, and secretions of gastrointestinal tract and bronchial tract
2. Accounts for 10 to 15 per cent of total human immunoglobulin
3. Serum concentration of 140 to 420 mg. per 100 ml.
4. Possesses antibody activity against viruses and such bacteria as *Escherichia coli*, *Corynebacterium diphtheriae*, *Brucella* species, and *Clostridium tetani*
5. Protects the mucous membranes in the respiratory and GI tract against invasion by microorganisms
6. Does not cross the placenta and is therefore absent in infants

IgM
1. Constitutes five to ten per cent of total human immunoglobulin
2. Serum concentration of 50 to 190 mg. per 100 ml.
3. First antibody to appear after antigens enter the body
4. Possesses antibody activity against gram-negative organisms and rheumatoid factors
5. Forms the natural antibodies such as the ABO blood group

6. Is a powerful activator of complement
7. Does not pass across the placenta and is therefore usually absent in the newborn

Explanation of Test

This test measures the levels of three classes of immunoglobulins (IgG, IgA, and IgM) in the blood. It is difficult to identify these immunoglobulins by conventional electrophoresis, and this test constitutes a special method of differentiation.

Procedure

1. A venous blood sample of 10 ml. is usually obtained.
2. Check with the individual laboratory requiring the sample. Quantities needed may vary from lab to lab.

Clinical Implications

A. *IgG*
   1. Increases in:
      (a.) Chronic granulomatous infections
      (b.) Infections of all types
      (c.) Hyperimmunization
      (d.) Liver disease
      (e.) Malnutrition (severe)
      (f.) Dysproteinemia
      (g.) Disease associated with hypersensitivity granulomas, dermatologic disorders, and IgG myeloma

B. *IgD*
   1. Biologic functions of these antibodies are still relatively unknown.
   2. Only small amounts are present in the blood but more than IgE.
   3. Increase in:
      (a.) chronic infections
      (b.) IgD myelomas

C. *IgE*
   1. Possesses antibody activity for hypersensitivity reactions and presence may be a protection against parasitic worms
   2. Increases in:
      (a.) Atopic skin diseases such as eczema
      (b.) Hay fever
      (c.) Asthma
      (d.) Anaphylactic shock
      (e.) E-myeloma
   3. Only very small amounts are present in the blood.
   4. Decreases in:
      (a.) Congenital agammaglobulinemia
      (b.) Hypogammaglobulinemia due to faulty metabolism or synthesis of immunoglobulins
D. *IgA*
   1. Increases in:
      (a.) Wiskott-Aldrich syndrome
      (b.) Cirrhosis of the liver (most cases)
      (c.) Certain stages of collagen and other autoimmune disorders
      (d.) Chronic infections not based on immunologic deficiencies
      (e.) IgA myeloma
   2. Decreases in:
      (a.) Hereditary ataxia telangiectasia
      (b.) Immunologic deficiency states (*e.g.*, dysgammaglobulinemia, congenital and acquired agammaglobulinemia, and hypogammaglobulinemia)
      (c.) Malabsorption syndromes
E. *IgM*
   1. Increases (in adults) in:
      (a.) Waldenström's macroglobulinemia
      (b.) Trypanosomiasis
      (c.) Actinomycosis
      (d.) Carrión's disease (bartonellosis)
      (e.) Malaria
      (f.) Infectious mononucleosis

(g.) Dysgammaglobulinemia (certain cases)

Note: In the newborn, a level of IgM above 20 ng. per dl. is an indication of *in utero* stimulation of the immune system and stimulation by the rubella virus or the cytomegalovirus.

2. Decreases in:
   (a.) Agammaglobulinemia
   (b.) Lymphoproliferative disorders (certain cases)
   (c.) Lymphoid aplasia
   (d.) IgG and IgA myeloma
   (e.) Dysgammaglobulinemia

CARCINOEMBRYONIC ANTIGEN (CEA) TEST

Normal Values

2.5–3.0 ng./ml.

Background

Carcinoembryonic antigen (CEA) is an antigen present in embryonic tissue. This antigen is designated "carcinoembryonic" because of its initial isolation from entodermally derived adenocarcinoma and fetal gastrointestinal tissue. It is believed that as a cancer disrupts normal tissue, CEA enters the vascular system in larger amounts than normal.

Explanation of Test

This test may be used to diagnose colon cancer and to manage patients with documented colon cancer for signs of recurrent tumor. However, it is a nonspecific test and is not used for a definitive diagnosis of carcinoma of the GI tract. It may also be an aid in following those inflammatory colon diseases which place the patient at high risk for developing particular malignant states.

Procedure

A venous blood sample of seven to ten ml. is obtained.

Limitations of the Test

1. It is not recommended as a screen to detect cancer.
2. CEA levels are not an absolute test for malignancies.
3. CEA titers less than 2.5 ng. per ml. are not proof of the absence of malignant disease.
4. In the management and diagnosis of the patient suspected or known to have cancer, all other tests and procedures must continue to be emphasized.

Clinical Implications

1. CEA levels are elevated in 66 to 75 per cent of patients with known carcinoma of the large intestine or pancreas. Levels are highest in patients with metastatic colon neoplasma.
2. Levels are also elevated in:
    (a.) Inflammatory bowel diseases, especially ulcerative colitis
    (b.) Cirrhosis
    (c.) Chronic cigarette smoking
    (d.) Other cancers:

(1). Breast	(6). Neuroblastoma
(2.) Lung	(7). Multiple myeloma
(3). Ovary	(8). Osteogenic sarcoma
(4). Prostate	(9). Leukemia
(5). Bladder	

    (e.) Without evident cause (at times)
3. If the level drops to near normal after treatment, this is an indication that there is either a complete surgical removal of the cancer or a favorable response to treatment. If the level remains high after treatment, it is an indication of either incomplete removal of the cancer or undetected metastasis.
4. Prognosis is better when the level is moderately increased initially as compared to those patients with greatly increased initial levels; the latter is often indicative of extensive metastasis.

FUNGAL ANTIBODY TESTS (HISTOPLASMOSIS [HP] AND COCCIDIOIDOMYCOSIS [CM])

Normal Values

Negative

Background

Certain species of fungi are associated with human respiratory diseases acquired by inhalation of spores from sources such as dust, soil, and bird droppings. Serologic tests may be used for diagnosis of these conditions.

Fungal diseases may be categorized as either "superficial" or "deep." For the most part, the superficial mycoses are limited to the skin, mucous membranes, nails, and hair. The deep mycoses involve the deeper tissues and internal organs. Histoplasmosis, coccidioidomycosis, and blastomycosis are three diseases caused by the deep mycoses.

Following are brief descriptions of the fungal diseases:
1. Coccidioidomycosis (Desert Fever, San Joaquin Fever, Valley Fever): a condition contracted from inhalation of soil or dust containing spores of *Coccidioides immitis.*
2. Blastomycosis: an infection caused by organisms of the genus *Blastomyces.*
3. Histoplasmosis: a granulomatous infection caused by *Histoplasma capsulatum.*

Explanation of Test

These tests are used to detect serum precipitin antibodies present in the fungal diseases coccidioidomycosis, blastomycosis, and histoplasmosis.

Procedure

A venous blood sample of at least seven ml. is obtained.

Clinical Implications

Antibodies to coccidioidomycosis, blastomycosis, and histo-plasmosis appear early in the disease (from the 1st to the 4th weeks) and then disappear.

Interfering Factors

1. Antibodies against fungi may be found in the blood of apparently normal people.
2. In tests for blastomycosis, there may be cross-reactions with histoplasmosis.

FEBRILE AGGLUTINATING ANTIGEN TEST

Normal Values

Negative

Explanation of Test

This test is ordered to detect and determine the level of bacterial antibodies in blood occurring in febrile conditions such as typhoid and Salmonella fever, typhus, brucellosis, and tularemia. Levels may vary in individuals, especially if they have been vaccinated. The client's history and clinical findings are essential in establishing a diagnosis. The test is a direct one, meaning that if the patient has antibodies against these organisms, agglutination occurs *in vitro*.

Procedure

A venous blood sample of seven ml. is obtained.

Clinical Implications

1. A titer of 1:60 or 1:80 is considered significant.
2. A single test is not diagnostically significant unless the titer

is unusually high. Tests must be given in pairs, that is, a second test must be administered seven to ten days later.
3. A four-fold rise in titer taken seven to ten days after initial test is almost absolute proof of infection.
4. A negative test does not necessarily exclude infection, as it will serve as a basis for the evaluation of subsequent tests.

Limitations of Test

1. The exact species of *Salmonella* responsible for the infection cannot be determined by this test.
2. No one test level can be considered diagnostic.

Interfering Factors

1. Recent vaccination may cause a false positive result.
2. Antibiotic therapy may cause decreased levels of bacterial antibodies. For this reason it is best to obtain the blood sample before specific therapy is instituted.

L.E. TEST

Normal Values

Negative

Background

L.E. cells are neutrophils which contain in their cytoplasm large masses of depolymerized DNA from the nuclei of polymorphonuclear leukocytes. The lupus erythematosus (L.E.) factor is present in the gamma globulin fraction of the serum protein of many patients with lupus erythematosus. The L.E. factor has the characteristics of an antinuclear (altered nucleus) antibody.

Explanation of Test

This test is ordered to diagnose lupus erythematosus. L.E. cells are produced on incubation of normal neutrophils with the serum of affected patients. The test is usually repeated on three consecutive days for thorough testing.

Procedure

A venous blood sample of five to ten ml. is obtained.

Clinical Implications

1. The test is positive in 75 to 80 per cent of patients with lupus erythematosus.
2. Positive results also are associated with:
   (a.) Rheumatoid arthritis
   (b.) Scleroderma
   (c.) Blood-sensitivity reactions
   (d.) Hepatitis (certain types)
3. A positive L.E. test should show frequent L.E. cells and bodies accompanied by rosettes. Rosette cells are rosette-shaped neutrophils grouped around a mass of nuclear protein; they are thought to be pre-L.E. cells.

Interfering Factors

1. Drugs that may cause positive test for L.E. cells:
   (a.) Acetazolamide
   (b.) Para-aminosalicylic acid (PAS)
   (c.) Chlorprothixene
   (d.) Chlorothiazide
   (e.) Diphenylhydantoin
   (f.) Griseofulvin
   (g.) Methyldopa
   (h.) Oral contraceptives
   (i.) Penicillin
   (j.) Phenylbutazone
   (k.) Procainamide
   (l.) Streptomycin
   (m.) Sulfonamides
   (n.) Tetracyclines

SYPHILIS DETECTION TESTS

Normal Values

Nonreactive: negative

Background

Syphilis is a venereal disease caused by *Treponema pallidum,* a spirochete is closely wound coils approximately 8 to 15 microns long. The untreated disease progresses through three stages which may extend over many years. These stages are as follows:

1. Primary Stage (3–6 weeks)

   A *chancre* forms. In the male this is usually on the penis. In the female it may be on the labia, clitoris, vaginal walls, or cervix. Other sites include the lips, rectum, and palm of the hand. The chancre heals spontaneously.

2. Secondary Stage

   This phase begins two to ten weeks after the disappearance of the chancre. The condition is marked by eruption of red papular lesions on the skin or pharynx. Lesions may also appear on other sites, such as the eyes and CNS. Spontaneous subsidence of this phase occurs and is followed by a period of dormancy lasting several years.

3. Tertiary Stage

   (Condition does not always progress to this stage, even if untreated.) Soft, granulomatous lesions called *gummas* form. Other changes include cardiovascular disease, CNS involvement, general paresis, deafness, blindness, and insanity.

Explanation of Tests

The major types of tests used in the diagnosis of syphilis are: (1) complement fixation, (2) flocculation, (3) fluorescent antibody test (FTA), (4) hemagglutination tests.

1. *Complement-Fixation Test*

   This type of test relies on the antigen-antibody reaction and resulting hemolysis to determine the presence of the spirochete, *Treponema pallidum,* in the blood. Complement, which is a complex series of proteins occurring in serum, becomes "used up" in the reaction, and then it is said to be "fixed."

The Reiter test is an example of a complement-fixation test in current use.

2. *Flocculation Test*

A flocculant material is any material that is downy or has flaky shreds. Positive results in a test of this type depend on the degree of flocculant material formed in the test substance. The VDRL is an example of a flocculation test in current use.

3. *Fluorescent Antibody Test*

FTA-ABS is an example of a fluorescent antibody test in current use.

4. *Hemagglutination Tests*

The TP-MHA is an example of a hemagglutination test in current use.

Testing for Serum Antibody

During the course of the infection, two types of antibodies may form: (1) reagin, and (2) treponemal antibody. Different serologic tests are available to show the presence of each of these antibodies:

Tests to show reagin: VDRL and RPR

Tests to show treponemal antibody: Treponemal immobilization test (TPI), fluorescent antibody (FTA) test, and Reiter complement-fixation test. In general, the serologic tests for detection of treponemal antibody are used only when the reagin tests are inconclusive.

Interpreting Tests for Syphilis

1. In interpreting tests for syphilis, several factors must be considered:
    (a.) Geographical area
    (b.) Ability of patient to produce reagin or treponemal antibodies
    (c.) Stage of the disease

TABLE 7–2. SEROLOGIC TESTS FOR SYPHILIS (STS)

Name of Test	Type/Description	Comments
FTA (fluorescent treponemal antibody)	Syphilitic serum is bound to surface of *Treponema pallidum:* antibody is made visible by using fluorescein-tagged antiserum	Fluorescent labeled antibody against human globulin is added to serum. Spirochetes combined with antibody will fluoresce.
FTA-ABS (fluorescent treponemal antibody absorption)	Fluorescent antibody	Detects treponemal antibodies. Differentiates biologic false positives from true syphilis positives and diagnoses syphilis when definite clinical signs of syphilis are present but other tests are negative.
RPR (rapid plasma reagin)	Flocculation	Reagin reacts with lipid antigens; used as screening test; shows presence of reagin.
TPI (Treponemal pallidum immobilization)	Uses living, motile *Treponema pallidum* as antigen	Shows presence of treponemal antibody; most sensitive and specific test for syphilis. Only performed at Center for Disease Control in Atlanta, Ga.
VDRL	Flocculation	Used as a screening test. Developed in the Venereal and Research Laboratories of the U.S. Public Health Service: shows presence of reagin.
TP-MHA (Micro-hemagglutination assay for *Treponema pallidum* antibodies)	Hemagglutination	Shows presence of treponemal antibody. Even more specific than an FTA-ABS.
Reiter	Complement-fixation	An antigen-antibody reagin that causes hemolysis. Detects the presence of Treponema antibody in the blood. Based on the outdated Wasserman test.

(d.) Previous antibiotic therapy

(e.) Manner in which serological tests are performed

(f.) Various conditions eliciting biologic false positive reactions

Procedure

1. A venous blood sample is obtained.
2. Fasting is usually *not* required.

Clinical Implications

1. These test results are considered *positive* for syphilis antibodies:
   - (a.) "Reactive"
   - (b.) "Weakly reactive"
   - (c.) "Borderline"
2. When the test is positive for syphilis it should be repeated. If the test is again positive, and none of the diseases which cause false positives are present, the diagnosis of syphilis is suggested if the history and symptoms of the patient point to the disease. A single nonreactive test *suggests* the absence of syphilis but does not *prove* it. The test requires repetition if the patient's medical history warrants it.
3. Treatment of syphilis may change both the clinical course and serological pattern of the disease. The effect of treatment during the three stages in relation to the VDRL, or any test for syphilis that shows the presence of reagin, are as follows:
   - (a.) If the patient is treated adequately before the appearance of the primary chancre, it is probable that the VDRL will remain nonreactive (negative).
   - (b.) If the patient is treated at the seronegative primary stage (*e.g.*, after the appearance of the chancre, but before the appearance of reaction or reagin), the VDRL will remain nonreactive.
   - (c.) If the patient is treated in the seropositive primary stage (*e.g.*, after the appearance of reaction) the VDRL usually becomes nonreactive within six months.
   - (d.) If the patient is treated during the secondary stage, the VDRL will usually become nonreactive within 12 to 18 months. If the patient is treated ten or more years after the onset of the disease, the VDRL can be expected to change little, if any. The longer the patient goes untreated, the longer it will take the VDRL to

become nonreactive after adequate treatment, if it ever does.

3. A negative serological test may indicate:
   (a.) The patient does not have syphilis.
   (b.) The infection is too recent to have allowed the patient to produce antibodies which give the reactions. Repeat tests should be performed one week, one month, and three months later to exclude syphilis in patients with typical symptoms of syphilis.
   (c.) The patient is temporarily nonreactive after treatment or because of other causes such as drinking of alcoholic fluids.
   (d.) The syphilis is in a latent or inactive phase.
   (e.) The patient has a faulty immuno-defense mechanism.
   (f.) The laboratory techniques were inferior.

False Positive Reactions

A positive reaction does not necessarily mean that the client has syphilis. Several conditions will give a biologically false positive (BFP) reaction for syphilis. Biological false positive reactions are by no means "false." They may reveal the presence of serious diseases other than syphilis. Little is known about the antibody or reaction concerned in the mechanism of BFP reactions. It is believed that reagin (reaction) is an antibody against tissue lipids. Lipids are presumed to be liberated from body tissue in the course of normal wear and tear, and these liberated lipids may induce the formation of antibodies within the same individual.

Interfering Factors

In tests for syphilis that detect reagin:
1. Alcohol decreases the intensity for the reaction.
2. Excess chyle in the blood interferes with the reaction. For this reason, blood sample should be drawn before a meal.

Patient Preparation

Instruct patient not to drink alcohol for 24 hours prior to taking of blood sample.

TABLE 7–3. NONSYPHILITIC CONDITIONS GIVING BIOLOGICAL FALSE POSITIVES (BFP'S) USING VDRL AND RPR TESTS

Disease	*Percentage (Approximate) BFP's*
1. Malaria	100
2. Leprosy	60
3. Relapsing fever	30
4. Active immunization in children	20
5. Infectious mononucleosis	20
6. Lupus erythematosus	20
7. Lymphogranuloma venereum	20
8. Pneumonia, atypical	20
9. Ratbite fever	20
10. Typhus fever	20
11. Vaccinia	20
12. Infectious hepatitis	10
13. Leptospirosis (Weil's disease)	10
14. Periarteritis nodosa	10
15. Trypanosomiasis	10
16. Chancroid	5
17. Chickenpox	5
18. Measles	5
19. Rheumatoid arthritis	5–7
20. Rheumatic fever	5–6
21. Scarlet fever	5
22. Subacute bacterial endocarditis	5
23. Pneumonia, pneumococcal	3–5
24. Tuberculosis, advanced pulmonary	3–5
25. Blood loss, repeated	?(low)
26. Common cold	?(low)
27. Pregnancy	?(low)

CLINICAL ALERT

1. Sexual partners of patients with primary, secondary, or early latent syphilis should be evaluated for signs and symptoms of syphilis and should have a blood test for syphilis. Social contacts of infants with symptomatic neonatal syphilis should be examined in a similar manner.

2. After treatment, patients with early syphilis should be tested at three-month intervals for one year. The reaction level declines in most patients followed for a year until little or no reaction is detected.

ANTINUCLEAR ANTIBODY (ANA), ANTI-DNA ANTIBODY TESTS

Normal Values

Negative

Background

Antinuclear antibodies are gamma globulins that react to specific antigens when mixed in the laboratory. These detectable antinuclear antibodies usually belong to more than one immunoglobulin classification. Such antibodies (anti-DNP, anti-DNA, extractable antibody) are produced in response to the nuclear part of white blood cells.

Explanation of Test

This test is used to detect the presence of antinucleoprotein factors associated with certain autoimmune diseases. A particular pattern is associated with systemic lupus erythematosus (SLE); another antibody pattern correlates with scleroderma, Raynaud's disease, Sjögren's syndrome, hepatitis, and tuberculosis.

Procedure

A venous blood sample of ten ml. is obtained.

Clinical Implications

1. A test is positive at a titer of 1:10 or 1:20, depending upon laboratory.
2. Appearance of a positive result does not necessarily indicate a disease process because anti-nuclear antibodies are present in some apparently normal individuals.
3. Some positive reactions have been reported to be related to patients with connective tissue disease or to persons who may develop such a disease at a later time.

4. Positive tests are associated with:

(a.) Systemic lupus erythematosus
(b.) Rheumatoid arthritis
(c.) Chronic hepatitis
(d.) Periarteritis nodosa
(e.) Dermatomyositis
(f.) Scleroderma
(g.) Atypical pneumonia
(h.) Tuberculosis
(i.) Anaplastic carcinomas or lymphomas
(j.) Raynaud's disease
(k.) Sjögren's syndrome

5. A negative test for total antinuclear antibody is strong evidence against the diagnosis of SLE.

Interfering Factors

1. Drugs that may cause positive tests for antinuclear antibodies include:

(a.) Acetazolamide
(b.) Para-aminosalicylic acid (PAS)
(c.) Chlorprothixene
(d.) Chlorothiazide
(e.) Oral contraceptives
(f.) Penicillin
(g.) Phenylbutazone
(h.) Procainamide hydrochloride
(i.) Griseofulvin
(j.) Hydralazine
(k.) Isoniazid
(l.) Methyldopa
(m.) Streptomycin
(n.) Sulfonamides
(o.) Tetracycline
(p.) Thiouracil
(q.) Trimethadione

2. Positive antibody patterns are also seen in the blood of:

(a.) Elderly patients (certain cases)
(b.) Normal adults (small number)

HUMAN TRANSFERRIN TEST (TOTAL IRON-BINDING CAPACITY [TIBC])

Normal Values

250–450 mg./dl.

Background

Transferrin, a protein and beta-globulin regulates iron absorption and transport in the body. Transferrin (also called siderophilin) is believed to contribute in some nonspecific manner to the body's defense against bacterial infection.

Explanation of Test

In the laboratory the quantity of transferrin is measured by the amount of iron with which it can bind. This ability is referred to as the "total iron-binding capacity." In conditions where the body is deficient in iron, the TIBC is increased. When the body has an excess of iron, the TIBC is decreased.

Procedure

A venous blood sample of ten ml. is obtained.

Clinical Implications

1. *Increased levels* are caused by:
   - (a.) Inadequate dietary iron
   - (b.) Iron-deficiency anemia due to hemorrhage
   - (c.) Acute hepatitis
   - (d.) Polycythemia
   - (e.) Oral contraceptives
2. *Decreased* levels are caused by:
   - (a.) Pernicious anemia
   - (b.) Thalassemia
   - (c.) Sickle cell anemia
   - (d.) Chronic infection
   - (e.) Cancer
   - (f.) Hepatic disease
   - (g.) Uremia
   - (h.) Rheumatoid arthritis

Interfering Factors

1. Transferrin is elevated in:
   - (a.) Children two and a half to ten years of age
   - (b.) Pregnant women during the third trimester
2. Drugs which may cause increased iron-binding capacity include:
   - (a.) Chloramphenicol
   - (b.) Fluorides

(c.) Iron dextran complex
(d.) Oxalate
(e.) Oral contraceptives
(f.) Tungstate
3. Drugs which may cause decreased iron-binding capacity include:
(a.) ACTH
(b.) Hydroxyurea
(c.) Steroids
(d.) Fluorides
(e.) Oxalate and tungstate may cause decreases or increases.

C-REACTIVE PROTEIN (CRP) TEST

Normal Values

Trace amounts

Background

During the course of an inflammatory process—whether due to infection or to tissue destruction—an abnormal specific protein, C-reactive protein (CRP), appears in the blood. This protein is virtually absent from the serum of healthy persons. CRP appears rapidly in the blood in response to many injurious stimuli. Almost any disease which brings about an inflammatory condition of any tissue will result in quantities of CRP being present in the blood and body fluids (*e.g.*, peritoneal fluid and synovial fluid).

CRP is thought to be synthesized mainly in the liver and is found in large amounts in inflammatory body fluids such as peritoneal, pleural, pericardial, and synovial. It is considered to be a transport protein for certain polysaccharides. From recent studies, it appears that a major function of CRP in health and disease involves its ability to interact with the complement system.

Explanation of Test

The CRP is an antigen-antibody reaction test that is a nonspecific method for evaluating the severity and course of inflammatory diseases and those conditions in which there is tissue necrosis, such as in myocardial infarction and malignancies, as well as in rheumatoid arthritis. The presence of C-reactive protein in the blood serum can be detected 18 to 24 hours after the onset of tissue damage. This is a useful test in following the progress of rheumatic fever under treatment and in the interpretation of the sedimentation rate.

Procedure

A venous blood sample of five ml. is obtained.

Clinical Implications

1. Any titer is significant, whether 1:2 or 1:64.
2. A positive reaction indicates the presence of an active inflammation, but not the cause of the process. The results of the test must be used in association with clinical judgment.
3. The test is positive with the following conditions.
    - (a.) Rheumatic fever
    - (b.) Rheumatoid arthritis
        Note: The test becomes negative with successful treatment, indicating that the inflammatory reaction has disappeared, even when the sedimentation rate continues.
    - (c.) Lupus erythematosus (disseminated)
    - (d.) Myocardial infarction
    - (e.) Malignancy (active, widespread)
    - (g.) Bacterial and viral infections (acute)
4. Demonstration of the presence of CRP has added significance over and above the finding of an elevated erythrocyte sedimentation rate (ESR) which may be influenced by changed physiological states unassociated with any actual tissue damage such as:
    - (a.) In the absence of inflammation
    - (b.) In anemia, beacuse of a decreased number of red blood cells

(c.) In pregnancy, because of increased fibrinogen
(d.) In multiple myeloma and other instances of hyperglobulinemia
(e.) In nephrosis, because of loss of albumin and the increase of globulin

Patient Preparation

1. Instruct patient to fast for eight to twelve hours before test if laboratory requires fasting. (Check the policy of the laboratory being used.)
2. Water is permitted.

MONOSPOT AND HETEROPHILE ANTIBODY TITER TEST; MONOSCREENING-MONO-DIFF

Normal Values

Negative

Background

Normal serum contains heterophile antibodies of the Forssmann type. A heterophile antibody is one which is capable of reacting with an antigen that is completely unrelated to the antigen originally stimulating its formation. Infectious mononucleosis, probably caused by the Epstein Barr virus, induces the formation of lymphocytes and monocytes in lymph nodes in increased numbers and in abnormal forms. It also stimulates an increase in antibody formation which is similar to the Forssmann type.

Explanation of Test

Monospot and Monoscreening tests are the routine presumptive diagnostic tests for infectious mononucleosis. The heterophile titer is done to differentiate this antibody of infectious mononucleosis from the Forssmann antibody and from those associated with serum sickness.

In the laboratory, the sheep RBC is commonly used to detect heterophile antibodies in the serum of patients (not Forsmann type) with suspected infectious mononucleosis. Such patients begin developing heterophile antibodies shortly after the appearance of symptoms, usually during the first two weeks.

Useful Tests

1. Screening tests:
    (a.) Monospot
    (b.) Monoscreen
2. Confirmatory tests or differential tube dilution:
    (a.) Heterophile antibody test
    (b.) Mono-Diff

Clinical Implications

1. A presumptive antibody titer of 1:56 is suspicious. A titer of 1:2224 or greater is diagnostic of infectious mononucleosis.
2. Positive reactions last four to eight weeks after appearance of symptoms.
3. The highest titers are usually found during the second and third weeks of illness.
4. The clinical symptoms of infectious mononucleosis disappear before the abnormal blood picture disappears.
5. When interpreting the significance of the titer from the presumptive test, certain points are important:
    (a.) Many normal persons have titers of 1:28 or 1:56.
    (b.) A titer of 1:1112 or 1:2224 may be present in various infections.
    (c.) A high titer may be present in persons who have received horse serum.

CLINICAL ALERT
A differential tube dilution must be carried out on all titers of 1:56 or higher.

HEPATITIS-ASSOCIATED ANTIGEN (HAA) TESTS

Normal Values

HAA: negative

Explanation of Test

These tests are done to detect the antibodies to hepatitis A and hepatitis B antigens, the hepatitis-associated antigens. Infectious hepatitis and serum hepatitis are caused by viruses that are possibly related. The virus/antigen causing infectious hepatitis has been called hepatitis virus A, and the virus/antigen causing serum hepatitis is called virus B. All donor blood must be screened to insure that only HAA negative blood is used.

Useful Tests

1. Immunofluorescence (p. 397)
2. Complement-fixation (p. 198)
3. Radioimmunoassay (p. 480)
4. Hemagglutination inhibition (p. 198)

Procedure

1. A venous blood sample of five ml. is obtained.
2. All blood specimens should be handled as if they are capable of transmitting viral hepatitis.
3. Wash hands after handling equipment.

Clinical Implications

1. If transfused, blood containing HAA carries a 40 to 70 per cent risk of causing hepatitis.
2. HAA is found in many patients with chronic active hepatitis whether or not prior acute hepatitis has occurred.
3. HAA is found frequently in:

TABLE 7–4. COMPARISON OF INFECTIOUS AND SERUM HEPATITIS

	Infectious Hepatitis (Infective/Epidemic)	Serum Hepatitis (Syringe Jaundice Transfusion Jaundice Post-Vaccine Hepatitis)
Virus	Virus A	Virus B
Incubation period days'	15–40	60–160
Type of onset	Acute	Insidious
Season prevalence	Winter, autumn	Year round
Age usually affected	Children, young adults	All ages
Susceptible host	Human	Human
Virus in blood	3 days before onset and in acute phase	Incubation period and acute phase
Route of infection	Oral and parenteral	Parenteral
Duration of carrier state in:		
blood	Unknown	Many years
feces	1–2 years	Not demonstrated
Immunity:		
Homologous	Present	Equivocal
Heterologous	None apparent	None apparent
Prophylactic value of gamma globulin	Good	Equivocal

    (a.) Patients receiving renal dialysis
    (b.) Institutionalized patients with Down's syndrome
    (c.) Patients receiving immunosuppressive medication (certain cases)
4. A small number of seemingly healthy individuals who have no history of acute illness have HAA in their blood serum. It may be that in these patients a very mild infection has occurred that is more likely to produce a carrier state than an acute illness and subsequent clearing.

REFERENCES

Barrett, James T.: BASIC IMMUNOLOGY AND ITS MEDICAL APPLICATION. St. Louis, The C. V. Mosby Company, 1976.

Bryant, Neville J.: LABORATORY IMMUNOLOGY AND SEROLOGY. Philadelphia, W. B. Saunders Company, 1978.

————: AN INTRODUCTION TO IMMUNOHEMATOLOGY. Philadelphia, W. B. Saunders Company, 1976.

Carpenter, Philip L.: IMMUNOLOGY AND SEROLOGY. 3rd Ed., Philadelphia, W. B. Saunders Company, 1975.

Erskine, Addine G., and Socha, Wladyslaw W.: THE PRINCIPLES AND PRACTICE OF BLOOD GROUPING. 2nd Ed., St. Louis, The C. V. Mosby Company, 1978.

Meyer, John S., et al.: REVIEW OF LABORATORY MEDICINE. 2nd Ed., St. Louis, The C. V. Mosby Company, 1975.

Ortho Research Foundation: BLOOD GROUP ANTIGENS AND ANTIBODIES AS APPLIED TO COMPATIBILITY TESTING. Raritan, N.J., Ortho Diagnostics, 1967.

Ortho Research Foundation: BLOOD GROUP ANTIGENS & ANTIBODIES AS APPLIED TO THE ABO & Rh SYSTEMS. Raritan, N.J., Ortho Diagnostics, 1969.

Pamahac, Patricia: LABORATORY METHODS IN CLINICAL SEROLOGY. Milwaukee County General Hospital, 1976 (unpublished).

8 □ □ RADIOISOTOPE STUDIES

INTRODUCTION

Radioisotopes, radioactive materials that emit atomic radiations of several different kinds, may be used in the diagnosis of many pathologic conditions. The radioactive material, consisting of *radionuclides* or *radiopharmaceuticals,* will distribute uniformly through normal tissue, but it will be picked up unevenly in tissue affected by pathologic activity. Since the radioisotope emits radiations, these radiations can be detected by scanning devices, and the distribution of the substance in various organs can then be determined. However, the success of a particular scan depends on there being significant differences in the concentrations of the radioisotopes in various areas of the tissue under study.

Radioisotopes exhibit tissue specificity; that is, certain radioisotopes are more likely to be concentrated in some organs than in others. Within these organs, the radioactive material shows distributions in normal tissue which differ from those in diseased tissue. The following are examples of tissue specificity:

Radioisotope	*Tissue*
1. Technetium tagged to sulfur colloid	1. Liver
2. Technetium tagged to phosphate	2. Bone
3. DTPA (Diethylenetriamine Penta-acetic acid)	3. Brain or kidneys
4. ^{131}I—rose bengal	4. Liver
5. ^{131}I—Hippuran (iodohippurate sodium)	5. Kidneys
6. Thallium 201 (^{201}Tl)	6. Heart
7. Krypton 81^m	7. Lung ventilation scan

Manufacture of Isotopes

Manufacture of isotopes can be explained in the following way:
1. The substance to be made radioactive is placed inside a reactor, where it is bombarded by the neutrons liberated by the fission process. This bombardment changes the material to an unstable, or "excited," state.
2. The bombarded material has a natural strong tendency to

return to its stable, or normal state. As it returns, or decays, it gives off energy in the form of particles or rays.

Principles of Scanning

In general, the gamma rays are those radioactive emissions used for imaging of organ systems or the specific functions of organs. Computerized radiation detection equipment, particularly *scintillation detectors*, show the presence of gamma rays by giving off a light flash, or "scintillation." The scanner outlines and photographs the organ under study and gives information on its size, shape, position, and functional activity. Isotope scans should be thought of as a crude form of measurement.

Diagnostic Use for Scanners

Scanning is used mainly to allow visualization of organs and regions within organs that cannot be seen on an ordinary x-ray. Space-occupying lesions, especially tumors, stand out particularly well. Generally, these lesions are represented by areas of reduced radioisotopic activity.

The diagnostic penetration of the inner spaces of the body by noninvasive scanning gives the clinician more information to allow for more accurate diagnosis and therapy. This information can be obtained very simply and usually without discomfort to the patient; it is for this reason that scanning is becoming a routine procedure.

Radioactive isotope procedures are used to study pathologic conditions of these organs:

1. Thyroid
2. Liver
3. Brain
4. Bone
5. Kidney
6. Spleen
7. Pancreas
8. Lung
9. Placenta (when echograms are not available)
10. Parathyroid
11. Myocardium and heart pool

Recordings of Scans

Two types of scanning devices are used most often: rectilinear camera (emits clicking noise) and gamma camera. The results of scanning may be recorded in the following ways:

1. *Black and White Dot* With black and white photoscanning, count rates appear as shades of gray rather than bunches of black dots lumped together. Its disadvantages are that it requires processing in subdued light and takes more than eight minutes to obtain a finished scan.

2. *Black and White Photos* The black and white dot scan does not give as much quantitative information, but the scan is visible while it is being made.

3. *Color Photo Scanning* Color photoscanning involves more complicated processing but gives the clearest readout of all three procedures.

General Procedure

1. A radioactive isotope is administered orally or intravenously to the patient.

   Note: A blocking agent that is not radioactive may be administered prior to administration of the radioisotope to prevent tissues other than the organ under study from concentrating the radioactive substance. Examples of blocking agents include:

   (a.) Lugol's solution is administered orally when iodine-tagged isotopes are used, except in thyroid studies.

   (b.) Potassium perchlorate is administered orally to patients who are allergic to iodine. Blocks choroid plexus in brain.

   (c.) Mercaptomerin is administered intravenously to block uptake of ^{197}Hg—chlormerodrin by the kidneys.

2. A sufficient time interval is allowed for the radioactive material to follow its specific metabolic pathway in the body and to concentrate in the specific tissue to be studied.

3. A scanner outside the body reflects and records the concentration of the penetrating radiation that emerges from the radioisotope.

4. Total length of examining time depends upon:

   (a.) Radioisotope used and time variable to allow for concentration in tissues

   (b.) Type of scanning equipment used

Limitations to Procedure

1. Localizing tumors by scanning can be difficult when normal tissues surrounding the lesion absorb the radioisotope and produce fuzzy or ambiguous outlines.
2. A radiation hazard to the patient always exists. In all isotope procedures, the value and importance of the information gained must be weighed against the potential hazard of radiation to the patient. If an isotope study will advance the solution of a difficult problem, or provide information which cannot be obtained in any other way, then it should be done. For example, some of the following factors may be considered:
    - (a.) If a liver scan can be used to demonstrate hepatic metastases in a patient with lung carcinoma—thus sparing the patient from an unnecessary thoracotomy—the procedure is indicated.
    - (b.) Doses of radiation are actually less than the radiation received by a patient undergoing diagnostic x-rays.
    - (c.) With a radioisotope scan, metastatic disease to bone can be found six months to a year before it can be detected with the usual bone x-ray.

Information Needed Prior to Radioisotope Scanning

1. Menstrual history of women of childbearing age:
   Pregnancy is a contraindication to most radioisotope studies.
2. Whether a young mother is breastfeeding her baby:
   Radioisotope studies are contraindicated in nursing mothers.
3. History of allergies:
   Certain allergic patients may have adverse reactions to some of the radioisotopes.
4. Knowledge of recent exposure to radioisotopes:
   Exposure could interfere with the interpretation of the results.
5. Presence of any prostheses in the body:
   Certain devices could absorb radioisotopes and thereby distort results.

☐ PART ONE ☐
Scintillation Scans

KIDNEY SCAN

Normal Values

Normal size, shape, and function of kidneys

Explanation of the Test

This test is done to determine anatomical outlines and renal plasma flow in each kidney. It is also used to detect renal masses and to localize the kidney prior to needle biopsy. It can reveal positive evidence of renal disease when other tests are normal. The scan will also reveal lesions produced by vascular occlusion in the kidney. A radioactive substance, technetium 99^m (^{99m}Tc), is injected intravenously and a short time later will be concentrated and held in the kidneys. Scanning will demonstrate the size, shape, and position of the kidneys as well as the distribution of the radioisotope in the kidneys. Renal scans and renograms can be done simultaneously, giving bone morphologic and functional data about the kidneys. The iodine-sensitive or azotemic patient who cannot tolerate an IVP can be evaluated in this way.

Procedure

1. Scanning of the kidney area is done 30 minutes after the intravenous injection of the radioisotope.
2. The patient must be still during the scanning period of 30 minutes to one hour.

Clinical Implications

1. Abnormal results will indicate:
   (a.) Space-occupying "cold" or nonfunctioning areas

    (b.) Congenital abnormalities
    (c.) Space-occupying lesions
    (d.) Nonfunctioning kidneys
    (e.) Infarction
    (f.) Status of postrenal transplant
    (g.) Severe renal insufficiency
    (h.) Tumors and cysts

2. In patients with uremia, the size, shape, and location of the kidneys can be demonstrated when no visualization occurs in the IVP.

Patient Preparation

1. Instruct the patient about the purpose and procedure of the test.
2. Alleviate any fears patient may have about radioisotope procedures.

RENOGRAM (RENOCYSTOGRAM)

Normal Values

1. Right and left kidney blood flow is compared. In healthy individuals, flow is equal in both kidneys.
2. In 10 minutes 50 per cent of isotope should be excreted.

Explanation of Test

This test is done to study flow and related functions in the kidney. This is a dynamic study; blood flow is recorded as it is occurring. The test is indicated under the following conditions:

1. To detect the presence or absence of unilateral kidney disease
2. To study the hypertensive patient to determine a renal basis for the disease

3. To study the hypertensive obstetrical patient
4. To study the azotemic patient and the patient in whom uretheral catheterization is contraindicated or impossible
5. To evaluate obstruction in the upper urinary tract
6. To study the kidney when an IVP cannot be done because of allergy to iodine.

The radioactive drug, ^{131}I-hippuran, is the radioisotope administered intravenously and is selectively excreted by the kidney. The placement of the radiation detectors over the kidneys permits the monitoring of the uptake and the disappearance of the radioactivity. This information is usually displayed with a chart recording or put into computer. The shape of this wave may be correlated with several measures of renal function.

Procedure

1. The radioisotope ^{131}I-hippuran is injected intravenously.
2. Scanning is done immediately.
3. A urine sample may be obtained at the end of the test.
4. Total examination time is about one hour.

Clinical Implications

1. Abnormal pattern results may be indicative of:
   (a) Hypertension
   (b) Obstruction
   (c) Renal failure in the urinary tract

Patient Preparation

1. Instruct patient about the purpose of the test and procedure.
2. The patient should eat and be well hydrated with two to three glasses of water (unless contraindicated) before undergoing scan.
3. Alleviate any fears patient may have about radioisotope procedures.

THYROID SCAN (See also Chapter Five, Protein-Bound Iodine Test)

Normal Values

Normal or evenly distributed concentration of radioactive iodine; normal size and position of thyroid

Explanation of Test

This test systematically measures the uptake of radioactive iodine (either ^{131}I or ^{123}I) by the thyroid. It is requested for the evaluation of thyroid size, position, and function. It is used in the differential diagnosis of masses in the neck, base of the tongue, or mediastinum. (Thyroid tissue can be found in each of these three locations.)

Benign adenomas may appear as nodules of increased uptake of iodine, the so-called "hot" nodules, or they may appear as nodules of decreased intake, the "cold" nodules. Malignant areas generally take the form of "cold" nodules. The most important use of thyroid scans is in the functional assessment of these thyroid nodules.

Iodine (and consequently, radioiodine) is actively transported by the thyroid gland, where it is incorporated into the production of thyroid hormone. The radioactivity of the gland is scanned by a scintillation scanning device, and this information is then plotted out visually on paper and film, thereby outlining the gland and any areas of abnormally concentrated iodine or of diminished concentration.

A thyroid scan is usually done in conjunction with a radioactive iodine uptake test, which is a common form of radioimmunoassay.

Procedure

1. The patient swallows a tasteless capsule of radioactive iodine.
2. Usually 6 or 24 hours later (or both), the neck area is scanned.
3. The patient lies on his back on the examining table with his neck hyperextended.

Clinical Implications

1. Cancer of the thyroid most often presents itself as a nonfunctioning "cold" nodule, which indicates an area of decreased uptake of radioiodine.
2. Abnormal results will indicate:
    - (a.) Hyperthyroidism represented by an area of increased uptake of radioiodine.
    - (b.) Hypothyroidism represented by an area of decreased uptake of radioiodine.
    - (c.) Graves' disease represented by an area of increased uptake of radioiodine.
    - (d.) Autonomous nodular thyroiditis represented by an area of decreased uptake of radioiodine.
    - (e.) Hashimoto's disease represented by an area of decreased uptake of radioiodine.

Interfering Factors

1. Iodine-substances can interfere for up to six months.
2. Anti-thyroid medication:
    Radioactive technetium is used when gallbladder x-ray or IVP has been done previously.

Limitations to the Test

Measurements of the total serum thyroxine (Total T_4) and the triiodothyronine uptake are much more reliable tests for function of the thyroid.

Patient Preparation

1. Instruct the patient about the purpose of the test, procedure, and special restrictions.
2. Since the thyroid gland responds to small amounts of iodine, the patient must eliminate iodine intake for at least one week before the test. Restricted items include:
    - (a.) All thyroid drugs
    - (b.) Weight control medicines
    - (c.) Multiple vitamins
    - (d.) Some oral contraceptives
    - (e.) Gallbladder and other x-ray dyes containing iodine

(f.) Cough medicine
(g.) Iodized salt
(h.) Iodine-containing foods, especially kelp, and "natural foods"

3. Alleviate any fears patient may have about radioisotope procedures.

CLINICAL ALERT
1. Thyroid scans are contraindicated in pregnancy. Thyroid testing in pregnancy is limited to blood testing.
2. Occasionally, scans are done purposely with iodine or some thyroid drug in the body. In these test patients the doctor is testing the thyroid response to drugs. These stimulation and suppression scans are usually done to determine the nature of a particular nodule and to determine if the tissue is functioning or nonfunctioning.

PANCREAS SCAN

Normal Values

Pancreatic normality is demonstrated by radioactivity in the upper jejunum.

Explanation of Test

This test is done to demonstrate pancreatic disease. A radioactive substance, selenomethionine (^{75}Se) or technetium sulfur (^{99m}Tc) is injected intravenously, and scanning is done. Scanning will demonstrate the size and position of the pancreas as well as the distribution of the radioisotope in the pancreas. Liver and spleen scans may be performed simultaneously with the pancreatic scan. Of all the organs examined by radioisotope scanning, the pancreas is the most difficult to completely and correctly visualize.

Procedure

1. A low-fat supper is eaten on the evening before the examination, and a low-fat breakfast is eaten on the day of the examination.
2. Morphine sulfate may be injected 20 minutes before scanning. Morphine constricts the sphincter of Oddi, which is the bile duct sphincter.
3. Four glasses of water are to be consumed before the radioactive isotope is injected intravenously.
4. Scanning follows the isotope injection. The patient is asked to lie very still on his back during scanning. The examination takes two hours, which is a long time to lie quietly.

Clinical Implications

1. Diagnosis of a normal pancreas is correct in 90 per cent of cases.
2. Diagnosis of an abnormal pancreas is correct in less than 60 per cent of cases.
3. Inability to demonstrate the pancreas to the most reliable sign of pancreatic disease.
4. Distortion of the shape of the pancreas is not always indicative of abnormality.

Patient Preparation

1. Instruct patient about the purpose and procedure of the test and his involvement.
2. Alleviate any fears patient may have about radioisotope procedure.

PAROTID OR SALIVARY GLAND SCAN

Normal Values

No evidence of tumor type activity or blockage of ducts

Explanation of Test

This scan is done to detect blocked ducts of the parotid and submaxillary glands, tumors of parotid or salivary glands, and to diagnose Sjogrens' syndrome in rheumatoid arthritis. The isotope injected intravenously is 99m Tc Technetium pertechnetate (^{99m}Tc). One of the limitations of the test is that it cannot furnish an exact preoperative diagnosis.

Procedure

1. A radioisotope (^{99m}Tc) is injected intravenously. Scanning is done immediately.
2. Patient is examined in a sitting position during examination.
3. Pictures of the gland are taken every five minutes for 30 minutes (2 anteroposterior and one oblique).
4. If a function test is being done to detect blockage of salivary duct, then three-fourths of the way through the test, the patient is asked to suck on a lemon slice. If the salivary gland is normal, it will cause the gland to empty. This is not done in tumor detection.

Clinical Implications

1. The reporting of a "hot" nodule amidst normal tissue which accumulates the radioisotope, is associated with tumors of the ducts as in:
   (a.) Warthin's tumor
   (b.) Oncocytoma
   (c.) Mucoepidermoid tumor
2. The reporting of a "cold" nodule amidst normal tissue which does not accumulate the radioisotope is associated with:
   (a.) Benign tumors or cysts, which are indicated by smooth, sharply defined outlines
   (b.) Adenocarcinoma, which is indicated by ragged, irregular outlines

Patient Preparation

1. Instruct patient about purpose of the test and procedure.
2. There is no pain or discomfort involved.
3. Alleviate any fears patient may have about radioisotope procedures.

ROSE BENGAL LIVER CELL FUNCTION SCAN (^{131}I-ROSE BENGAL EXCRETION TEST)

Normal Values

Normal size, shape, and position on the abdomen; normal size of cardiac impression on liver; normally functioning liver, gallbladder, and upper intestine.

Explanation of Test

This test is used to demonstrate the functions and anatomy of the liver cells, gallbladder, and upper intestine. Alterations in function may indicate an obstruction, hepatitis, toxicity, gallbladder disease, and the cause of jaundice.

A radioactive dye, rose bengal tagged with radioactive iodine, is injected intravenously. The basis of the test is that the dye is of no use to any tissue, since the liver cells remove all rose bengal within 10 to 20 minutes (blood clearance) and the dye is excreted into the bile. After storage in the gallbladder, the bile is excreted into the intestines during the next few hours (liver clearance). The scanner, or radioactive detector, is slowly passed back and forth over the liver area. Wherever there are functioning cells, a dot is recorded on photographic film. This scan of the radioactive area shows the size, shape, and position of the functioning liver. This type of scan is preferred for younger patients who develop sudden liver diseases. Occasionally, both types of liver scans are necessary.

Limitations of Test

1. The scan is not specific.
2. A rose bengal scan is not as good in the presence of jaundice, since excretion is dependent on liver function.
3. Rose bengal has a short transit time through the liver with the advantage of a low radiation dose, but the scan must be done quickly, for the radioisotope, excreted by the hepatic parenchymal cells, is concentrated in the gallbladder and excreted into the gastrointestinal tract. For this reason, the background radioactivity obscures the liver, and the scan cannot be conveniently repeated.

Procedure

1. The rose bengal tagged with radioactive iodine is injected intravenously.
2. After administration of radioisotope, the client lies on his back on an x-ray table for anterior pictures to determine liver uptake.
3. Scanning is usually done two, four, six, and 24 hours after injection to determine liver uptake, gallbladder uptake, and bile excretion into the intestine.
4. Patient must lie quietly during the scanning procedure and return for several scanning exams (as above).

Clinical Implications

1. Abnormal results will reveal:
    (a.) A diffuse nodular pattern of decreased uptake as in:
        (1.) Cirrhosis
        (2.) Hepatitis
        (3.) Fatty metamorphosis
        (4.) Diffuse cancer
        (5.) Sarcoidosis
    (b.) A solitary filling pattern caused by:
        (1.) Tumor (primary or metastatic)
        (2.) Cyst
        (3.) Perihepatic abscess
        (4.) Gumma

(5.) Tuberculoma
(c.) If the dye is not seen in the intestines after a few hours, obstructive jaundice will occur.

Patient Preparation

Explain purpose and procedure of test to patient.

LIVER SCAN; BLOOD VESSEL STRUCTURAL SCAN

Normal Values

Normal size, shape, and position of the liver and spleen; evidence of filling defects

Explanation of Test

This test of liver function is ordered to detect structural defects of the liver and is used to evaluate the size, shape, and position of the liver and the spleen. Commonly, the radioactive substance used is a colloidal sulfur compound tagged with radioactive technetium-99m. pertechnetate (^{99m}Tc). Liver scans can demonstrate the location of space-occupying lesions and help in the estimation of severity of parenchymal disease. The majority of liver scans are performed as part of the search for metastatic tumors. They may also be done to locate lesions prior to needle biopsy.

Liver scans have proved of great value in the differential diagnosis of jaundice, especially in the preoperative and postoperative evaluation of patients with known malignant tumors, and in the differential diagnosis of jaundiced patients. There is a good correlation between liver function studies and scan results.

The wide variety of information offered by a liver scan is comparable to the information obtained from a chest roentgenogram. The liver scan, like the chest roentgenogram, should therefore become a routine procedure. This test of liver function is based on phagocytosis of radioactive colloidal particles that have been injected intravenously. Within 30 minutes these colloidal particles are trapped in the reticuloendothelial cells of the liver and spleen; then scanning or visualization of both organs is obtained. Very simply, within a short time after injection, all scavenger cells in the blood vessels, especially those in the spleen, bone marrow, and liver, will pick up the particles from the blood stream.

During the next 12 hours the spleen and bone marrow will slowly release these particles back into the blood stream. The particles are then picked up for final removal from the blood by the liver scavenger cells (Kupfer's cells), which are lodged in the walls of the blood vessels.

Procedure

1. The radioisotope is injected intravenously 30 minutes before scanning is done.
2. The patient is asked to assume the following positions: He will lie on his back so that the front half of the liver can be checked; halfway on his left side to check the right surface; and on his abdomen to check the rear half of the liver. This last position is uncomfortable for some patients.
3. This procedure will take about one hour.
4. If the spleen is to be examined, scanning can be done immediately after injection of the radioisotope.

Clinical Implications

1. Abnormal results may reveal defects of concentrations that are indicative of:
   - (a.) Cysts
   - (b.) Tumors
   - (c.) Abscesses
   - (d.) High portal pressure
   - (e.) Cirrhosis
2. A liver structure scan is most commonly done for middle-aged and older patients in whom the liver is more likely to be functioning on an abnormal timetable. When the liver has already attempted to repair itself, there may be testable changes in the structure of the liver. ^{99m}Tc is adequate for repeat structural scans.

Patient Preparation

1. Instruct patient about the purpose and procedure of the test.
2. Alleviate any fears patient may have about radioisotope procedure.

HEART MUSCLE SCAN

Normal Values

Normal heart; no areas of ischemia
Normal stress test (E.C.G. and blood pressure)

Explanation of Test

Two types of myocardial scans may be performed. These scans are noninvasive and involve the intravenous injection of a radioisotope followed by scanning.

1. *Myocardial Infarction Detection.* Technetium 99m, tagged to pyrophosphate (^{99m}Tc-pyrophosphate), is the radioactive imaging agent used to demonstrate the general location and extent of myocardial infarction (MI) 24 to 48 hours after suspected myocardial infarction. In some instances the test is sensitive enough to detect MI 12 hours to six days after its occurrence. This test is useful when ECG and enzymes studies are not definitive.

2. *Ischemic Heart Disease Detection.* Thallium 201 (^{201}Tl) is the radioactive imaging agent used in conjunction with the treadmill-stress-ECG test and is used to diagnose ischemic heart disease. It is commonly called the *stress thallium myocardial scan.* When thallium is injected near the end of the stress test and scanning is done immediately, areas of myocardial ischemia can be detected. A completely normal stress test and normal stress myocardial scan may eliminate the need for cardiac catheterization in the evaluation of chest pain and nonspecific abnormalities of the ECG.

Procedure for Technetium Myocardial Scan

1. The technetium myocardial scan involves a 30 minute to one hour waiting period for the patient after the intravenous injection of the radioisotope. During this waiting period, the radioactive material will accumulate in the heart muscle.
2. The scanning period takes 15 to 30 minutes, during which time the patient must lie quietly on an examining table.

Procedure for Stress Thalium Myocardial Scan

1. Before the treadmill stress test is begun an IV is started, and ECG leads and blood pressure cuff are attached.
2. When the cardiologist has determined that the patient has reached maximum heart stress using the treadmill, an injection of radioactive thallium is given. The patient then lies down on the scanning table.
3. After a waiting period of 10 to 15 minutes for the imaging substance to concentrate in the heart muscle, the scanning is begun and polaroid pictures are taken. The scan period is about one hour.

Clinical Implications

1. Abnormal myocardial scans will reveal myocardial infarction and ischemic heart disease.
2. Specific and significant abnormalities in the stress ECG or myocardial scan are usually indications for cardiac catheterization or further studies.

Patient Preparation

Instruct patient about purpose and procedure. (There are no other special preparations or aftercare.)

CLINICAL ALERT
The isolated treadmill stress test is contraindicated in patients who:
1. Have right and left bundle-branch block
2. Have left ventricular hypertrophy
3. Are using Digitalis and quinidine
4. Are hypokalemic (results are difficult to evaluate)

LUNG SCAN

Normal Values

Normal functioning lung
Normal pulmonary vascular supply

Explanation of Test

This test is done for three major purposes: to detect the percentage of the lungs functioning normally in order to detect the regions of lung functioning abnormally; to diagnose and locate pulmonary emboli; and to assess the pulmonary vascular supply. It is a simple method for following the course of embolic disease, since an area of ischemia will persist after apparent resolution on chest x-ray. Only three tests are positive immediately following pulmonary embolus: pulmonary arteriogram, measurement of physiological dead space, and lung scan. Assessment of the adequacy of pulmonary artery perfusion in areas of known disease can also be done reliably.

Following the IV injection of a radioactive iodinated human serum albumin (RISA), assessment of the pulmonary vascular supply can be done by scanning. Krypton 81^m is used in the ventilation lung scan. In effect, multiple radioactive microemboli are introduced immediately into the minor circulation, allowing an assessment of the pulmonary vascular supply by scanning. If many particles slightly larger than red blood cells are injected into the bloodstream, they will be trapped throughout the entire functioning lung, except in areas already blocked by disease. If each particle is radioactive, a highly sensitive scanner van will produce a picture of which areas are and are not functioning normally.

There are three types of lung scans:

Perfusion scan: Blood is injected through a tissue.

Ventilation scan: Passage of blood to air is shown.

Inhalation scan: Path of the movement of air in the airways is shown.

Certain limitations exist with this test. With a positive chest film and a positive scan, the differential possibilities are multiple: pneumonia, abscess, bullae, ateliosis, and carcinoma, among others. A pulmonary arteriogram is still necessary before an embolectomy can be attempted.

Procedure

1. The patient may or may not be given a drink of iodinated water as a blocking agent. It is not necessary for the lung scan, but if further tests are considered, it will prevent thyroid uptake.
2. Five minutes later the radioisotope is injected intravenously, followed by the scan. Four projections equal one scan.
3. Examining time is about 30 minutes. During this time, the patient must be still.

Clinical Implications

1. Abnormal test results may indicate the possibility of:
   (a.) Tumors   (c.) Pneumonia
   (b.) Emboli   (d.) Atelectasis
2. If an embolus is present, a diminished or absent area of radioactive uptake is visible.

Patient Preparation

1. Instruct patient about purpose and procedure of the test.
2. Alleviate any fears patient may have about radioisotope procedure.

CLINICAL ALERT
Lung scans are restricted in pregnancy.

BRAIN SCAN

Normal Values

Normal distribution and uptake in all regions of the brain

Explanation of Test

A brain scan is a diagnostic procedure which follows a careful neurological history and exam. It is valuable in visualizing and localizing intradural lesions for *early* evaluation of patients with suspected intracranial pathology or subdural hematoma and for postoperative or postirradiation follow-up. The procedure is nonspecific, since neoplasms, vascular accidents, or malformations and extracerebral hematomas all present areas of increased activity on the scan. The brain scan is usually negative during the first week after a cerebrovascular accident. Most strokes will cause a positive scan in the third or fourth week.

A radioactive isotope, usually ^{99m}Tc or Diethylenetriamine penta-acetic acid, is injected intravenously. When it is introduced into the circulation it will concentrate in or about a variety of intracerebral lesions, allowing visualization on scanning.

The detection of a lesion rests on the differential between its uptake of radioactive materials and that in surrounding tissue.

Brain scanning is one of the testing systems in which lesions appear as an area of high radioactivity within the surrounding zone of low activity found in normal tissues. This relative increase in the concentration of radioactivity in brian lesions compared to surrounding normal brain occurs since most tracers fail to penetrate into normal brain tissue as a result of the blood-brain barrier. Tumors and other lesions of the brain interfere with the barrier, allowing a relatively high concentration of radioactive material to be attained. A change in the endothelium is one of the earliest changes in brain tumors. The blood-brain barrier is not a specific anatomical structure, but a complex system including capillary endothelium with closed intracellular clefts, a small or absent extravascular fluid space between endothelium and glial sheaths, and the membrane of the neurons themselves. To the extent that the blood-brain barrier is absent or has been rendered inoperative, the concentration of blood around a lesion increased, or the normal channels of flow altered, the existence and source of trouble is made apparent.

Procedure

1. An oral blocking agent taken in the form of stale-tasting liquid or a tasteless capsule may be given prior to testing. The blocking agent reduces uptake of the isotope in the thyroid, choroid plexus, salivary glands, and mucosa of mouth and sinuses.
2. Scanning will be done from 30 minutes to two hours after blocking agent is given.
3. Examining time is about two hours. Patient must be quiet during this time with hands at sides of the body.

Clinical Implications

1. Abnormal results are indicative of:
   - (a.) Brain tumors, such as astrocytomas, gliomas, and meningiomas
   - (b.) Aneurysms
   - (c.) Cerebral vascular accident (CVA)
   - (d.) Hematomas
   - (e.) Malformations
2. Lesions appear as areas of high radioactivity; normal surrounding tissue shows low radioactivity.
3. Scan does not reveal ventricular system, blood supply, or tumor type.

Interfering Factors

1. If the patient coughs or changes position, the scan picture is altered.
2. Immediately after the injection of the radioisotope, the patient's saliva, tears, and urine become radioactive for a few hours. More ^{99m}Tc goes into saliva than the brain tissues. If the patient coughs into his hand and then scratches his head, he might contaminate his scalp. The scan will record a false marking if this occurs. However, it is not harmful to the patient.

Patient Preparation

1. Explain purpose and procedure of test to patient.
2. Reassure patient that the test is safe, nontoxic, and painless. The only discomfort is that he must remain very quiet and still.

BONE SCAN

Normal Values

No areas of greater or lesser concentration of radioactive material in bones

Explanation of Test

This test is used most commonly to confirm the presence of metastasis to the skeletal system in cases of known carcinoma when the suspected metastasis is not visible on x-rays. It is also common practice to do this test on every person with a suspected malignancy of any body system. This scan is used in the evaluation of patients with unexplained bone pain; patients who have had breast or prostate cancer, primary bone tumors, arthritis, osteomyelitis, abnormal healing of fractures, and compression fractures of the vertebral column; patients with chronic renal failure in whom it is necessary to detect soft tissue calcification; and pediatric patients with hip pain (Legg-Calvé-Perthes disease).

A radioactive substance, technetium 99 m polyphosphate (^{99m}Tc), is injected intravenously. Two hours later scanning is done. Scanning will demonstrate the distribution and concentration of the substance in the bone (greater concentration occurs in diseased than in normal bone). The radioactive substance mimics calcium physiologically and will, therefore, concentrate less heavily in normal bone than in bone undergoing abnormal change.

Procedure

1. Radioactive technetium 99m polyphosphate is injected intravenously.
2. A two hour waiting period is necessary for the radioisotope to concentrate in the bone. During this time, the patient may be asked to drink four to six glasses of water.
3. Before the scan begins, the patient is asked to urinate, for a full bladder will mask the pelvic bones.
4. The scan takes about 30 to 60 minutes to complete. The patient must be still during scanning. The table or the scanner will slowly move the patient under and over a sensitive radiation detector.

Clinical Implications

1. Abnormal concentrations will indicate:
    (a.) Very early bone disease and healing. This is detectable by radioisotopic scan long before it is visible on x-ray. X-rays are positive for bone lesions only after 30 to 50 per cent decalcification (bone calcium decreased) has occurred.
    (b.) Many disorders can be detected but not differentiated by this test, e.g., cancer, arthritis, benign bone tumors, fractures, osteomyelitis. The findings must be interpreted in the light of the whole clinical picture, since any process inducing an increased calcium excretion rate will be reflected by an increased uptake in the bone.

Patient Preparation

1. Instruct the patient about the purpose and procedure of the test and his involvement. Alleviate any fears he may have about the procedure.
2. Laxatives may be given the evening before the exam, and an enema may be given just prior to scanning if the area of the suspected bone involvement is at or near the level of the abdomen or pelvis.
3. The patient can be up and about during the waiting period.
4. If the patient is in pain or debilitated, assist him to void prior

to the test. Otherwise, give a reminder about emptying the bladder prior to the test.
5. A sedative should be ordered and administered to any patient who will have difficulty lying quietly during the scanning period.

DEEP VEIN THROMBOSIS (DVT) SCAN

Normal Values

No areas of abnormal concentration

Explanation of Test

This scan is done to detect deep venous thrombosis in the legs from the ankle to the groin. These studies will demonstrate the early development of thrombi so that they can be managed with anticoagulant therapy before clots of significant size can form and, in some cases, embolize. The DVT scan is indicated in surgical patients and in high-risk medical patients where immobility and medical problems may be conducive to the formation of deep venous thrombosis. The radioisotope injected intravenously is ^{125}I-fibrinogen.

Procedure

1. The radioisotope ^{125}I-fibrinogen is injected intravenously. In surgical patients, it is usually injected in the recovery room.
2. The lower extremities are marked from the ankle to the groin.
3. Daily readings are taken over these marked areas to determine whether the injected fibrinogen is being incorporated in the formation of clots.
4. The examination is done at the bedside with a portable scanner.
5. The scan is done daily, seven days a week, for as long as two weeks.

Clinical Implications

1. Abnormal concentration will reveal:
   - (a.) Deep venous thrombosis formation
   - (b.) Recurrence of thrombosis

Patient Preparation

1. Explain the purpose and procedure to the patient. (In hospitals where these studies are done routinely, such instruction should be part of the preoperative teaching.)
2. Reassure patient that there is no discomfort or inconvenience and that the scan is safe and non-toxic.

CLINICAL ALERT
Do not wash markings off thighs and legs when patient is bathed.

GALLIUM (^{67}Ga) SCANS
(LIVER, BONE, BRAIN, BREAST SCAN)

Normal Values

No evidence of tumor-type activity.

Explanation of Test

This test is used to detect the presence, location, and size of tumors, adhesions, abscesses, and inflammation in body cavities, primarily of liver, bone, brain and breast. The lymph nodes are also scanned for involvement. Tumors of Hodgkin's disease, lymphomas, tumors of the lymph structures, abscesses and inflammation can be detected. These studies are also used to record tumor regression following radiation or chemotherapy, thereby noting the body response to therapy. The radioisotope injected intravenously is gallium citrate (^{67}Ga).

Areas of the body examined most often by this method are the liver, bone, brain, and breast. Only five per cent pathological activity is necessary for detection by this technique, while 45 per cent activity is required for x-ray examination.

Procedure

1. A laxative is usually given the evening before the scanning is done.
2. Tap water enemas are often ordered one to two hours before scanning.
3. The patient must lie quietly without moving during the scanning procedure.

Clinical Implications

1. An abnormal gallium concentration usually implies the existence of underlying pathology.
2. Further diagnostic studies are done usually to distinguish benign from malignant lesions.

Interfering Factors

1. A negative study cannot be definitely interpreted as ruling out the presence of disease (40 per cent false negative results in gallium studies).
2. It is difficult to detect a single, solitary nodule such as in adenocarcinoma.
3. Because gallium does collect in the bowel, there may be an abnormal concentration in the lower abdomen. For this reason, enemas are ordered prior to testing.

Patient Preparation

1. Explain the purpose of the test and the test procedure.
2. Reassure the patient that there is no pain involved.
3. Alleviate any fear patient may have about radioisotope procedure.

WHOLE BODY SCAN

Normal Values

Normal whole body scan; no evidence of tumor type activity or any evidence of suspected pathologic condition.

Explanation of Test

The scans are done primarily to identify tumor growth. A "whole body" scan means that the following organs will be examined for tumor growth over a period of days or weeks: brain, lung, liver, spleen, brain, and bone.

Whole body radioisotope scanning can also mean a head to toe scan of the patient in six to 22 minutes, while at the same time recording an accurate body outline image. In this type of whole body scanning, the patient lies on a moving table under a scanning camera. Type of scan differs from a body CT Scan, which is discussed in Chapter 9.

More than one scan can be done at a session, but it is preferred to study organ systems that are not located within the same region of the body. For example, the lungs and liver could be studied at the same session, but the kidney and liver would not since they are too close to each other. The skull and brain should not be studied on the same day. The type of isotope administered is dependent upon which organs are to be specifically examined.

Procedure

1. If many parts of the body are to be examined, the scans are done over a period of days.
2. A radioisotope is injected intravenously prior to examination. The radioisotope used depends on the organs to be studied during that session.
3. Two scanners are used, with pictures being taken above and below the body part. This procedure results in pictures of several layers of tissue. Two types of scanners are used:
   (a.) A moving scanner with a stationary examining table
   (b.) A moving examining table with a fixed scanner

4. The length of time of the scan depends on the organ examined:
   - (a.) If the lung is identified as the primary area, the scan can be done immediately after injection. The test takes ½ hour to complete.
   - (b.) In liver examination, injection is done 10 to 15 minutes prior to scanning, which is completed in 30 minutes.
   - (c.) An injection is given 1 to 3 hours before a bone scan and takes 1 hour to complete.
   - (d.) In scanning of the brain, injection is given 30 minutes to two hours prior to exam and is completed in one hour.
   - (e.) A gallium scan requires injection 30 minutes to two hours before scanning and is completed in one hour.
5. The patient must lie quietly on an examining table during the examination.

Clinical Implications

Abnormal results will indicate tumor activity or metastasis in organs studied.

Interfering Factors

1. Barium and the gas produced interfere with these tests.
2. Any tests that require the use of iodine; *e.g.*, thyroid function tests, IVP, and gallbladder tests) interfere with these studies. For this reason, whenever possible, these scans should be scheduled before the test that interferes.

Patient Preparation

1. Instruct the patient about the purpose and procedure of the test.
2. The procedures are the same as for specific organ radioisotope scans (See brain, lung, liver, bone,). Tap water enemas may be given prior to some scans.

□ PART TWO □
Radioisotope Laboratory Procedures

INTRODUCTION

Minute quantities of radioactive materials may be detected in blood, urine, other body fluids, and glands. Therefore, very small amounts of radioactive substances may be administered to patients, and then their body fluids and glands may be assayed for concentrations of radioactivity.

The majority of isotope procedures check the ability of the body to absorb the administered radioactive compound. An example of this type of study is the fat absorption test (radioactive triolein uptake test). Other procedures, such as radioactive iodine uptake or blood volume determination, test the ability of the body to localize or dilute the administered radioactive substance. In some isotope procedures no radioactive compounds are administered to the patient, but are used in the laboratory testing procedure. An example of this type of study is the T_3 test.

The use of radioisotopes in analysis depends on the fact that the radioactive atoms of a substance such as iodine react chemically just as nonradioactive iodine does, but the radioisotope can be readily detected because of its radioactivity.

Part II of this chapter includes a sampling of tests that employ the use of radioisotopes in the laboratory.

SCHILLING TEST

Normal Values

Excretion of 8 per cent or more of test dose of Cobalt-tagged Vitamin B_{12} in urine

Explanation of Test

This 24-hour urine test is used to diagnose macrocytic anemia, pernicious anemia, and malabsorption syndromes. It is an indirect test of the intrinsic factor and is based upon the anticipated urinary excretion of radioactive Vitamin B_{12}. In this test the fasting patient is given an oral dose of Vitamin B_{12} tagged with radioactive cobalt (^{57}Co). One hour later an I.M. injection of Vitamin B_{12} (1 mg.) is given to saturate the liver and serum protein–binding sites and to allow radioactive B_{12} to be absorbed in the GI tract and to be excreted in the urine. A 24-hour urine specimen is then collected. The amount of excreted radioactive B_{12} is determined and expressed as a percentage of the given dose. Normal individuals will absorb (and therefore excrete) a large proportion of the radioactive Vitamin B_{12} for they can absorb Vitamin B_{12} from the GI tract. Patients with pernicious anemia absorb little of the oral dose and thus have little radioactive material to excrete in the urine.

Procedure

1. Patient must fast for 12 hours before test. (Breakfast is delayed two hours or until the intramuscular injection of Vitamin B_{12} is administered.)
2. A tasteless capsule of radioactive Vitamin B_{12} is administered orally by a medical technician.
3. One hour later, nonradioactive B_{12} is given via intramuscular injection by R.N.
4. Urine is collected for 24 hours from the time the patient receives the injection of Vitamin B_{12}.
   - (a.) Obtain a special 24-hour urine container from the laboratory. No preservative is needed.
   - (b.) Take care that there is no contamination of the urine with stool.
   - (c.) Follow procedure for 24 hour urine collection (see Chapter 2).

Clinical Implications

1. An abnormally low value (*e.g.*, 0–3%) allows two interpretations:

(a.) Absence of intrinsic factor

(b.) Defective absorption in the ileum

2. When the absorption of radioactive Vitamin B_{12} is low, the test must be repeated with intrinsic factor to rule out intestinal malabsorption (confirmatory Schilling test).

   (a.) If the urinary excretion then rises to normal levels, it indicates a lack of intrinsic factor, suggesting the diagnosis of pernicious anemia.

   (b.) If the urinary excretion does not rise, malabsorption is considered the cause of the patient's anemia.

Interfering Factors

1. Renal insufficiency may cause reduced excretions of radioactive Vitamin B_{12}. If renal insufficiency is suspected, a 48- to 72-hour urine collection is advised since eventually nearly all the absorbed material will be excreted and urine specific gravity and volume are checked.

2. The single most common source of error in performing the test is incomplete collection of urine. Some laboratories may require a 48-hour collection to allow for a small margin of error.

3. Urinary excretion of B_{12} is depressed in elderly patients, diabetics, patients with hypothyroidism, and those with enteritis.

Patient Preparation

1. Instruct patient about the purpose and procedure of test.

2. Give a written reminder to patient about fasting and collection of urine specimen.

3. Food and drink is permitted after the intramuscular dose of Vitamin B_{12} is given.

4. Be certain the patient receives the nonradioactive B_{12}. If the IM Vitamin B_{12} is not given, the radioactive Vitamin B_{12} will be found in the liver.

CLINICAL ALERT

1. No laxatives are to be used during the test.

2. Bone marrow aspiration should be done before the Schilling test, since the Vitamin B_{12} administered in the Schilling test will destroy the diagnostic characteristics of the bone marrow.

RADIOACTIVE TRIOLEIN UPTAKE
(TRIOLEIN ^{131}I ABSORPTION TEST)

Normal Values

8–12% tagged triolein in blood in 3–4 hours
Less than 2% tagged triolein in feces in 48 hours

Explanation of Test

Triolein, a fat, is tagged with radioactive iodine (^{131}I) and is given orally to the patient with symptoms of poor fat absorption who is suspected of having pancreatic malfunction or malabsorption syndromes. In this fat-absorption test, samples of blood are drawn at intervals, and the absorbed radioactivity is measured. Absorption of the fat in this test depends on adequate lipolytic enzyme activity and adequate bowel absorption. The pancreas plays a major role in fat absorption. Its enzymes are essential for hydrolysis of nonabsorbable dietary fat into absorbable fractions. It has been suggested that neutral fats are dependent on pancreatic enzymes for absorption, while fatty acids are handled by the small bowel.

Procedure

1. An overnight fast is required; water is permitted.
2. A blocking agent such as Lugol's solution or SSKI (saturated solution of potassium iodide) is administered prior to the test to prevent thyroidal concentration of the radioactive iodine.
3. The radioactive acid is administered orally in a tasteless capsule. Stool collection is begun immediately after administration of the capsule and continued for at least 24 hours.
4. Venous blood samples are drawn at four, five, and six hours after the administration of the tagged triolein.

Clinical Implications

1. Decreased values occur in:
   - (a.) Pancreatic insufficiency
   - (b.) Chronic pancreatitis
   - (c.) Malabsorption syndrome
2. If abnormal results occur, an oleic acid ^{131}I absorption test is often ordered.

Note: Test results are not generally accepted as reliable.

Patient Preparation

1. Explain purpose and procedure of test to patient.
2. Give a written reminder about fasting and stool collection.
3. Collect all stools for 24 hours. Use 24-hour stool collection procedure.

CLINICAL ALERT
1. This test should be done before any x-ray requiring barium sulfate.
2. Patient should receive *no* drugs affecting gastric motility.

OLEIC ACID TEST (^{131}I ABSORPTION TEST)

Normal Values

8–12% in blood in 3–4 hours.

Explanation of Test

This blood-and-stool collection test is performed when the triolein absorption test is abnormal. The test is ordered because the patient exhibits symptoms of poor fat absorption and malfunctioning of the small bowel is suspected.

Oleic acid, which is a sample fatty acid, is tagged with radioactive iodine and given orally. Absorption of the radioactive fatty acid is independent of enzymatic activity and dependent on small bowel absorption only. Absorbed radioactivity is measured in blood samples drawn at intervals and a 24-hour stool collection.

Procedure

1. Patient must fast overnight; water is permitted.
2. A blocking agent such as Lugol's solution or saturated solution of potassium iodine is administered just prior to the test to prevent thyroidal concentration of the radioactive iodine.
3. The radioactive acid is administered orally in a tasteless capsule. After administration of the radioactive tasteless capsule, the patient may be instructed to either fast for four more hours or eat a breakfast which includes buttered toast and whole milk.
4. Stool collection is begun immediately after administration of the capsule and continued for 24 hours.
5. Venous blood samples are drawn at four, five and six hours after the administration of the isotope.

Clinical Implications

Decreased values occur in malabsorption syndromes.
Note: Test results are not generally accepted as reliable.

Interfering Factors

Oily laxatives may cause false positive results.

Patient Preparation

1. Explain purpose and procedure of test to patient.
2. Collect all stools for at least 24 hours (Check with your laboratory for specific time, and follow the 24-hour stool collection procedure. See Chapter 3)
3. Give a written reminder about fasting and stool collection.

CLINICAL ALERT
1. This test must be done before any x-ray requiring barium sulfate.
2. Administer no laxatives during the test.

BLOOD VOLUME DETERMINATION

Normal Values

Total blood volume: 55–80 ml./kg.

Red cell volume: 20–35 ml./kg. (Greater in men than in women)

Plasma volume: 30–45 ml./kg.

Note: Since adipose tissue has a sparser blood supply than lean tissue, the patient's body type can affect the proportion of blood volume to body weight.

Explanation of Test

The purpose of this test is to determine circulating blood volume, to help evaluate the bleeding or debilitated patient, and to determine the origin of hypotension in the presence of anuria or oliguria when dehydration may be the cause. This determination is one way to monitor blood loss during surgery; it is used as a guide in replacement therapy following blood or body fluid loss and in the determination of whole body hematocrit. The results are useful in determining the most appropriate blood component for replacement therapy, *e.g.*, whole blood, plasma, or packed red cells. Blood volume determinations are of value in the following situations:

1. To evaluate gastrointestinal and uterine bleeding
2. To aid in the diagnosis of hypovolemic shock
3. To aid in the diagnosis of polycythemia vera
4. To determine the required blood component for replacement therapy

This test will reveal a decreased blood or plasma volume and decreased total red cell mass. A sample of the patient's blood is mixed with a radioactive substance, incubated at room temperature, and reinjected. Another blood sample is obtained 15 minutes later. The most commonly used tracers in blood volume determination are serum albumin tagged with ^{131}I or ^{125}I and patient or donor RBC's tagged with ^{51}Cr. The total red cell mass and blood volume are calculated, based on hematocrit. The computation is done by an automatic instrument that gives blood volume determinations within 15 minutes to an accuracy of five per cent.

Procedure

1. Record the patient's height and weight. A blood sample is then obtained.
2. A venous blood sample is obtained and then mixed with a radioisotope.
3. Fifteen to 30 minutes later, the blood is reinjected.
4. About 15 minutes later, another venous blood sample is obtained.

Clinical Implications

1. A normal total blood volume with a decreased red cell content would indicate the need for a transfusion of packed red cells.
2. Polycythemia vera may be differentiated from secondary polycythemia:
   - (a.) Increased total blood volume, plasma volume and red cell mass suggest polycythemia vera.
   - (b.) Normal or decreased total blood volume and plasma volume suggest secondary polycythemia.

CLINICAL ALERT
If intravenous therapy is ordered for the same day, the blood volume determination should be done before the IV is started.

Patient Preparation

Instruct patient about purpose and procedure.

RED BLOOD CELL SURVIVAL TIME TEST

Normal Values

RBC survival time of 25 to 35 days. However, a normal value is determined by the nuclear medicine physician/radiologist.

Explanation of Test

This blood test has its greatest use in the evaluation of known or suspected hemolytic anemia and is also indicated when there is an obscure cause for anemia. A sample of the patient's red blood cells is mixed with a radioactive substance (^{51}Cr), incubated at room temperature and reinjected. Blood specimens are drawn at the end of a 24-hour period and at regular intervals for at least three weeks. After counting, the results are plotted and the red cell survival time calculated.

Scanning of the spleen is often done as part of this test. RBC survival is usually ordered in conjunction with blood volume determination.

Procedure

1. A venous blood sample of 20 ml. is obtained.
2. Ten to 30 minutes later, the blood is reinjected after being tagged with a radioisotope, ^{51}Cr.
3. Blood samples are usually obtained at 24 hours, 48 hours, 72 hours, 96 hours, and weekly intervals for three weeks. Time may be shortened depending on the outcome of the test.
   As part of this procedure, a radioactive detector may be used over the spleen, sternum, and liver to assess the relative concentration of radioactivity in these areas. This external counting helps to determine if the spleen is taking part in excessive sequestration of red blood cells as a causative factor in anemia.
4. In some instances a stool collection may be ordered.

Clinical Implications

1. Shortened red cell survival may be the result of:
   (a.) Blood loss
   (b.) Hemolysis
   (c.) Removal of red blood cells by the spleen
2. Prolonged red cell survival time may be the result of abnormality of red cell production
3. If hemolytic anemia is diagnosed, further studies are needed to establish whether RBC's have intrinsic abnor-

malities or whether anemia results from immunologic effects of the patient's plasma.

Patient Preparation

Explain purpose and procedure of the test.

CLINICAL ALERTS
1. The test is usually contraindicated in an actively bleeding patient.
2. Record and report signs of active bleeding.
3. Transfusions should not be given when the test is in progress.
4. Test is contraindicated if there is a history of recent transfusions.

RADIOACTIVE IODINE (RAI) UPTAKE TEST

Normal Values

1–13% absorbed by thyroid gland after 2 hours
2–25% absorbed by thyroid gland after 6 hours
15–45% absorbed by thyroid gland after 24 hours

Explanation of Test

This direct test of the function of the thyroid gland measures the absorption of radioactive iodine (^{131}I) by the thyroid gland. (The test may also measure radioactivity in saliva, urine, and other body fluids.) When radioactive iodine is administered, it is rapidly absorbed into the bloodstream. This procedure measures only the first step in the production of the hormones of the thyroid gland (thyroxin and triiodothyronine). The rate of absorption of the radioactive iodine (which is determined by an increase in radioactivity of the thyroid gland) is a measure of the ability of the thyroid gland to concentrate iodide from the blood plasma.

The patient who is a candidate for this test may have a lumpy or swollen neck or complain of pain in the neck. He may be jittery and ultrasensitive to heat or may be sluggish and ultrasensitive to cold. The test is more useful in the diagnosis of hyperthyroidism than in hypothyroidism.

Procedure

Note: The test is usually done in conjunction with a thyroid scan.

1. A fasting state is preferred. Water, coffee and tea without sugar and cream are permitted.
2. A tasteless capsule of radioiodine or a liquid is administered orally. However, it can be administered intravenously if a quick test is desired. The patient is usually instructed not to eat for one hour after isotope administration.
3. Two, six, and 24 hours later the amount of radioactivity is measured by a scan of the radioactivity in the thyroid gland. There is no pain or discomfort involved.
4. The patient will have to return to the laboratory at the designated time, for the exact time of measurement is crucial in determining uptake.

CLINICAL ALERT
^{131}I uptakes are restricted during pregnancy. Thyroid testing is restricted in pregnancy to blood tests that expose neither the mother or the baby.

Clinical Implications

1. Increased uptake (*e.g.*, 20% in 1 hr; 25% in 6 hrs.; 50% in 24 hrs.) suggests hyperthyroidism.
2. Decreased uptake (*e.g.*, 9% in 2 hrs.; 7% in 6 hrs.; 15% in 24 hrs.) may be caused by hypothyroidism, but it is not diagnostic for hypothyroidism.
   (a.) If the administered iodine is not absorbed as in severe diarrhea or intestinal malabsorption syndromes, the uptake may be low even though the gland is functioning normally.
   (b.) Rapid diuresis during the test period may deplete the

supply of iodine, causing an apparently low percentage of iodine uptake.

(c.) In renal failure the uptake may be high, even though the gland is functioning normally.

3. The test is contraindicated in pregnant or lactating women, children, and infants.

Interfering Factors

1. The chemicals, drugs, and foods that interfere with the test by *lowering uptake* are:

(a.) Iodized salt and iodine-containing drugs, such as Lugol's solution, expectorants (S.S.K.I.); saturated solution of potassium iodide; vitamin preparations that contain minerals; suntan lotions and nail polish. (1–3 weeks duration time of the effect of these substances in the body)

(b.) Radiographic contrast media such as Diodrast (iodopyracet), Hypaque (sodium diatrizoate), Renografin, Lipiodal, Ethiodol, Pantopaque (isophendylate), Telepaque (iopanoic acid) (one week to a year or more). Consult with Nuclear Medicine Laboratory for specific times.

(c.) Antithyroid drugs, such as propylthiouracil and related compounds (2–10 days)

(d.) Thyroid medications such as desiccated thyroid, thyroxine (1–2 weeks)

(e.) Miscellaneous drugs: thiocyanate, perchlorate, nitrates, sulfonamides, orinase, corticosteroids, PAS, isoniazid, Butazolidin (phenylbutazone), Pentothal (thiopental), antihistamines, ACTH, aminosalicylic acid, amphenone, cobalt, coumarin anticoagulants.

(f.) Foods:
  (1.) Cabbage
  (2.) Enriched breakfast cereals

2. The compounds and conditions that interfere by *enhancing uptake* are:

(a.) TSH (d.) Barbiturates
(b.) Estrogens (e.) Lithium carbonate
(c.) Cirrhosis (f.) Phenothiazines (1 week)

Patient Preparation

1. Instruct the patient about the purpose of the test and the test procedure.
2. Advise him that iodine intake is restricted for at least one week before testing.

THYROID STIMULATION TEST;
TSH (THYROID STIMULATING HORMONE) TEST

Normal Values

TSH: Less than $5\mu U/ml$.

In normal individuals, T_4 and RAI uptake is increased within 8 to 10 hours after TSH is given.

Explanation of Test

This is a radioimmunoassay test that is used in conjunction with the RAI uptake test. It is done to differentiate primary from secondary hypothyroidism and to determine the level of thyroid gland activity. The thyroid gland may have impaired RAI uptake because of intrinsic disease (primary hypothyroidism) or insufficient stimulation by the pituitary gland (secondary hypothyroidism). Patients who have a decreased amount of functioning thyroid gland, as in subtotal thyroidectomy radiation therapy or thyroiditis, may have a normal RAI uptake and still fail to respond to TSH stimulation. Such persons have a low thyroid reserve and need continued observation to prevent myxedema.

The responsiveness of the thyroid gland to the administration of TSH (thyrotropin) is measured. The TSH test can be used even if the patient is receiving thyroid replacement therapy, but iodine intake will invalidate ^{131}I uptake results and may antagonize TSH stimulation.

Procedure

1. An intramuscular injection of TSH (bovine) is given.
2. Blood samples will be obtained at intervals. Check with your laboratory for specific procedure.

Clinical Implications

1. Thyroid-Stimulating Hormone (TSH) is increased in the following conditions:
    - (a.) Primary untreated hypothyroidism (increase ranges from 3 times normal to 100 times normal in severe myxedema).
    - (b.) Hashimoto's thyroiditis
2. TSH is normal in the following conditions:
    - (a.) Secondary hypothyroidism
        - (1.) Hypothalamic hypothyroidism
        - (2.) Pituitary hypothyroidism
3. TSH cannot be detected in thyrotoxicosis.
4. There is no response to TSH administration in cases of diminished thyroid reserve.

Interfering Factors

Iodine intake will invalidate ^{131}I uptake results.

T_3 AND T_4 RESIN UPTAKE TEST
AND THYROID BINDING GLOBULIN (TBG) TEST

Normal Values

T_3	25–35%
TBG	0.9–1.1
T_4	3.8–11.4%

Explanation of Test

These *in vitro* tests are used to diagnose thyroid disorders using radioimmunoassay techniques in the laboratory. (No radioactive substance is administered to the patient.)

Triiodothyronine (T_3) and thyroxine (T_4) are hormones synthesized and released by the thyroid gland to influence metabolic processes and the rate of growth by increasing oxygen consumption and heat production in the tissue. The levels of T_3 and T_4 in the blood regulate the thyroid stimulating hormone (TSH) secreted by the anterior pituitary gland. In a healthy individual a checks and balances system of negative feedback is established.

The TBG test follows the clinical state of the patient very closely. As the hyperthyroid patient improves with treatment, the TBI increases to more normal levels.

Procedure

A venous blood sample is obtained.

Clinical Implications

1. T_3 (Triiodothyronine) is increased in hyperthyroidism.
   T_3 level is decreased in hypothyroidism.
2. T_4 (thyroxine) levels are decreased in myxedema.
   T_4 levels are increased in hyperthyroidism.
3. TBG is decreased in hyperthyroidism.
   TBG is increased in hypothyroidism.

Interfering Factors

1. Triiodothyronine (T_3) Levels
   (a.) Conditions that have been shown to *decrease the levels of T_3* include menstruation, normal pregnancy, and liver disease. Drugs that may *increase the levels of T3* include ACTH, anabolic agents, androgens, anticoagulants (oral, corticosteroids, dextrothyroxine, diphenylhydantoin, heparin, phenylbutazone, salicylates (high doses) thyroid therapy.
   (b.) Drugs or conditions that have been shown to *increase the levels of T_3* include liver disease, severe nephrosis, atrial arrhythmias and fibrillation, metastatic cancer, COPD with CO_2 retention, polycythemia vera, uremia, threatened abortion, infancy, heparin, heroin withdrawal, methadone, dicumarol, salicylates, prednisone, phenylbutazone, diphenylhydantoxin, large doses of penicillin, testosterone, dextrothyroxine, and thyroid.

(c.) Drugs that may *decrease the levels of T_3* include ACTH, antithyroid drugs, BAL, chlordiazepoxide, corticosteroids, estrogens, ipodate, perphenazine, oral contraceptives, thiazide diuretics, and sulfonylureas.
2. Thyroxine (T_4) Levels
   (a.) Drugs or conditions that have been shown to *increase T_4 levels* include pregnancy, residual radioactivity from other tests, clofibrate, diethylstilbestrol, estradiol, estrogens, oral contraceptives, progestins, perphenazine.
   (b.) Drugs that have been shown to *decrease T_4 levels* include aminosalicylic acid, cortisone, lithium, methylthiouracil, sulfonamides, chlorpromazine, reserpine, prednisone, testosterone, heparin, tolbutamide, and diphenylhydantoin.
3. Thyroid binding globulin (TBG) levels:
   (a.) Drugs that have been known to *increase TBG levels* include Chlormadinone and oral contraceptives.
   (b.) Drugs that have been known to *decrease TBG levels* include anabolic agents and androgens.

REFERENCES

Belcher, E. H., and Vetter, H. (eds.): RADIOISOTOPES IN MEDICAL DIAGNOSIS. London, Butterworths, 1971.

Berkow, Robert (ed.): THE MERCK MANUAL OF DIAGNOSIS AND THERAPY. 13th Ed., Rahway, N.J., Merck Sharp & Dohme Research Laboratories, 1977.

Brucer, Marshall: WHAT EVERY YOUNG NURSE SHOULD KNOW ABOUT NUCLEAR MEDICINE. St. Louis, Malinckrodt, Inc., 1974.

Brucer, Marshall: WHAT YOU CAN EXPECT FROM YOUR BRAIN SCAN. St. Louis, Malinckrodt, Inc., 1974.

Brucer, Marshall: WHAT YOU CAN EXPECT FROM YOUR BONE SCAN. St. Louis, Malinckrodt, Inc., 1974.

Collins, R. Douglas: ILLUSTRATED MANUAL OF LABORATORY DIAGNOSIS. 2nd Ed., Philadelphia, J. B. Lippincott Company, 1975.

Freeman, Leonard, M., and Blaufox, Donald, M. PHYSICIAN'S DESK REFERENCE FOR RADIOLOGY AND NUCLEAR MEDICINE. Oradell, N.J., Medical Economics, 1975.

Spencer, Richard P.: NUCLEAR MEDICINE—FOCUS ON CLINICAL DIAGNOSIS. Flushing, N.Y., Medical Examination Publishing Company, Inc., 1977.

Wallach, Jacques: INTERPRETATION OF DIAGNOSTIC TESTS—A HANDBOOK SYNOPSIS OF LABORATORY MEDICINE. 3rd Ed., Boston, Little, Brown and Company, 1978.

Watner, Henry N. (ed.): NUCLEAR MEDICINE. New York, H. P. Publishing Company, Inc., 1975.

9 □ □ COMMON X-RAY PROCEDURES

INTRODUCTION

General Principles

X-ray studies (also known as radiographs or roentgenograms) are used to examine the soft and bony tissues of the body. X-rays (roentgen rays) are electromagnetic vibrations of very short wavelength produced when fast-moving electrons hit various substances. They are similar to light rays except that their wavelength is only 1/10,000 the length of visible light rays. Because of their short wavelength, x-rays have the ability to penetrate very dense substances and to produce an image or shadow that can be recorded on photographic film. The entire principle of radiography depends on differences between different body structures, which produce shadows of varying intensity on the x-ray film.

In x-ray examinations (radiographic studies), a high-voltage electric current is passed through a "target" made of tungsten in a vacuum tube. Less than one per cent of the high-speed electrons (cathode rays) are transformed into x-rays; the rest of the energy is transformed into heat.

X-rays travel in straight lines at the speed of light. When a beam of rays passes through matter, its intensity is reduced by absorption. The denser the matter, the greater the absorption. A photographic film is affected by x-rays the same as it is affected by light. The sensitive silver emulsion of the film turns black when it has been exposed to the radiation. The film is subsequently processed by development and fixation. When an x-ray beam of suitable intensity and wavelength is passed through the part of the body being studied, an image will be produced and brought out by the developing process. This image will be an accurate representation of the variable densities of the tissue through which the beam has passed.

Use of Contrast Media

Many radiographic techniques can utilize the natural contrasts that exist in body tissue—air, water (in soft tissue), fat, and bone. The lungs and gastrointestinal tract normally contain gases; certain body structures are encased in a fatty envelope, and bone has naturally occurring mineral salts. However, diagnosis of certain pathologic conditions at times requires the visualization of details not revealed through plain film radiography. These details can be highlighted through administration of *contrast media,* which can be inserted orally, rectally, or through injection.

The ideal contrast medium should be harmless, inert, and should not interfere with any physiologic function. It may be either radiopaque (not permitting the transmission of x-rays) or radiolucent (permitting the transmission of x-rays but still offering some resistance).

Certain contrast media are used routinely in radiographic studies:

1. Barium sulfate (radiopaque)
   - (a.) Used in gastrointestinal studies
   - (b.) Prepared in a colloidal suspension
   - (c.) Effectively demonstrates small filling defects
2. Organic iodides (radiopaque)
   - (a.) Examples: Sodium diatrizoate, meglucamine diatrizoate
   - (b.) Used for studies of the kidney, liver, blood vessels, urinary bladder, and urethra.
3. Iodized Oils (radiopaque)
   - (a.) Used in myelography (study of the spinal cord after contrast media have been injected) or bronchography (study of the lung after contrast media have been injected).
4. Oxygen, helium, air, carbon dioxide, nitrous oxide, and nitrogen (radiolucent substances)
   - (a.) Used for visualization of the brain, joints, subarachnoid space, pleural space, peritoneal cavity, and pericardial space

Adverse Reactions to Contrast Media

The administration of contrast media can sometimes cause allergic reactions in certain individuals. The degree of reaction may range from mild (causing such symptoms as nausea and vomiting) to severe (causing cardiovascular collapse, CNS depression, and death, if untreated).

Below is a table indicating the range of possible adverse reactions to contrast media:

TABLE 9–1. SIGNS AND SYMPTOMS OF REACTIONS TO CONTRAST MATERIAL*

Type	Cardio-vascular	Respira-tory	Cutaneous	Gastro-intestinal	Nervous	Urinary
Mild	Pallor Diaphoresis	Sneezing Coughing	Erythema Feeling of	Nausea Vomiting	Anxiety Head-ache	
	Tachycardia	Rhinorrhea	warmth	Metallic taste	Dizziness	
Interme-diate	Bradycardia Palpitations Hypotension	Wheezing Acute asthma attack	Urticaria Pruritus	Abdominal cramps Diarrhea	Agitation Vertigo Slurred speech	Oliguria
Severe	Acute pulmonary edema Shock Congestive heart failure Cardiac arrest	Laryngo-spasm Cyanosis Laryngeal edema Apnea	Angio-neurotic edema	Paralytic ileus	Disorien-tation Stupor Coma Convul-sions	Acute renal failure

*From Daffner, Richard H.: Introduction to Clinical Radiology—A CORRELA-TIVE APPROACH TO DIAGNOSTIC IMAGING. St. Louis, The C. V. Mosby Co., 1978.

CLINICAL ALERT
If a patient experiences a *severe* reaction to contrast media, his cardiopulmonary status must be determined, and the technical staff in attendance must be able to give cardiopulmonary resuscitation (CPR).

The patient who has had an allergic reaction to contrast media should have this fact noted on his medical records. Such a patient can possibly have subsequent adverse reactions.

Tomography: Overview

Tomography is also known as *body section radiography, planigraphy, laminography,* and *stratigraphy.* These terms refer to a method of x-ray examination that is based on geometric principles. With this method it is possible to examine a single layer, plane, or level of tissue and to blur the tissues above and below this level by motion to make the other tissues (above and below) almost invisible. This effect is obtained by moving the x-ray tube in one direction while the film is moved simultaneously in the other, with the patient remaining still. The technique allows more detail to be visualized such as when there is a small cavity within a mass. Tomography is commonly used in examination of the chest and bones.

The most common organs and structures now examined by tomography are the chest and lung, the paranasal sinuses, the spine, the hands, the ankles, the cardiovascular system, the biliary system, the kidney, the mastoids, the optic canal, and the lacrimal passages. Surgeons use it as an aid in surgery, especially for small areas.

Most of the tests take at least 45 minutes to complete. The biliary system examination is the lengthiest, requiring one to three hours. This examining time depends on the person examined and the function of the biliary tract. Since barium interferes with tomographic studies, tomograms should be scheduled prior to x-rays using barium contrast. Tomograms may be ordered with an IVP or IV cholecystogram in which a radiopaque iodine substance is injected intravenously sometime during the exam.

Xeroradiography: Overview

Xeroradiography differs from traditional x-ray examinations in that the image is created on a photoconductive surface of selenium rather than on a silver halide film. The selenium plate is housed in a cassette to protect it from rough handling and from light.

Xeroradiography is a photoelectric process; traditional film radiography is primarily a photochemical process. This relatively new technique uses the technology of the Xerox office copier to process x-ray images on paper.

Several distinct advantages exist in the use of this method: (1) it is more accurate, for there is greater resolution of the image; (2) small point densities can be easily distinguished because of greater contrast; and (3) the xeroradiographs are easily interpreted.

Xeroradiography has been found useful in radiography of the extremities and especially in soft-tissue studies. Radiographic study of the breast is the prime use of this technique. Patient exposure during a xeromammogram is less than 1 rad (radiation absorbed dose). Prior to the discovery of this technique, mammograms were taken using industrial film which resulted in a much higher radiation dosage for the patient.

Computed Tomography (CT): Overview

Computed tomography (CT), also called CT scanning, computerized axial tomography (CAT) and EMI scanning, uses x-rays similar to those used in conventional radiography but with a special machine having a scanner system. The x-rays in conventional radiography pass through the body, and an image of bone, soft tissues, and air is projected onto film. In CT scans, a computer provides rapid complex calculations determining the degree of multiple x-ray beams that are not absorbed by all the tissue in its path. The single most valuable function of CT scanning is to provide the geography and characteristics of tissue structures within solid organs.

Computed tomography may eventually replace isotope scanning of all organs and structures of the body. This will occur when enough special machines* are built to meet the demand and when adequate funds exist to pay for the machines.*

RISKS OF RADIATION

Exposure of the human body to x-rays carries certain risks. These risks are of two types: (1) genetic, and (2) somatic. If the genital organs are exposed to radiation, the reproductive cells (specifically, the chromosomes) may undergo mutations. These mutations can cause changes in the offspring of the patient. Somatic changes (those occurring in body tissue other than the

---

*The first company to develop the technology for CT scanning was Emitronics Limited of England (1972). By 1974, the Pfizer Medical Systems in the U.S. was also manufacturing scanners. By now, over 15 companies throughout the world are in the field of producing these devices.

reproductive cells) may occur in parts of the patient's body receiving excessive doses of radiation or receiving repeated exposure of the same bodily structures.

The dangers of exposure to radiation arise not only from the absorption of relatively large amounts of radiation received over a short period of time, but also from the cumulative effects of very small amounts received over months or years. Moreover, the cumulative effects of radiation may not become evident for several years.

A woman in the first trimester of pregnancy is especially at risk. A developing embryo or fetus that is exposed to ionizing radiation is very likely to be born with abnormalities.

Safety Measures

Certain precautions must be taken to protect medical/nursing personnel, patients, and any technical staff assisting in the x-ray examination from unnecessary exposure to radiation.

General Precautions

1. Patients, radiologists, and other staff in the radiology laboratory should wear lead aprons and gloves. The lead aprons may be full-body aprons or may cover the genital organs.
2. The x-ray tube housing should be checked periodically to prevent leakage.
3. The patient's medical records should be carefully checked to determine the frequency of diagnostic radiologic examinations and the dosage received with each study.
4. X-ray tubes should have additional layers of aluminum to act as a filtering device that will reduce the exposure to radiation without sacrificing detail.
5. Fast film as well as a screen enhancing the action of x-rays should be used.
6. Adjustable or fixed cones as well as diaphragms can be used to reduce exposure to the lowest possible level. These devices will restrict the area being radiated, avoiding excessive peripheral exposure.

Precautions to be Used with Pregnant Patients

1. Women of childbearing age who could possibly be in the first trimester of pregnancy should *not* have x-ray exam-

inations. A brief menstrual history should be taken to determine if the woman is or could be pregnant. If any doubt exists about whether the woman is pregnant, she should *not* risk having the exam.

2. Some radiology departments apply the *"ten-day rule"* to all female patients between the ages of 13 and 45: They consider such patients pregnant unless proven otherwise. These patients can be x-rayed only during the interval of not more than ten days following the onset of the menstrual period. If this rule is adhered to, the radiologist nearly eliminates the risk of irradiating a vulnerable embryo or fetus.

3. Pregnant patients (at any time during the pregnancy) should avoid radiographic studies of the pelvic region, lumbar spine, abdomen, or procedures involving serial film or fluoroscopy.

4. If films are made for obstetric reasons, *repeat films* should be avoided.

5. If x-ray studies are made of body parts other than the pelvic area (*e.g.*, x-rays of the teeth), the woman should wear a lead apron to cover the abdominal and pelvic regions.

CHEST RADIOGRAPHY

Normal Values

Normal chest:
1. Normal bony thorax (all the bones present position and symmetry and shape)
2. Normal soft tissues
3. Normal mediastinum
4. Normal lungs (proper number of lobes, position and alteration)
5. Normal pleura
6. Normal heart (aortic arch and abdominal arteries)

Explanation of Test

The chest x-ray is the radiograph requested most freauently. More than half the x-ray studies done are of the chest. This type of x-ray is very important in the diagnosis of pulmonary disease and diseases of the mediastinium and bony thorax. The chest x-ray is also a record of the presence or absence of disease on the date it was taken and any x-rays that follow this date determine progress or development of the disease. This study can also give valuable information on the condition of the heart, lung, gastrointestinal tract, and thyroid gland.

Procedure

1. Routine x-ray consists of at least a front and side view of the chest. It is usually performed with the patient in a standing position. Upright films of the chest are of utmost importance, for films taken with the patient supine will not demonstrate fluid levels. This is especially important to observe when testing persons confined to bed.
2. Clothing is removed to the waist.
3. The patient is asked to take a deep breath and exhale; then he is required to take a deep breath and hold it while the picture is taken.
4. The procedure takes only a few minutes.

Clinical Implications

1. Abnormal results will indicate these conditions of the lungs:
   - (a.) Aplasia
   - (b.) Hypoplasia
   - (c.) Cysts
   - (d.) Lobar pneumonia
   - (e.) Bronchopneumonia
   - (f.) Aspiration pneumonia
   - (g.) Pulmonary brucellosis
   - (h.) Viral pneumonia
   - (i.) Lung abscess
   - (j.) Middle lobe syndrome
   - (k.) Pneumothorax
   - (l.) Pleural effusion
   - (m.) Atelectasis
   - (n.) Pneumonitis
   - (o.) Congenital pulmonary cysts
   - (p.) Pulmonary tuberculosis
   - (q.) Sarcoidosis
2. Abnormal results will indicate these conditions of the bony thorax:
   - (a.) Scoliosis
   - (b.) Hemivertebrae
   - (c.) Kyphosis
   - (d.) Trauma
   - (e.) Sarcoma
   - (f.) Bone destruction

Interfering Factors

An important consideration in interpreting chest radiographs is whether the film is in "full inspiration." Certain conditions do not allow the patient to inspire fully. The following conditions should be considered when radiographs are evaluated:
1. Obesity
2. Severe pain
3. Congestive heart failure
4. Scarring of lung tissue

CHEST TOMOGRAPHY

Normal Values

Same as for chest x-ray

Explanation of Test

Chest tomograms are particularly useful in the study of patients with pulmonary tuberculosis, the compressed lung beneath a thoracoplasty, and study of lung abscess. It is also used to outline detailed anatomy of the lung, mediastinum, and thoracic structures in which an abnormality is observed in the chest film and to outline the vascular pattern in emphysema, pulmonary hypertension, and pulmonary vascular abnormalities.

Clinical Implications

1. Abnormal results will reveal:
    (a) Cavities and nodular infiltration in tuberculosis that is not visible in routine x-rays
    (b) Bronchiectasis associated with tuberculosis
    (c) Outline of tumor in patients with bronchogenic carcinoma
    (d) Calcium in small parenchymal nodules
    (e) Site of a bronchial occlusion

PARANASAL SINUSES RADIOGRAPHY AND TOMOGRAPHY

Normal Values

Normal sinuses are radiolucent because of their air content. The paranasal sinuses are paired cavities lined by mucous membranes that arise as outpouchings from the nasal fossa and extend into the maxillary, ethmoid, sphenoid, and frontal bones. They are named according to the bones in which they develop.

Explanation of Test

Radiographs of the sinuses are to detect the unilateral or bilateral diseases which may affect them and which may cause detectable alterations. Tomograms of the sinuses are usually done to outline foreign bodies, to determine the presence or extent of bony tumor involvement, and to determine the extent and location of fractures of the bony walls of the sinuses and nasal bones.

Procedure

1. If possible, the patient should be in an upright sitting position during the examination of the sinuses. This will allow demonstration of fluid levels when they are present.
2. The patient is usually required to have his head put into a vise during the exam. This does not hurt; the braces are generally comfortable.
3. The exam may take 10 to 15 minutes to complete.

Clinical Implications

1. Abnormal results will reveal
   (a) Acute sinusitis
   (b) Chronic sinusitis
   (c) Cysts (retention and nonsecreting)
   (d) Mucocele
   (e) Polyps
   (f) Tumors of the bone and soft tissue
   (g) Allergic reactions
   (h) Trauma
   (i) Foreign bodies

Patient Preparation

Explain purpose and procedure of test.

CARDIAC RADIOGRAPHY

Normal Values

Normal size and shape of heart, aorta, pulmonary arteries, and pulmonary vascularity

Explanation of Test

Diagnosis of cardiovascular disorders may involve a wide range of diagnostic procedures. There are, however, three routine radiographic imaging techniques that are used for the evaluation of the heart:
1. Plain film radiography
2. Fluoroscopy
3. Cardiac series

The heart may also be evaluated by more sophisticated radiographic studies (*e.g.*, cardiac catheterization) or by procedures that are discussed in more detail in other chapters (*e.g.* ultrasound studies; radioisotope scans).

Use of Routine Procedures

Plain Film Radiography:
1. Routine screening technique with all suspected cardiac patients
2. Useful for determining cardiac size

Fluoroscopic Examination:
1. For assessing heart motion and dynamics
2. For determining whether calcification exists in heart
3. For investigating suspected pericardial effusion
4. For verifying position of pacemaker electrodes
5. For guiding movement of catheter in cardiac catheterization

Cardiac Series:

This radiographic procedure is a four-view exam. Generally,

the patient will be asked to swallow barium during the following views:

1. Posteroanterior view
2. Lateral view
3. Right anterior oblique view
4. Left anterior oblique view

Cardioangiography (Angiography of the Heart):

This procedure is technically very difficult and places the patient at risk. A large quantity of contrast material must be introduced rapidly into the blood vessels, and films must be rapidly exposed so that the blood vessels can be visualized. A radiopaque contrast material containing iodine is injected directly into one of the heart chambers, the greater vessels, or the coronary arteries via a catheter.

Note: Cardioangiography is the most invasive, and thus the most potentially dangerous of all the diagnostic procedures. In many medical facilities, the technique is being replaced by CT scanning and by echocardiography.

Procedure

1. The procedure entails the catheterization of a blood vessel, usually in the arm, under fluoroscopy.
2. The catheter is guided into the heart chamber.
3. Once positioned, contrast is rapidly injected while serial films or motion films are taken.
4. If the chambers and valves of the right side of the heart are to be demonstrated, a vein is catheterized.
5. If the left side of the heart is to be studied, an artery is catheterized. (Also, see p. 695 in Chapter 14 on special tests of cardiovascular system.)

Clinical Implications

1. Abnormal results will indicate:
    (a.) Enlargement of the heart
    (b.) Congenital heart disease
    (c.) Anomalies of the aortic arch and its large branches

(d.) Congenital anomalies of the pulmonary artery and its branches
(e.) Mitral valve disease
(f.) Aortic valve disease
(g.) Pulmonary valve disease
(h.) Tricuspid valve disease
(i.) Hypertensive cardiovascular disease
(j.) Arteriosclerotic heart disease
(k.) Cor pulmonale
(l.) Condition of heart and lungs in congestive failure
(m.) Cardiac injuries
(n.) Tumors of the heart
(o.) Arteriosclerosis of aorta
(p.) Aortic aneurysm
(q.) Syphilitic aortitis
(r.) Traumatic aneurysm
(s.) Dissecting aneurysm
(t.) Pericarditis
(u.) Spontaneous pneumopericardium

Patient Preparation

(for cardioangiography)
1. The patient is not allowed any food or liquid for 12 hours prior to the examination.
2. Advise the patient that he may experience headache and discomfort at the site of the puncture.
3. The patient must sign a written consent form for administration of anesthetic.

Patient Aftercare

(for cardioangiography)
1. The patient's activities must be limited for 12 hours after the examination.
2. The patient's vital signs must be checked every 15 minutes until his condition has stabilized.
3. Check for bleeding at the site of the puncture.

CLINICAL ALERT
Emergency equipment should be available for resuscitation.

ABDOMINAL PLAIN FILM
or
KUB (KIDNEY, URETERS, AND BLADDER)

Normal Values

Normal abdominal structures

Explanation of Test

This radiographic study, which does *not* use contrast media, is done to diagnose intra-abdominal diseases such as nephrolithiasis, intestinal obstruction, soft tissue masses, or a ruptured viscus. It is also the preliminary step in the examination of the gastrointestinal tract, the gallbladder, or the urinary tract. The study is done before an IVP or before any renal study. It is also useful in the study of abnormal accumulations of gas and of ascites within the GI tract and of the size, shape, and position of the liver, spleen and kidneys. This type of x-ray is also called a "scout film" and was formerly called the "flat plate."

Procedure

1. Patient is not required to fast.
2. During the test the patient lies on his back on an x-ray table. He may also have a second film taken when he is standing or sitting.
3. If the patient cannot sit or stand, he is asked to lie on his left side with his right side up.
4. There is no discomfort involved, and the x-ray takes only a few minutes.

Clinical Implications

1. Abnormal results will reveal:
   - (a.) Calcium in blood vessels, lymph nodes, cysts, tumors, or stones
   - (b.) Ureters cannot be defined, but calculi may be detected along the course of the ureters.
   - (c.) The shadow cast by the urinary bladder can often be identified, especially when it contains urine of a high specific gravity along with fusion anomalies and horseshoe kidneys.
   - (d.) Abnormal size, shape, and position of kidney
   - (e.) Presence of appendicolithiasis
   - (f.) Presence of foreign bodies
   - (g.) Abnormal fluid; ascites

Interfering Factors

Because of the interference of barium, this exam should be done prior to any barium studies.

Patient Preparation

Explain the purpose and procedure of the test to the patient.

CLINICAL ALERT
Abdominal plain films are not useful with conditions such as esophageal varices and bleeding peptic ulcer.

GASTRIC RADIOGRAPHY (INCLUDING UPPER GI EXAMINATION)

Normal Values

Normal size, contour, motility and peristalsis of the stomach

Explanation of Test

This x-ray and fluoroscopic examination is done to visualize the form and position, mucosal folds, peristaltic activity, and motility of the stomach.

Preliminary film without contrast media is useful in detecting perforation, presence of metallic foreign substances, thickening of the gastric wall, and displacement of the gastric air bubble, indicating a mass outside of the stomach wall.

The use of an oral contrast substance such as barium sulfate or Gastrografin (meglucamine diatrizoate), will demonstrate a hiatal hernia, pyloric stenosis, gastric diverticulitis, undigested food, gastritis, congenital anomalies (*e.g.*, dextroposition and duplication), and diseases of the stomach (*e.g.*, gastric ulcer, cancer, and stomach polyps).

If this exam includes the esophagus and upper part of the jejunum, it is called the upper GI examination.

Procedure

1. The patient lies on the examining table in the x-ray department while a preliminary film is made.
2. The patient swallows the chalk-flavored contrast substance while standing in front of the fluoroscopy machine. All of the chalky substance must be swallowed.
3. The contrast agent swallow is followed by x-rays. 24 hour films may also be taken.
4. Examining time is 45 minutes.

Clinical Implications

1. Abnormal results will reveal:

   (a) Congenital anomalies   (f) Foreign bodies
   (b) Gastric ulcer   (g) Gastric diverticula
   (c) Carcinoma of stomach   (h) Pyloric stenosis
   (d) Gastric polyps   (i) Hiatus hernia
   (e) Gastritis   (j) Volvulus of the stomach

   Note: Displacement of the gastric air bubble may indicate the existence of an extrinsic mass, or the normal contour of it may be deformed by intrinsic tumor.

Interfering Factors

1. Because of poor physical condition of the patient, examination is sometimes difficult, and it may be impossible to adequately visualize all parts of the stomach.
2. Retention of food and fluid residues may cause difficulty and lead to errors.

Patient Preparation

1. Instruct patient about the purpose and procedure of the test. Give a written reminder.
2. No food or liquid is permitted from midnight until the examination is completed.

Patient Aftercare

1. Provide fluids, food, and rest after the test.
2. Administer laxatives if ordered. If barium sulfate or meglucamine diatrizoate is used during the exam, a laxative should be taken after the procedure.
3. Observe and record stools for color and consistency to determine that all of the barium has been evacuated.

SMALL INTESTINE RADIOGRAPHY AND FLUOROSCOPY

Normal Values

Normal contour, position, and motility of the small intestine.

Explanation of Test

This radiographic and fluoroscopic study is done to diagnose diseases of the small bowel (*e.g.*, ulcerative colitis, tumors, active bleeding, or obstruction). The patient swallows a contrast material such as barium sulfate or meglucamine diatrizoate to aid in the diagnosis of Meckel's diverticulum, congenital atresia, obstruction, filling defects, regional enteritis, lymphoid hyperplasia, tuberculosis of small intestine (malabsorption syndrome), sprue, Whipple's disease, intussusception, and edema. This test is usually scheduled in conjunction with an upper GI exam.

The mesenteric small intestine begins at the duodenojejunal junction and ends at the ileocecal valve. The mesenteric small intestine is not included routinely as part of the upper gastrointestinal study (upper GI).

Procedure

1. A preliminary plain film study is made while the patient lies on the examining table.
2. While in a standing position in front of the fluoroscopy machine, the patient swallows a chalky contrast material. (All of the chalky substance must be swallowed.)
3. The contrast agent swallow is followed by x-rays. Timed films are taken, usually every 30 minutes.
4. Examining time is variable. The exam is not completed until the ileocecal value has filled with contrast. This may take several minutes (for those patients having a bypass) or several hours.

Clinical Implications

1. Abnormal results will indicate
   - (a.) Anomalies of the small intestine
   - (b.) Errors of rotation
   - (c.) Meckel's diverticulum
   - (d.) Atresia
   - (e.) Neoplasms
   - (f.) Regional enteritis
   - (g.) Tuberculosis
   - (h.) Malabsorption syndrome
   - (i.) Intussusception
   - (j.) Round worms (ascariasis)
   - (k.) Intra-abdominal hernias

Interfering Factors

1. Delays in motility in the small intestine can be due to:
   (a.) Use of morphine
   (b.) Patients with severe or poorly controlled diabetes
2. Increases in motility in the small intestine can be due to:
   (a.) Fear
   (b.) Excitement
   (c.) Nausea

Patient Preparation

1. Instruct patient about purpose of the test and the procedure. Give a written reminder.
2. Advise patient that no food or liquids are permitted from midnight until the examination is completed.

Patient Aftercare

1. Provide fluids, food, and rest after the examination.
2. Administer laxatives if ordered. If a barium sulfate swallow is used during the exam, a laxative should be taken after the exam is finished.
3. Check stools for color and consistency to determine that all the barium has been evacuated.

BARIUM ENEMA COLON RADIOGRAPHY; AIR-CONTRAST STUDY

Normal Values

Normal position, contour, filling, rate of passage of barium, movement, and patency of colon.

Explanation of Test

This examination of the large intestine, or colon uses x-rays and fluoroscopy to visualize the position, filling, and movement of the divisions of the colon. It is an aid in determining the presence or absence of disease such as diverticulitis, cancer, polyps, colitis, any form of obstruction, and active bleeding. Barium or hypaque are used as contrast media and are instilled through a rectal tube. The radiologist observes the barium through a fluoroscope as it flows into the large intestine. X-rays are taken.

For a satisfactory examination the colon must be cleansed thoroughly of fecal matter. This is most important if a search is being made for a source of bleeding. The accurate identification of small polyps is possible only when there are no confusing shadows caused by retained lumps of stool.

If polyp formation is suspected, an "air contrast colon" exam may be ordered. The procedure for this test is basically the same as the barium enema. However, it does require that more complex radiographs be taken in several positions. A "double contrast" of air and barium are instilled into the colon under fluoroscopy.

Procedure

1. In the x-ray department, the patient is asked to lie on his back while a preliminary film is made.
2. The patient lies on his side, and the barium is introduced by enema.
3. The patient is instructed to retain barium until x-rays are taken. Following fluoroscopic examination, which includes several "spot films, conventional x-ray films are taken. After completion of the films, the patient is asked to go into the bathroom to expel the barium. After evacuation, another film is made.
4. Total examining time is one and one quarter hours.

Clinical Implications

1. Abnormal results will indicate:

   (a.) Lesions
   (b.) Obstructions
   (c.) Megacolons
   (d.) Fistulae
   (e.) Inflammatory changes
   (f.) Diverticulae
   (g.) Chronic ulcerative colitis
   (h.) Stenosis
   (i.) Right-sided colitis
   (j.) Hernias
   (k.) Polyps
   (l.) Intussusception
   (m.) Carcinoma

2. Size, position, and motility of the appendix can be determined by this examination, however, a diagnosis of chronic appendicitis *cannot* be made from x-ray findings. A diagnosis of appendicitis is made from the presence of typical signs and symptoms.

Interfering Factors

A poorly cleansed bowel is the most common interfering factor. Unless fecal matter is satisfactorily cleansed from the colon, small polyps or a source of blockage will not show up well on the x-ray.

Patient Preparation

1. Explain the purpose and procedure of the test to the patient.
2. Give a written reminder of the following instructions:
    (a.) A clear liquid diet is taken at the evening meal.
    (b.) Laxatives and enemas will be given in order to obtain the clearest possible x-rays.
    (c.) No food is to be eaten after the evening meal, and no liquids are to be taken from midnight until the examination is completed. Oral medications are not permitted.

Patient Aftercare

1. Provide food, fluids, and rest after the examination is completed. This examination is the most fatigue producing of all x-ray studies. Patients may be weak, thirsty, or tired after the test is finished.
2. A laxative should be given for at least two days following the x-ray studies or until stools are normal in consistency and color.
3. Stools must be checked and recorded for color and consistency for at least two days in order to determine whether all the barium has been evacuated. Stools will be light in color

until all barium has been expelled. Outpatients should be given a written reminder to inspect stools for two days.

CLINICAL ALERT
1. When barium studies are ordered, constipating narcotics, especially codeine, should be avoided, if possible, because of the tendency of these drugs to interfere with the elimination of barium from the gastrointestinal tract. Check with physician about the possibility of using nonconstipating analgesics during the examining period.
2. Barium studies may interfere with many other studies. Check with radiology department for sequence of exams. Many abdominal exams, including some x-rays, radioisotope scans, and ultrasound studies and proctoscopy must be scheduled prior to barium x-rays.
3. A judgment should be made about the administration of cathartics or enemas in the presence of acute abdominal pain, ulcerative colitis, or obstruction. Consult the physician or radiology department and consider the following points:
   (a.) When giving enemas, remember that introducing large quantities of water into the bowel should be avoided in patients with megacolon because of the danger of water intoxication. In general, patients with toxic megacolon should *not* be given enemas.
   (b.) If any obstruction is suspected in the colon, the water from large enemas may be reabsorbed and impaction can occur.
   (c.) If there is an obstruction in the rectum, it will be difficult or impossible to give the cleansing enemas, for the fluid will not flow into the colon. Consult the physician or radiology department in these matters.
4. Strong cathartics in the presence of obstructive lesions and in the presence of acute ulcerative colitis can be hazardous or life-threatening.
5. The danger of introducing barium into the colon and the preparation for the procedure should always be considered.
6. Barium may aggravate acute ulcerative colitis or cause a partial to complete obstruction.
7. "NPO" also includes oral medications.
8. Preparations for the test will vary from one x-ray department to another.

CHOLECYSTOGRAPHY
(GALLBLADDER RADIOGRAPHY)

Normal Values

Normal functioning gallbladder and ducts without stones

Explanation of Test

This x-ray involving the use of an oral iodine contrast substance such as Telepaque (iopanoic acid) Oragrafin (Sodium spodate), and Priodax (iodoalphionic acid), is done to evaluate the functioning of the gallbladder (filling, concentration, contraction, and emptying) and to determine the presence of disease or gallstones. Since gallstones are not usually radiopaque, it is necessary to fill the gallbladder with a radiopaque dye which permits stones to show up as shadows. After administration of the dye, it takes about 13 hours for it to reach the liver and be excreted into the bile where it is stored in the gallbladder. This test is effective only if the liver cells are functioning normally and are capable of excreting the radiopaque dye into the bile.

Procedure

1. A series of at least three x-ray examinations is made with the patient assuming the following positions: lying on his abdomen, lying with the right side of his body elevated away from the table; sitting or standing. Total examining time is one hour.
2. In some instances, a high-fat drink may be given to make the gallbladder contract and after 20 minutes to an hour another x-ray is conducted.

Clinical Implications

1. Abnormal results will reveal:
    (a.) Cholelithiasis (gallstones)
    (b.) No evidence of gallbladder
    Note: If the gallbladder is chronically inflamed or contains stones, it may not show up at all. This will

provide presumptive evidence of disease if on two different occasions the gallbladder cannot be demonstrated.

(c.) Presence of gas within the gallbladder or ducts, which is always abnormal

(d.) Papillomatous or adenomatous tumors of the gallbladder

(e.) Congenital anomalies

(f.) Obstruction of cystic duct

Scheduling of Test

1. Thyroid scans, I^{131} uptake, and protein-bound iodine (PBI) must be performed before a gallbladder examination.
2. Barium studies should be performed after gallbladder studies are completed, since barium may interfere with the results.
3. When a series of GI x-rays are made in a single day, the usual order of examination is (1) gallbladder, (2) barium enema, and (3) upper GI x-ray.

Patient Preparation

1. Explain the purpose and procedure of the test.
2. Tell patient that this test often has to be repeated, so that if it is requested again there is no need to be alarmed.
3. Emphasize the importance of drinking a large amount of water with the dye capsules. Give a written reminder.
4. Be familiar with the procedures of your medical facility. Prepare the patient with the following information:

   (a.) A low-fat meal is eaten the evening before the x-ray.

   (b.) An oral laxative or stool softener is given after the meal.

   (c.) The iodine dye is given orally, usually in the form of six tasteless capsules to be swallowed every five minutes with a full glass of water.

   (d.) Some x-ray departments require the patient to have an enema.

   (e.) No food is permitted from the time the dye is given until the exam is completed. Usually water and coffee

or tea without cream and sugar are permitted if the
exam is not done in conjunction with intestinal
studies.

Patient Aftercare

1. Provide fluids, food, and rest after the examination is completed.
2. Observe the patient for allergic reaction to the iodine contrast substance.

CLINICAL ALERT
1. This examination is contraindicated in:
    (a.) Jaundice patients who will be unable to metabolize and concentrate the dye in the gallbladder because of liver disease.
    (b.) Patients sensitive to iodine
    (c.) Vomiting patients
    (d.) Patients with diarrhea
2. Observe for reactions to iodine dye.

T-TUBE CHOLANGIOGRAPHY; INTRAVENOUS CHOLANGIOGRAPHY

Normal Values

Patent common duct.

Explanation of Test

The intravenous cholangiogram is an exam done to study the
biliary ducts. It is usually performed after non-visualization of
the GB following an oral choledochogram. A contrast is injected
intravenously and followed by radiographic and tomographic
evaluation.

The T-tube cholangiogram is done after gallbladder surgery
to evaluate the patency of the common bile duct prior to re-

moval of the T-tube (a T-tube is a self-retaining drainage tube that is attached to the common bile duct during surgery). An iodine contrast dye is injected into the T-tube; then a fluoroscopic examination is made. This test is usually done about ten days after the operation.

Procedure

For T-tube cholangiogram:
1. The patient lies on the x-ray table while a contrast medium such as Hypaque is injected into the T-tube.
2. No pain or discomfort is involved.
3. The procedure takes at least ten minutes. On leaving the x-ray department, the T-tube should be unclamped and draining freely unless otherwise ordered. This avoids prolonged, often irritating, contact of the residual dye with the bile duct.

For intravenous cholangiogram:
1. A "scout film" of the right upper quadrant is made.
2. The patient lies on the x-ray table while a contrast agent, usually Cholografin is injected. This process will take about 15 minutes.
3. Films are taken every 15 to 30 minutes until the common bile duct visualizes.
4. Following visualization of the biliary ducts, tomographic studies are performed.
5. If the patient's GB has not been removed, the exam may include fluoroscopy of the gallbladder with the patient standing.

Clinical Implications

Results will reveal whether the lower end of the duct is clear.

Patient Preparation

1. Instruct the patient about the purpose and procedure of the test.
2. The meal before the x-ray is held. If the exam is in the morning, hold breakfast. If the exam is in the afternoon, hold

lunch. Decrease patient's fluid intake as well. A laxative may be administered the afternoon before the examination, and after midnight nothing can be eaten. Fluids are usually allowed upon completion of infusion.
3. The intravenous cholangiogram is a lengthy procedure, requiring two to four hours, and in some instances, longer.

Patient Aftercare

1. After the test, nausea, vomiting, and transient elevated temperature may occur as a reaction to the dye.
2. Record observations and notify physician.

CLINICAL ALERT
Persistent fever, especially with chills, may signify inflammation of the bile duct.

ESOPHAGEAL RADIOGRAPHY

Normal Values

Normal size, contour, swallowing, movement of material through the esophagus; peristalsis of esophagus

Explanation of Test

Usually the esophagus is examined together with the stomach, duodenum, and upper part of the jejunum. By common usage, this examination is referred to as an Upper GastroIntestinal series (UGI series). In addition, the esophagus may be examined separately because of specific complaints pertaining to this region of the GI tract.

   This x-ray and fluoroscopic examination is done to visualize the position, patency, and contour of the esophagus. The technique of examination will vary, depending on such factors as the presence or absence of a lesion and the amount of obstruction. Preliminary films without contrast media are done to identify opaque foreign bodies in the neck and thorax, displacement of trachea, air or fluid in mediastinal tissues or pleural cavities.

The use of an oral contrast medium, barium sulfate or meglucamine diatrizoate will permit visualization of the lumen of the esophagus. Meglucamine diatrizoate is a chalky material used as a contrast medium. Swallowing small pledgets of cotton soaked in barium is useful when the esophagus is being examined for the presence of small or sharp foreign bodies such as fish bones. Congenital abnormalities of the esophagus can be detected by this method as well as esophageal involvement in scleroderma, diverticulae, cancer, stricture with inflammation, and spasms. It is difficult to identify esophageal varies, but if present they are an indication of cirrhosis of the liver.

Procedure

1. The patient lies on the examining table in the x-ray department while a preliminary plain film study is made.
2. Barium sulfate or meglucamine diatrizoate is swallowed while the patient is in a standing position in front of the fluoroscope. All of the chalky substance must be swallowed.
3. The barium swallow is followed by x-rays. Twenty-four hour films may also be done.
4. Examining time is 45 minutes.

Clinical Implications

1. Abnormal results will indicate:
    - (a.) Congenital abnormalities
    - (b.) Esophageal involvement in scleroderma
    - (c.) Diverticulae
    - (d.) Cancer
    - (e.) Stricture with inflammation and spasm
    - (f.) Acute ulcerative esophagitis
    - (g.) Chronic fibrosing esophagitis
    - (h.) Peptic ulcer of the esophagus
    - (i.) Achalasia (cardiospasm)
    - (j.) Chalasia (cardioesophageal relaxation)
    - (k.) Polyps
    - (l.) Foreign bodies

(m.) Rupture

(n.) Paralysis

2. Esophageal varices may be difficult to identify, but if present they are an indication of cirrhosis of the liver.

Patient Preparation

1. Instruct patient about the purpose and procedure of the test. Give a written reminder. Since barium has a chalky taste, it is often flavored.
2. No food or liquids are permitted from midnight until the examination is completed.

Patient Aftercare

1. Provide food and fluids after the test is completed.
2. If barium is used during the exam, a laxative should be given after the exam is completed.
3. Check stool for barium (color and consistency) to determine that all the barium has been evacuated.

INTRAVENOUS PYELOGRAPHY (IVP) (EXCRETORY UROGRAPHY OR IV UROGRAPHY)

Normal Values

1. Normal size, shape, and position of the kidneys, ureters, and bladder. Normal kidneys are approximately as long as three and one-half vertebral bodies. Size of kidneys is estimated in relation to the shadows cast against the vertebra on the x-ray film.
2. Normal renal function:
    (a.) Two to five minutes after the injection of the contrast material the kidney outline will appear. Thread-like strands of the contrast material will be seen in the calyces.
    (b.) When the second film is taken five to seven minutes after the injection the renal pelvis can be noted.

(c.) In the last stages of film-taking, the ureters and bladder can be visualized as the contrast material makes it way down the lower urinary tract.
3. No signs of residual urine should be found on the postvoid film.

Explanation of Test

An intravenous pyelogram (IVP) is one of the most frequently ordered tests in instances of suspected renal disease or urinary tract dysfunction. A radiopaque iodine contrast substance, such as sodium diatrizoate (Hypaque) or n-methylglucamine iothalamate (conray) is injected intravenously, concentrating the contrast substance in the urine. Then a series of x-rays are taken at set intervals over a 20 to 30 minute period. A final postvoid film is taken after the patient has been asked to empty his bladder.

The resulting x-rays allow for visualization of the size, shape, and structure of the kidneys, ureters, and bladder, and the ability of the bladder to empty sufficiently. Renal function is reflected by the length of time it takes the contrast material to appear and be excreted in each kidney. Kidney disease, ureteral or bladder stones, and tumors can be detected via this test.

An IVP is indicated in the initial investigation of any suspected urologic problem, especially in the diagnosis of lesions of the kidney and ureters and in the determination of renal function.

Timed-Sequence Pyelogram

In a timed-sequence, or "rapid-series" pyelogram, a series of x-ray films are taken at one-minute intervals over a five-minute period. The purpose of the rapid series is to identify unilateral kidney disease as evidenced by the normal kidney concentrating the dye faster than the abnormal kidney. This type of pyelogram is frequently used as a screening test for renovascular hypertension.

Tomography of the kidney may also be done at this time to obtain better visualization of renal pathology and tumors. This will increase the exam time, for more films will be taken. If kidney tomography or nephrotomogram is ordered separately, the procedure and preparation are the same as for IVP.

Procedure

1. A preliminary x-ray is taken with the patient in a supine position in order to assure that the bowel has been properly emptied and that kidney placement can be visualized.
2. The dye or contrast material is injected intravenously usually via the antecubital vein.
3. During and following the IV injection, the patient should be forewarned that he may experience the following sensations: warmth, flushing of the face, salty taste, and nausea.
    (a.) Should these sensations occur, the patient should be instructed to take slow deep breaths.
    (b.) As a precaution, an emesis basin should be handy.
    (c.) Other untoward signs should be watched for such as respiratory difficulty, heavy sweating, numbness, and palpitations.
4. Following injection of the contrast material, at least three x-ray films are taken at set intervals.
5. The patient is then asked to go to the bathroom to void, after which another film is taken to determine bladder emptying.
6. Total examination time is about 45 minutes.

Clinical Implications

1. Abnormal IVP findings will reveal:
    (a.) Altered size, form, and position of the kidneys, ureters, and bladder.
    (b.) Duplication of the pelvis or ureter
    (c.) The presence of only one kidney
    (d.) Hydronephrosis
    (e.) A supernumerary kidney
    (f.) Renal or ureteral calculi (stones)
    (g.) Tuberculosis of the urinary tract
    (h.) Cystic disease
    (i.) Tumors
    (j.) The extent of renal injury following trauma
    (k.) Very large kidneys suggesting obstruction or polycystic disease

(l.) Evidence of renal failure with kidneys of normal size, suggesting an acute rather than a chronic process

(m.) Irregular scarring of the renal outlines, suggesting chronic pyelonephritis

2. A delay in the appearance time of the radiopaque dye indicates renal dysfunction. No dye may indicate very poor function or no function at all.

Interfering Factors

1. Feces or gas not cleared from the intestinal tract will obscure the view of the urinary tract.
2. Retained barium and the resulting gaseous distention from a previous barium examination can obscure the kidneys. (For this reason, barium tests should be scheduled to follow an IVP when possible.)

Patient Preparation

1. Instruct patient about the purpose and procedure of the test. Give a written reminder.
2. Since dehydration is necessary for the contrast material to be concentrated in the urinary tract, instruct the patient that no food, liquid, or medication is to be taken 12 hours before the examination. This usually means NPO after the evening meal.

   Note: Elderly or debilitated patients with poor renal reserves may not tolerate dehydration procedures (NPO, laxatives, enemas). In such instances, consult with the radiologist or the patient's physician to see if these procedures are contraindicated and if the patient should be given fluids during the normal NPO period.

   For infants and small children the NPO time will usually vary from six to eight hours preceding the test. However, be sure to obtain specific orders since each child will require different limits.
3. Usually, a laxative is prescribed for the evening before the examination and an enema the day of the examination.

   (a.) Patients with intestinal disorders such as ulcerated colitis, probably should not be given a cathartic. Special orders should be obtained in such instances.

(b.) Elderly patients need special attention for possible assistance to the bathroom.

4. Children under seven should not be given cathartics or enemas prior to the exam. Should the preliminary X-ray show gas obscuring the kidneys, a few ounces of formula or carbonated drink may help push the gas aside.

5. Check stool and abdomen for distention to assure that barium from previous enema has been eliminated and that the bowel evacuation efforts have been successful.

Patient Aftercare

1. Provide fluid and food immediately after the examination.
2. Inform patient about the importance of drinking fluids to overcome dehydration and feelings of weakness.
3. Encourage bedrest following the examination, up to eight hours for elderly and debilitated patients.
4. Observe and record any of the following mild reactions to the iodine material: hives, skin rashes, nausea, swelling of the parotid glands (iodinism).
    (a.) Consult with the physician if the signs and symptoms persist.
    (b.) Administration of oral antihistamines may relieve the more severe symptoms.

CLINICAL ALERT
1. Contraindications to an IVP include:
    (a.) Hypersensitivity to iodine preparation
    (b.) The presence of combined renal and hepatic disease
    (c.) Oliguria
    (d.) A BUN of more than 40 mg. per 100 ml. (40 mg. per dl.)
    (e.) Multiple myeloma, unless the patient can be kept well hydrated during and after the study.
    (f.) Advanced pulmonary tuberculosis
    (g.) Patients receiving drug therapy for chronic bronchitis, emphysema or asthma
2. Whenever a radiopaque iodine substance is injected, some physiologic changes can be expected. Hypertension, hypotension, tachycardia, arrhythmia or other ECT changes are the types of conditions expected to occur.

3. Radiopaque contrast media containing iodine are given with caution to patients with hyperthyroidism or a history of asthma, hay fever, or other allergies.
4. Patients should be observed for any anaphylactic or severe reaction to iodine as evidenced by signs of shock, respiratory distress, a precipitous drop in blood pressure, fainting or convulsions.
5. In all cases, except emergencies, the contrast media should not be injected sooner than 90 minutes after eating.
6. Intravenously injected iodine can be highly irritating to the intima of the veins and may cause a painful vascular spasm.
   (a.) Intravenous injection of one per cent procaine solution may help relieve vascular spasm and pain.
   (b.) Sometimes local vascular irritation is severe enough to induce thrombophlebitis. The area may be treated with warm compresses to relieve pain. The attending physician should be notified. In some cases, anticoagulant therapy is prescribed.
7. Patients should be observed for local reaction to iodine as evidenced by extensive redness, swelling and pain at the injection site. A leakage of even a small amount of iodine contrast into the subcutaneous tissues can ultimately cause sloughing of the area, which may require skin grafting.
   (a.) When extravasation is recognized, the local injection of hyaluronidase may hasten reabsorption of the iodine and resolution of the reaction.
   (b.) The use of local applications of warm saline packs may alleviate discomfort, but it does not prevent sloughing.

RETROGRADE PYELOGRAPHY

Normal Values

Normal contour and size of ureters and kidneys

Explanation of Test

This test is generally used to confirm findings suspected on the intravenous pyelogram (IVP). This test is also indicated when the IVP yields insufficient results because of nonvisualization of kidney (congenital absence of the kidney), decreased renal blood flow which restricts renal function and obstruction, when the IVP shows that one kidney is not working properly or provides evidence of a stone, or when the patient is allergic to intravenous contrast material. This x-ray examination of the upper urinary tract uses cystoscopy to introduce catheters into the ureters to the level of the renal pelvis. An iodine contrast dye is injected into the catheter and films are taken. The chief advantage or retrograde pyelography is that a dense contrast substance can be injected directly under controlled pressure so that visualization is good. The extent of impairment of renal function that may be present does not influence the degree of visualization.

Procedure

1. The examination is usually done in the surgical department and in conjunction with cystoscopy.
2. The examination is preceded by sedation and analgesia and insertion of a local anesthetic into the urethra (see cystoscopy). General anesthesia may be used.
3. Total examination time is less than one and one-half hours.

Clinical Implications

1. Abnormal results will reveal:
   (a.) intrinsic disease of ureters and pelvis of the kidney
   (b.) extrinsic disease of the ureters such as obstructive tumor or stones

Interfering Factors

Because of the tendency of barium to interfere with the test results, these studies must be done before barium x-rays.

Patient Preparation

1. Instruct patient about purpose and procedure of test.
2. A legal consent form must be signed by patient prior to examination.

3. The patient is allowed no foods or liquids after midnight prior to test.
4. Cathartics, suppositories, or enemas are usually ordered before the exam.

Patient Aftercare

1. Observe for allergic reaction to iodine contrast dye.
2. Following examination, check vital signs for at least 24 hours (every 15 minutes times 4, then every hour times 4, then every 4 hours times 4) If general anesthetic was used, care is the same following any general anesthetic.
3. Record accurate urine output and appearance for 24 hours. Hematuria and dysuria are common for several days after the examination.
4. Administer analgesics if necessary. Pain the first few days following exam is common and may require something stronger than aspirin (e.g., codeine).

CLINICAL ALERT
If ordered, renal function tests of blood and urine must be completed before this exam is done.

LYMPHANGIOGRAPHY

Normal Values

Normal lymphatic vessels and nodes

Explanation of Test

This x-ray examination of the lymphatic channels and lymph nodes uses a radiopaque iodine contrast oil, such as Ethiodol, injected into the small lymphatics of the foot. The test is commonly ordered for patients with Hodgkin's disease and cancer of the prostate to check for nodal involvement. Lymphography is also indicated in diagnosing edema of an extremity with an unknown cause, in evaluating the extent of adenopathy and the staging of lymphomas, and in localizing affected nodes for treatment planning, either surgery or radiotherapy.

Because of the dye's persistance in the nodes for six months to a year, repeat studies can be used to confirm disease activity and to follow the results of treatment.

Procedure

1. The patient is asked to lie on the examining table in the x-ray department.
2. A blue dye is injected intradermally between each of the first three toes of each foot in order to stain the lymphatic vessels.
3. Under local anesthesia, a one to two inch incision is made in the dorsum of each foot about fifteen to thirty minutes later.
4. The lymphatic vessel is identified and a cannula attached for an extremely *low* injection of the iodine contrast medium.
5. When the contrast medium reaches the level of the third and fourth lumbar vertebra (as seen in fluoroscopy), the injection is discontinued.
6. Films taken of the abdomen, pelvis, and upper body demonstrate the filling of the lymphatic vessels.
7. A second set of film is obtained in 24 hours to demonstrate filling of the lymph nodes.
8. The nodes in the equinal, external iliac, common iliac and para-aortic areas, as well as the thoracic duct and supra-clavicular nodes can be visualized.
9. When the injection is made in a lymphatic of the hand, the axillary and supraclavicular nodes are demonstrated.
10. Because the dye persists in the nodes for six months to a year, repeat studies can be used to confirm disease activity and follow the results of treatment without injection of dye.
11. The total examination time may take up to three hours, which can be very tiring.
12. The patient returns to the x-ray department for additional films in 24 hours.

Clinical Implications

1. Abnormal results will indicate:
   (a) Retroperitoneal lymphomas in patients with Hodgkin's disease
   (b) Metastasis to lymph nodes
   (c) Abnormal lymphatic vessels

Patient Preparation

1. Patient must sign legal permit.
2. Instruct patient about purpose and procedure of the test.
3. No fasting is necessary; the patient can eat and drink during the procedure if he desires.
4. There may be some discomfort when the local anesthetic is injected into the feet.
5. An oral antihistamine is administered to any patient whom the physician suspects may be allergic to the iodized oil used as a contrast medium.

Patient Aftercare

1. Check temperature every four hours for 48 hours after examination.
2. Allow patient to rest after test.
3. If ordered, elevate the legs to prevent swelling.
4. Be aware of complications such as delayed wound healing or infection at site of incision, edema of legs, allergic dermatitis, headache, sore mouth and throat, skin rashes, transient fever, lymphangitis, and oil embolism.

CLINICAL ALERT
1. The test is usually contraindicated in:
   (a) Known iodine hypersensitivity
   (b) Severe pulmonary insufficiency
   (c) Cardiac disease
   (d) Advanced renal or hepatic disease
2. The major complication of the procedure is related to embolization of the contrast media into the lungs. This will diminish pulmonary function temporarily and in some patients may produce lipid pneumonia.

MAMMOGRAPHY

Normal Values

Essentially normal breasts

Explanation of Test

Soft tissue mammography is the securing of an x-ray image of the breast on photographic film or on paper using the technology of the Xerox office copier. Its primary use is to discover cancers that escape detection by all other means. Cancers of less than one cm. in size cannot be regularly detected by routine clinical examination. Since the average cancer has probably been present in a woman's breast for six to eight years before it reaches the clinically palpable size of one cm., the prognosis for cure is excellent if breast cancer is detected in this pre-clinical or presymptomatic phase. Breast cancer can be detected as early as two years prior to clinical appearance.

Mammography x-ray diagnosis of breast disease is based on gross characteristics. A low energy x-ray beam is required to delineate the breast structures on mammograms. This radiation dose is quite acceptable for use in frequent re-examination, particularly when one considers that only a relatively small volume of tissue is in the low energy x-ray beam and that the radiation to the eyes and gonads of the patient is too small for measurement.

Benign lesions push breast tissue aside as they expand while malignant lesions invade the surrounding breast tissues. The x-ray criteria for diagnosing lesions of the breast are 85 per cent accurate in identifying carcinomas and giving less than 10 per cent false positive diagnosis.

Background

1. Most breast lumps are not malignant. Eight out of ten are benign.
2. For women at high risk of developing breast cancer, the benefits of using low-dose mammography to find early, curable cancers outweigh a possible risk from radiation 20 years later.

Risk factors in order of their importance are:
1. Personal history of breast cancer in the woman herself
2. Over 50 years of age
3. Lumps and thickenings in the breast
4. Nipple discharge
5. Family history of breast cancer on mother's or father's side or in sisters
6. Late menopause
7. No childbirth
8. First child at age 30 or older
9. Early onset of menstruation

Indications for Mammography

1. Signs and symptoms of breast cancer
2. Skin changes
3. Breast pain
4. Nipple or skin retraction
5. "Lumpy" breast; multiple masses or nodules
6. Pendulous breats that are difficult to examine
7. Survey of opposite breast after mastectomy
8. Patients at risk for having breast cancer (*e.g.* having family history of breast cancer)
9. Adenocarcinoma of undetermined site
10. Previous breast biopsy
11. Nipple discharge or erosion
12. Examination of tissue biopsied from breast

Procedure

1. A chest film is usually taken first.
2. The patient is asked to identify the area of lumps or thickening, if any.
3. The breasts are exposed and held in position on the film holder to reduce air pockets, skin folds, and wrinkles in order to get the clearest films.
4. The position is changed several times and two or three films are taken of each breast.
5. Following x-ray examination, the radiologist will often come in to palpate the breasts.
6. Total examining time is about one-half hour.

Clinical Implications

1. Abnormal findings will reveal:
    - (a.) Benign breast mass. On mammogram it appears as a round smooth mass with definable edges. If there are calcifications in the mass, they are usually coarse.
    - (b.) Cancerous mass. On mammogram it appears as an irregular shape with extensions into the adjacent tissue. An increased number of blood vessels are present. Calcification is frequent and occurs in the form of fine, sandlike granules or small deposits (calcium pungtate deposits).
    - (c.) Comedocarcinoma. A large number of comedocarcinomas (intraductal carcinomas) are diagnosed by soft tissue mammography because of their characteristic picture of grouped, punctate calcifications.
    - (d.) Intraductal papilloma. *Contrast mammography is a* most valuable aid in diagnosing intraductal papillomas. In contrast mammography, about one cc. of a radiopaque dye such as 50 per cent sodium diatrizoate is injected after careful cannulation of a discharging duct in the breast with a blunt #25 gauge needle.
2. Difficult diagnoses:
    - (a.) Colloid (gelatinous or mucinous) and medullary (circumscribed) carcinomas are difficult to diagnose by mammography.
    - (b.) Soft-tissue mammography is notoriously poor in the localizing of nonpalpable intraductal papillomas.

Patient Preparation

1. Explain the purpose and procedure to the patient.
2. Instruct the patient not to use any deodorant, perfume, powders, or ointment in the underarm area of the breasts on the day of the examination. Residue on the skin from these preparations can obscure the mammograms.
3. Advise the patient to wear a blouse with a skirt or slacks rather than a dress, since it is necessary to remove the clothing from the upper half of the body.

THERMOGRAPHY; MAMMOTHERMOGRAPHY

Normal Values

Normal temperature pattern in ranges of gray leading to extremes of black and white. Middle gray is considered the middle temperature.

Explanation of Test

Thermography is a technique that measures and records heat energy emanating from the body's surface, giving a pictorial representation of the infrared radiation of the skin surface of the breasts.

Due to increased metabolism and increased blood supply to a cancerous lesion, the presence of a malignant lesion increases the skin temperature and vascularity. A cancer thus appears as a "hot spot" on a thermogram.

The overall accuracy of thermography is about 85 per cent, but about 35 per cent of patients with benign breast lesions and about 15 per cent of thermograms give false-positive heat pattern elevations.

Thermography serves a useful purpose in screening programs. Mammography is then scheduled for patients with suspicious temperature changes. The test is valuable in studying clinical areas of suspicion and definite lesions in the breast to determine whether there is a temperature increase in those areas. Unfortunately, thermography can not be used to diagnose small or deep cancers. Therefore, this procedure is of greatest value when performed in conjunction with clinical examination of the breast and with mammography. It can be done as an office procedure.

Thermography must be done in conjunction with mammography and a physical exam. The actual value of thermography is debatable. Limitations of thermography:
1. Has a variable accuracy
2. Should not be relied upon for a definitive diagnosis

Clinical Implications

1. Thermograms are evaluated for possible changes from three basic patterns and for asymmetrical changes that will indicate the abnormal presence of breast tumors.
    (a.) There are three *normal* thermogram patterns:
        (1.) An avascular pattern and an even tissue temperature
        (2.) A mottled pattern with small areas of increased temperature
        (3.) A vascular pattern showing long linear areas of increased temperature

Procedure

1. Patient disrobes to waist and waits about ten minutes in a cooling area (temperature of 20° C [68° F] free of drafts and sunlight) to promote individual infrared heat emission.
2. During the test, the patient is seated in an upright position with the arms elevated.
3. A hand thermoscope with an instantaneous reading is used to measure the control temperature of the breast. The unit is then set to scan over the rest of the breast to determine temperature variations. Pictures are taken from the front and side of each breast.
4. The test takes only five to ten minutes.

Interfering Factors

1. Accuracy of test is decreased during menstruation because of vascular engagement and ductal changes in breast tissue.

2. Fluctuations in room temperatures will often cause faulty diagnosis.

Patient Preparation

1. Explain purpose and procedure of test.
2. Reassure patient that there is no pain or discomfort involved.
3. Advise patient to have thermogram taken after the menstrual period. When there is a minimum of vascular engorgement of breast tissue.

HYSTEROSALPINGOGRAPHY (UTEROSALPINGOGRAPHY)

Normal Values

Essentially normal uterus and fallopian tubes

Explanation of Test

This is an x-ray and fluoroscopic procedure requiring use of a contrast agent. It is undertaken to determine the position of the uterus and whether an obstruction exists in the fallopian tubes that may cause sterility. The radiopaque oil, Ethiodol, or the water-soluble medium, Salpix, may be used for contrast purposes. This procedure is valuable in identifying defects in the uterine cavity that may interfere with implantation, alterations in the tubal structures, and in the diagnoses of adhesions of the fallopian tubes. This test may also be done to confirm that the tubes have been adequately surgically ligated so that future pregnancies can be prevented.

Procedure

1. Some type of sedative is often ordered prior to procedure.
2. Patient is asked to remove all clothing from the waist down

and to lie down on an examining table in the lithotomy position.
3. The procedure is done by a radiologist and by a gynecologist who introduces a speculum into the vagina to expose the cervix.
4. A special type of cannula that occludes the external opening of the cervix and prevents escape of the contrast medium into the vagina is inserted through the speculum.
5. Six to 12 cc. of a contrast substance is injected into the uterine cavity under fluoroscopic control. X-rays are taken.
6. Total time of examination is 30 minutes.

Clinical Implications

1. Results of the examination will help in identifying:
   (a.) Causes of abnormal uterine bleeding
   (b.) Outline anomalies
   (c.) Pelvic masses and intrauterine tumors
   (d.) Extrauterine pregnancy when the fetus is dead

Patient Preparation

1. Instruct patient about purpose and procedure of test.
2. Warn the patient that she may experience cramping and transient dizziness.

Patient Aftercare

Instruct the patient that a vaginal discharge, sometimes bloody, may be present one to two days after the test.

CLINICAL ALERT
Contraindications to the examination include:
(a) Active infection of the genital tract
(b) Recent or active bleeding
(c) Pregnancy or suspected pregnancy
(d) Tuberculosis of genital organs
(e) Severe systemic disease involving the cardiorespiratory system
(f) The week preceding and the week following menstruation

COMPUTED TOMOGRAPHY (CT) OF THE BRAIN
(also called computerized axial tomography, CAT, and EMI scanning)

Normal Values

No evidence of tumor or pathologic activity

Explanation of Test

By means of a device called an Emitronics Head Computed Tomographic (C/T) Unit, a patient suspected of having intracranial pathology can have four to six detailed pictures of the internal structure of the cranium, brain tissue, and surrounding cerebrospinal fluid produced on polaraoid paper. The patient's upper head is slipped into a large circular device and the cranium is then scanned in successive layers by a narrow beam of x-rays so that the transmission of x-ray beams across a particular section of tissue can be measured. Destructive, atrophic, space-occupying intracranial pathology and such congenital abnormalities as hydrocephalus may be diagnosed. The x-ray dose per exam is the same as in a routine skull film.

Computed tomography, now generally called "CT scanning" uses computerized scanning of the brain. This is a noninvasive diagnostic technique that has virtually eliminated the use of pneumoencephalography and angiography. The scope of the information afforded by CT scanning is such that a large number of patients requiring investigation for neurological complaints will need to be subjected only to plain skull x-ray, a radioisotope brain scan, or a computerized brain scan. In neurologic practice, the common lesions that require identification are cerebral neoplasms, inflammation, hematomas, infarctions, infections, and cerebral edema which often accompany these lesions. The CT scan is the best screening test for this purpose.

In interpreting the scan, the radiologist identifies structures by their shape, size, symmetry, position, and color. On a typical CT brain scan, CSF appears black, bones appears white, and brain appears to be various shades of gray. Changes in the tissue density are then looked for. Usually a space-occupying lesion will produce a characteristic displacement or deformity of some part of the ventricular system and the extent of tissue change is defined.

Procedure

1. Each scan takes 30 to 60 minutes to complete. During this time the patient must lie perfectly still, but there is no other discomfort involved.
2. The patient lies on a motorized couch with his head resting in a stationary box (large empty circle) set in a movable frame (gantry) that revolves around the head. No movement is experienced by the patient. A monotonous sound is heard that some people compare to a dulled sound of a broken washing machine. The face is not covered and the head is enclosed and braced as if the patient were sitting under a hair dryer in a beauty salon.
3. If tissue density enhancement is desired (a questionable area that needs further clarification), sodium-iodine radio opaque substance may be injected intravenously. This contrast material can induce vomiting in some patients.
4. More pictures are taken after a short waiting period.
5. During and following the IV injection, the patient may experience the following sensations: warmth, flushing of the face, salty taste, and nausea.
   (a.) If these sensations occur, instruct the patient to take slow, deep breaths.
   (b.) Have an emesis basin ready as a precaution.
   (c.) Watch for other untoward signs, such as respiratory difficulty, heavy sweating, numbness, and palpitations.

Clinical Implications

1. *Tissues with Increased Density.* Tissues abnormalities can be identified by the tissue density alterations they exhibit in the scan pictures. Calcium is an important factor contributing to the increased density of a lesion. Meningiomas and low-grade astrocytomas are neoplasms that may show up as white areas because of their high tissue density. Calcium

also collects in angiomas, aneurysms, degenerative and infected tissue. Any hematoma can be easily distinguished. In intracranial hemorrhage, once clotting has occured, serum is absorbed and tissue density is much higher than in the normal brain. Hemoglobin and calcium ions play an important part in this increase of average density. From a surgical point of view, the demonstration of a hematoma, its size, relationship to deep structures or the point of nearest approach to the surface of the brain or the extent of surrounding edema, may be very valuable. In subarachnoid hemorrhage, the method may be used to locate a small hematoma. Where aneurysms are multiple, this may be a valuable means of identifying or confirming which aneurysm has, in fact, ruptured. In craniocerebral trauma, computerized scanning provides an easy method distinguishing between extradural, subdural, or intracerebral hematoma and cerebral edema resulting from brain damage.

2. *Tissues with Decreased Density.* Diminished tissue density on scanning is caused by large number of pathological conditions. The breakdown of cell structure in infarctions, infections, necrosis in malignant tumors, cyst formation, degenerative processes and collection of fluid and edema are the main changes that will reduce tissue density and are observed as darker areas on the scan pictures.

3. *Tissues Requiring Contrast Media.* Lesions having tissue densities that are the same as those of the surrounding normal brain are difficult to identify in the ordinary scan. Artificially raising the density of abnormal tissue or enhancement of tissue density is possible by intravenously injecting a contrast substance. The basis for use of this contrast enhancement is that the breakdown of the blood-brain barrier in an abnormal area should permit small amounts of specially selected circulating substances to pass into abnormal tissue. Contrast enhancement is indicated when there is evidence of a tumor, blood clot, aneurysm or vascular abnormality. Contrast enhancement is used in 80 to 85 per cent of patients with a history of headache and seizures. A quantity of 300 ml. of a radiopaque sodium iodine solution is given either by an IV injection or infusion. Another scan must be completed after the IV injection.

Patient Preparation

1. Instruct patient about the purpose and procedure of the test. Provide written explanation and reminders.
2. Generally, the patient should not eat or drink for three to four hours before the test.
3. Reassure patient that scanning results in no more radiation than that used in conventional x-rays.
4. If a contrast iodine intravenous substance is administered during the test (indications are usually not present prior to testing), nausea and vomiting may occur. Advise patient that he may experience a salty taste, nausea, vomiting, warmth, and flushing of the face.
5. Reassure patient that claustrophobic fears of being in the machine are common. Show a picture of the scanner.
6. Administer analgesics and sedatives to those patients with painful neck stiffness, injuries to the back of the head, or who are unable to cooperate by lying still. Any movement by the patient will give poor results.

Patient Aftercare

1. Determine whether or not an iodine contrast substance was used during the test. If the contrast material was used, observe and record any of the following mild reactions to the iodine material: hives, skin rashes, nausea, swelling of parotid glands (iodism).
   - (a.) Consult with the physician if the signs and symptoms persist.
   - (b.) Administer oral antihistamines to possibly relieve the more severe symptoms

COMPUTED TOMOGRAPHY (CT) OF THE BODY
(also called "Computerized Axial Tomography (CAT) Body Scan; Computerized Transaxial Tomography (CTT) Body Scan")

Normal Values

1. No tumor or pathological activity is not evident.
2. Air appears black on CT scans; bone appears white; soft

tissue appears in shades of gray. The pattern of shades and their correlation to different densities in the body with the added dimension of depth assist in identifying normal body structures and organs.

Explanation of Test

The body scanner is used primarily to give a clear image of the chest and abdomen and as an important diagnostic aid in the identification of cysts and tumors. The body scanner is 100 times more sensitive than the traditional x-ray machine in critical areas. Ordinary x-rays take a flat picture, with organs in the front of the body appearing to be superimposed over organs at the back. The result is a two-dimensional picture of a three-dimensional object. The scanner also produces a two-dimensional picture, but by taking many cross-section views of organs of the body and displaying the pictures in turn on the television screen, a three-dimensional appearance is created. Typical x-rays show only major contrasts between body densities such as bones, soft tissue, and air. Fine density differences, as between structures within the liver, do not usually register on an x-ray film but will appear on a body scan.

Procedure

1. The patient lies on his back in a comfortable position in the scanner. The head remains outside of the scanning unit.
2. Instructions are given to lie as motionless as possible.
3. No movement is felt by the patient as the x-ray beam makes a 180 degree scan of the body, one degree at a time, in three or four different planes.
4. A television picture of the inside of the living body is seen almost immediately.
5. Photographs are taken of tissue density and depth images are provided by a computer.
6. If there is a questionable area that needs further clarification, such as unusual tissue densities, a contrast iodine substance is injected intravenously and more pictures are taken after a short waiting period.
7. During and following the IV injection, the patient may experience warmth, flushing of the face, salty taste, and nausea.

(a.) If these sensations occur, instruct the patient to take slow, deep breaths.

(b.) Have an emesis basin available as a precaution.

(c.) Watch for other untoward signs, such as respiratory difficulty, heavy sweating, numbness, and palpitations.

8. The total examination time is as long as three hours.

Clinical Implications

1. Abnormal CT scan findings will reveal:
   (a.) Tumors, nodules, and cysts of the whole body (below the neck)
   (b.) Ascites
   (c.) Abscessed or fatty liver
   (d.) Aneurysm of abdominal aorta
   (e.) Lymphoma
   (f.) Enlarged lymph nodes
   (g.) Pleural effusion
   (h.) Radioactive iodine used in previous testing
   (i.) Cancer of pancreas
   (j.) Liver metastasis
   (k.) Retroperitoneal lymphadenopathy
   (l.) Collection of blood, fluid, or abnormal fat
   (m.) Skeletal metastasis
   (n.) Cirrhosis of liver

Interfering Factors

1. Retained barium can obscure organs in the upper and lower abdomen. (Barium tests should be scheduled to *follow* a CT scan when possible.)
2. Inability of patient to lie quietly. Movement will result in inaccurate pictures.

Patient Preparation

1. Instruct patient about the purpose and procedure of the test. Provide written explanation and reminders.
2. Reassure patient that CT scanning results in no more radiation than that used in conventional x-rays.

3. Caution patient not to eat three to four hours before the exam.
4. Warn patient that if a contrast iodine intravenous substance is administered during the test (indications are usually not present prior to testing), he may experience warmth, flushing of the face, salty taste, and nausea.
5. Reassure patient that claustrophobic fears of being in the machine are common. Show a picture of the scanner.
6. Sedation and analgesics may be ordered if it will be difficult for patient to lie quietly for a long period of time.

Patient Aftercare

1. If an iodine contrast material was used, observe the patient and record any of the following mild reactions to the iodine material: hives, skin rashes, nausea, swelling of parotid glands (iodism).
   (a.) Consult with the physician if the signs and symptoms persist.
   (b.) Administer oral antihistamines to relieve the more severe symptoms.

REFERENCES

Chesney, D. Noreen, and Chesney, Muriel O.: CARE OF THE PATIENT IN DIAGNOSTIC RADIOGRAPHY. 5th Ed., Oxford, Blackwell Scientific Publications, 1978.

Daffner, Richard H.: INTRODUCTION TO CLINICAL RADIOLOGY—A CORRELATIVE APPROACH TO DIAGNOSTIC IMAGING. St. Louis, The C. V. Mosby Company, 1978.

Eklöf, Ole (ed.): CURRENT CONCEPTS IN PEDIATRIC RADIOLOGY. Berlin, Springer International, 1977.

Greenfield, George B.: RADIOLOGY OF BONE DISEASES. 2nd Ed., Philadelphia, J. B. Lippincott Company, 1975.

Gyll, Catherine: A HANDBOOK OF PAEDIATRIC RADIOGRAPHY. Oxford, Blackwell Scientific Publications, 1977.

Meschan, Isadore: SYNOPSIS OF RADIOLOGIC ANATOMY —WITH COMPUTED TOMOGRAPHY. Philadelphia, W. B. Saunders Co, 1978.

Potchen, E. James: CURRENT CONCEPTS IN RADIOLOGY. Vol. 3, St. Louis, The C. V. Mosby Company, 1977.

10 □ CYTOLOGY AND CYTOGENETICS
□

INTRODUCTION

Cytologic Study

Exfoliated cells in body tissues and fluid are studied to (a) count the cells, (b) determine the type of cells present, and (c) detect and diagnose malignant and premalignant conditions. The staining technique developed by Dr. George N. Papanicolaou has been especially useful in diagnosis of malignancy and is now routinely used in the cytologic study of the female genital tract.

Some cytologic specimens (*e.g.*, smears of the mouth, genital tract, and nipple discharge) are relatively easy to obtain for study. Other samples are from less accessible sources (*e.g.*, amniotic fluid, pleural effusions, and cerebrospinal fluid) and special techniques are required for collection. Tissue samples obtained in surgery are also examined. In all studies, the source of the sample and its method of collection must be noted so that the evaluation can be based on complete information.

Specimens for cytologic study are usually composed of many different cells. Some are normally present, while others indicate pathologic conditions. Under certain conditions, cells normally observed in one sample may be indicative of an abnormal state when observed elsewhere. All specimens are examined for the number of cells, cell distribution, surface modifications, size, shape, appearance and staining properties, functional adaptations, and inclusions. The cell nucleus is also examined. Any increases or decreases from normal values are noted.

Most specimens are collected in containers partially filled with 70 per cent alcohol. Some, however, are collected without preservative and they must be handled carefully to prevent any drying out. (Check with your individual laboratory for collection requirements.) It is important for all cytology specimens to be sent to the laboratory as soon as they are obtained to prevent disintegration of cells or any other process that could cause alteration of the material for study.

CLINICAL ALERT
The test is only as good as the specimen received.

In practice, cytologic studies will be commonly be reported as:
1. Inflammatory
2. Benign
3. Atypical
4. Suspicious for malignancy
5. Positive for malignancy
   (a.) *In situ* versus invasive

Clinical Cytogenetics

Cytogenetics is the branch of genetics dealing with the microscopic study of chromosomes, the cellular constituents of heredity. This chapter will include two tests used in *clinical cytogenetics,* which is the application of cytogenetic techniques to the diagnosis of genetic abnormalities in humans.

Analysis of the structure and number of chromosomes in blood cells, epithelial cells, fibroblasts, or bone marrow cells, makes it possible to diagnose or confirm certain clinical disorders including Down syndrome, Turner syndrome, Klinefelter syndrome and others. Study of the karyotype, which is the arrangement by size of homologous chromosomes, may provide diagnosis and aid in treatment of patients presenting a variety of abnormalities, such as multiple malformations, growth failure, mental retardation, ambiguous genitalia, primary amenorrhea, or history of spontaneous abortions. Cytogenetic analysis of amniotic fluid from a woman in her fourteenth to sixteenth week of pregnancy can confirm or rule out the presence of a fetus with a chromosomal disorder.

At times, chromosomal disorders are inherited through normal individuals, who, because of a chromosome rearrangement, are at high risk of having abnormal children. Such high risk individuals include couples who have children with chromosomal abnormalities, persons who have relatives with certain chromosomal disorders, women with a history of miscarriages, and women who are over 35 and have not yet borne a child.

The usual body tissue used in cytogenetics is blood, bone marrow, skin, buccal smears, or amniotic fluid. Cells from these tissues are grown in a culture medium. Cultures are examined for the number of rapidly dividing cells. When the number is high enough, cell growth is halted chemically. The culture is then stained and examined under a high powered oil-immersion microscope so that the chromosomes can be visualized and photographed. Prints are made of the photomicrographs. Individual chromosomes are cut apart and assembled to form the karyotype, the arrangement of chromosomes pairs, according to their size. The karyotype is then evaluated for any structural or numerical deviations from the normal. Diagnosis of many genetic conditions are aided by this evaluation.

CYTOLOGIC STUDY OF THE RESPIRATORY TRACT
(see also Chapter 6, under "Respiratory Tract Cultures")

Normal Values

Negative

Background

The lungs and the passages that conduct air to and from the lungs form the respiratory tract, which is divided into the upper and lower respiratory tracts. The upper respiratory tract consists of the nasal cavities, the nasopharynx, and the larynx; the lower respiratory tract consists of the trachea and the lungs. Cytologic studies of sputum and bronchial secretions are very important as diagnostic aids because of the frequency of cancer of the lung and the relative inaccessibility of this organ. Also detectable are cell changes that may be related to the future development of malignant conditions and to inflammatory conditions.

Sputum is composed of mucous and cells and is the secretion of the bronchi, lungs, and trachea and is therefore obtained from the lower respiratory tract (bronchi and lungs). Sputum is ejected through the mouth but originates in the lower respiratory tract. Saliva produced by the salivary glands in the mouth is *not* sputum. A specimen can be correctly identified as sputum in microscopic examination by the presence of dust cells (carbon dust-laden macrophages). Although the glands and secretory cells in mucous lining of the lower respiratory tract produce up to 100 ml. of fluid daily, the healthy person does not cough up sputum.

Procedure

For Obtaining Bronchial Secretions:
1. Bronchial secretions are obtained during bronchoscopy (see Chapter 11, p. 584). Bronchoscopy involves removal of bronchial secretions and tissue for cytologic and microbiologic studies.

2. Fresh bronchial secretions or washings should be sent immediately to the cytology laboratory. Collection of post-bronchial sputum in the 24 hours after bronchoscopy can be of great value for a more definitive interpretation.

For Obtaining Sputum:

1. The preferred material is an early-morning specimen. Three specimens are usually collected on three separate days.
2. Patient must inhale air to full capacity of the lungs and then exhale the air with an expulsive deep cough.
3. Specimen should be coughed directly into a wide-mouthed sterile container.
4. Specimen should be covered with a tight-fitting sterile lid.
5. Specimen should be labeled with patient's name, age, date, diagnosis, and number of specimens (1, 2, or 3) and sent immediately to the laboratory.

Patient Preparation

1. Explain purpose and procedure of test.
2. Emphasize that sputum is not saliva.
3. Advise patient to brush teeth and rinse mouth well prior to obtaining specimen to avoid introduction of saliva to specimen.

Clinical Implications

Abnormalities in sputum and bronchial secretions may sometimes be helpful in detecting:

1. Benign atypical changes in sputum, as in:
   - (a.) Inflammatory diseases
   - (b.) Asthma (creola bodies)
   - (c.) Lipid pneumonia (Lipophages are found, but they are not diagnostic of the disease.)
   - (d.) Asbestosis (ferruginous or asbestos bodies)
   - (e.) Viral diseases
   - (f.) Benign diseases of lung such as bronchiectasis, atelectasis, emphysema, and pulmonary infarcts.
2. Metaplasia, which is substitution of one adult cell type for another. Severe metaplastic changes are found in patients with:

(a.) History of chronic cigarette smoking
(b.) Pneumonitis
(c.) Pulmonary infarcts
(d.) Bronchiectasis
(e.) Healing abscess
(f.) Tuberculosis
(g.) Emphysema
(Metaplasia often adjoins a carcinoma or a carcinoma *in situ*.)
3. Viral changes and presence of virocytes as in (viral inclusions may be seen):
    (a.) Viral pneumonia
    (b.) Acute respiratory disease caused by adenovirus
    (c.) Herpes simplex
    (d.) Measles
    (e.) Cytomegalic inclusion disease
    (f.) Varicella
4. Degenerative changes, as seen in viral diseases of lung
5. Fungal and parasitic diseases (In parasitic diseases ova or parasite may be seen.)
6. Tumor (benign and malignant)

Interfering Factors

False negatives can be due to:
Delays in preparation of specimen, causing a deterioration of tumor cells.
Note: Incidence of false negatives is about 15 per cent, in contrast to about 1 per cent in studies for cervical cancer. This high incidence occurs even with careful examination of multiple deep cough specimens.

CYTOLOGIC STUDY OF THE GASTROINTESTINAL TRACT

Normal Values

Negative. Squamous epithelial cells of the esophagus may be present.

Explanation of Test

Exfoliative cytology of the gastrointestinal tract is useful in diagnosis of benign and malignant diseases. However, it is not a specific test for these diseases. Many benign diseases, such as leukoplakia of the esophagus, esophagitis, gastritis, pernicious anemia, and granulomatous diseases, may be recognized because of their characteristic cellular changes. Response to radiation may also be noted from cytologic studies.

Procedure

1. For esophageal studies, a nasogastric Levin's tube is passed approximately 40 cm. (to the cardio-esophageal junction) with the patient in a sitting position.
2. For stomach studies, a Levin's tube is passed into the stomach (approximately 60 cm.) with the patient in a sitting position.
3. For pancreatic and gallbladder drainage, a special double lumen gastric tube is passed orally to 45 cm. with the patient in a sitting position. Then the patient is placed on his right side and the tube is passed slowly to 85 cm. It takes about 20 minutes for the tube to reach this distance. Tube location is confirmed by biopsy. Lavage with physiologic salt solution is done during all upper GI cytology procedures.
4. Specimens can also be obtained during endoscopy procedures (see p. 586).
5. Specimens for colon cytology involve use of the proctoscope and saline enema. See your laboratory for special instructions.

Patient Preparation

1. Patient should be told purpose of test, nature of the procedure, and to anticipate some discomfort from the procedure.
2. A liquid diet is usually ordered 24 hours prior to testing. The patient is encouraged to take fluids throughout the night and in the morning before the test.
3. No oral barium should be administered for the 24 preceding hours.
4. Laxatives and enemas are ordered for colon cytology studies.

5. Since insertion of the nasogastric tube can cause considerable discomfort, the patient and clinician should devise a system (*e.g.*, raising a hand) to indicate discomfort.
6. The patient should be informed that panting, mouth-breathing, or swallowing can help to ease the insertion of the tube.
7. Sucking on ice chips or sipping through a straw also makes insertion of the tube easier.

> **CLINICAL ALERT**
> Immediately remove tube if the patient shows signs of distress: coughing, gasping, or cyanosis.

Patient Aftercare

1. Patient should be given food, fluids, and rest after the tests are completed.
2. Provide rest. Patients having colon studies will be feeling quite tired.

Clinical Implications

1. The characteristics of benign and malignant cells of the gastrointestinal tract are the same as for cells of the rest of the body.
2. Abnormal results in cytologic studies of the esophagus may be a non-specific aid in the diagnosis of:
    - (a.) Acute esophagitis, which is characterized by increased exfoliation of basal cells with inflammatory cells and polymorphonuclear leukocytes in the cytoplasm of the benign squamous cells.
    - (b.) Vitamin B_{12} and folic acid deficiencies, which are characterized by giant epithelial cells.
    - (c.) Malignant diseases characterized by typical cells of esophageal malignancy.
3. Abnormal results in studies of the stomach may be a non-specific aid in the diagnosis of:
    - (a.) Pernicious anemia characterized by giant epithelial cells. An injection of vitamin B_{12} will cause these cells to disappear within 24 hours.

(b.) Granulomatous inflammations seen in chronic gastritis and sarcoid of the stomach which are characterized by granulomatous cells.

(c.) Gastritis which is characterized by degenerative changes and an increase in the exfoliation of clusters of surface epithelial cells.

(d.) Malignant disease, most of which are gastric adenocarcinomas. Lymphoma cells can be differentiated from adenocarcinoma. The Reed-Sternberg cell, a multinucleated giant cell, is the characteristic cell found along with abnormal lymphocytes in Hodgkin's disease.

4. Abnormal results in studies of the pancreas, gallbladder, and duodenum may reveal:

(a.) Malignant cells (usually adenocarcinoma) but is sometimes difficult to determine the exact site of the tumor.

5. Abnormal results in examination of the colon may reveal:

(a.) Ileitis, characterized by large multinuclear histocytes (bovine tuberculosis commonly manifests itself in this area).

(b.) Ulcerative colitis, characterized by a hyperchromic nuclei surrounded by a thin cytoplasmic rim.

Interfering Factors

Barium and lubricant used in Levin's tubes will interfere with good results, because their presence will distort the cells and prevent accurate evaluation.

CYTOLOGIC STUDY OF THE FEMALE GENITAL TRACT (PAPANICOLAOU SMEAR)

Normal Values

Normal: no abnormal cells

Maturation Index (MI): The MI is a ratio of parabasal to

intermediate to superficial cells. Following are representative ratios:

Normal Child	80/20/0
Preovulatory adult	0/40/60
Premenstrual adult	0/70/30
Pregnant adult (2nd mo.)	0/90/10
Postmenopausal adult (age 60)	65/30/5

Explanation of Test

The Papanicolaou (Pap) smear is used priniciply for diagnosis of precancerous and cancerous conditions of the genital tract, which includes the vagina, cervix, and endometrium. This test is also used for hormonal assessment and for diagnosis of inflammatory diseases. Because the Pap smear is of great importance in the early detection of cervical cancer, it is recommended that all women over the age of 20 have the test at least once a year.

The value of the Pap smear depends on the fact that cells readily exfoliate (or can be easily stripped) from genital cancers. Cytologic study can also be used for assessing response to the effect of administered sex hormones. It should be noted that the microbiologic exam on cytology samples is not as accurate as bacterial culture, but it can provide valuable information.

Specimens for cytologic examination of the genital tract are usually obtained by vaginal speculum examination or by colposcopy with biopsy. Material from the cervix, endocervix, and posterior fornix is obtained for most smears. Smears for hormonal evaluation are obtained from the vagina.

All Papanicolaou smears are usually reported on a five-point scale. The meaning of the classes vary, however, and are not universally agreed upon. Following is the scale:

1. Absence of atypical or abnormal cells, negative
2. Atypical cytology, dysplastic, borderline but not neoplastic
3. Cytology suggestive of, but not inclusive of malignancy
4. Cytology strongly suggestive of malignancy
5. Cytology conclusive of malignancy; cancer cells present

CLINICAL ALERT

It is important to remember that cytologic findings alone do not form the basis of a diagnosis of cancer or other diseases. Often they are used to justify further procedures, such as biopsy.

Cells are also examined for hormonal effect and organisms. Cells examined for effect are reported on a six-point scale.

1. Marked
2. Moderate
3. Slight
4. Atrophic
5. Compatible with pregnancy
6. No evaluation—specimen too bloody or inflammed or scanty

Cells can also be examined for microorganisms using routine staining techniques. These cells are also reported on a five-point scale.

1. Normal flora
2. Scanty or absent
3. *Trichomonas*
4. *Monilia*
5. Other (cocci, coccobacilli, mixed bacteria)

Background

Characteristic physiologic cellular changes occur in the genital tract from birth through the postmenopausal years. Hormonal evaluation by cytologic examination should be performed only on vaginal smears taken from the lateral vaginal wall or from the vaginal fornix. Smears from the ectocervix or endocervix cannot be used for hormonal evaluation because certain conditions, such as metaplasia and cervicitis, interfere with a correct assessment. There are three major cell types occurring in a characteristic pattern in vaginal smears:

1. Superficial squamous cells
2. Intermediate squamous cells that appear as a result of bacterial cytolysis
3. Parabasal cells that appear as a result of degeneration or necrosis. Deviation from physiologic cell patterns may be indicative of pathologic conditions.

Hormonal cytology is valuable in the assessment of many endocrine-related conditions, especially ovarian function.

Procedure

1. The patient is usually asked to remove clothing from the waist down.
2. The patient is placed in a lithotomy position on an examining table.
3. A speculum lubricated only with water is inserted into the vagina to expose the cervix.
4. The posterior fornix and external os of cervix are scraped with a wooden spatula and obtained material is spread on slides and placed in preservative or fixative.
5. Label specimen with name, date, woman's age, reason for examination, last menstrual period, and area from which specimen is obtained.
6. Examination only takes about five minutes.

Note: The best time to take a Pap smear is five to six days after the end of the menstrual period.

Procedure for Hormonal Smears, "Maturation Index"

Obtain specimen by scraping the proximal portion of the lateral wall of the vagina, avoiding the cervical area. Otherwise same as above.

Clinical Implications

1. Abnormal cytology responses can be classified as protective, destructive, reparative (regenerative), or neoplastic.
2. Inflammatory reactions and microbes can be identified to help in diagnosis of vaginal diseases.
3. Precancerous and cancerous lesions of the cervix can be identified. The stages of neoplastic disease can be arbitrarily classified as dysplasia (mild, moderate, and severe), carcinoma *in situ* (preinvasive carcinoma), microinvasive carcinoma, and invasive carcinoma.
4. Hormonal cytology reports will include several factors:
     (a.) Hormonal cell pattern. Report will state that the pat-

tern is, or is not, compatible with the age and menstrual history of the patient. The reason for non-compatibility is given.

(b.) Maturation Index (MI)

MI is a proportion of the major cell types (parabasal, intermediate, and superficial) in each 100 cells counted. The MI will be expressed as a ration (*e.g.,* MI = 100/0/0). See "Normal Values" for representative MI's.

5. The following facts should be kept in mind when hormonal cytology reports are reviewed:

(a.) The degree of maturity of the epithelium cannot be expressed in degrees of estrogenic effects or estrogen deficiencies, since more than one hormonal stimulus is involved (estrogen, progesterone, and adrenal hormones.)

(b.) Surgical removal of the ovaries does not necessarily result in epithelial atrophy.

(c.) Only two cell types can be identified with accuracy if the age and menstrual history of the patient are not known:

(1.) Abundant superficial squamous cells, indicative of unequivocal estrogenic effect.

(2.) Parabasal cells, indicative of lack of cell maturation due to lack of hormone stimulation

(d.) From a single specimen it is impossible to predict whether ovulation will occur, whether it has recently occurred, or what stage of menstrual cycle the patient is in. Serial specimens must be examined to obtain above results.

(e.) An intermediate cell type is always intermediate, regardless of its size.

(f.) No hormonal assessment should be made without knowing the age of the patient, her menstrual history, and her history of hormone administrations.

Interfering Factors

1. Medications such as tetracycline and digitalis, which affect the squamous epithelium, will alter test results.

2. The use of lubricating jelly in the vagina and recent douching will interfere with test results because the jellies will distort the cells and prevent accurate evaluation.
3. The presence of infection will interfere with hormonal cytology.
4. Heavy menstrual flow may make the interpretation of the results difficult and may obscure atypical cells.

Patient Preparation

1. Explain test purpose and procedure.
2. Instruct patient not to douche for two to three days before the test because this may remove the exfoliated cells.
3. Have patient empty her bladder and rectum prior to examination.
4. Ask patient to give following information:
   (a.) First day of last menstrual period
   (b.) Use of hormone therapy or birth control pills
   (c.) All medications taken
   (d.) Any radiation therapy
   This information must be sent to laboratory along with specimens for cytology.

CYTOLOGIC STUDY OF ASPIRATED BREAST CYSTS AND NIPPLE DISCHARGE

Normal Values

Negative for neoplasia

Background

Nipple discharge is normal only during the lactation period. Any other nipple discharge is abnormal and when it occurs, breasts should be examined for mastitis, duct papilloma, or intraductal cancer. Certain situations increase the possibility of finding a normal nipple discharge, such as pregnancy, perimenopause, and use of birth control pills. About three per cent of breast cancers and ten per cent of benign lesions of the breast are associated with abnormal nipple discharge.

The contents of all breast cysts obtained by needle biopsy are examined to detect malignant cells.

Procedure

1. Breast Cyst
   The contents of the identified breast cyst is obtained by percutaneous aspiration.
2. Nipple Discharge
   - (a.) The nipple should be washed with a cotton pledget and patted dry.
   - (b.) The nipple is gently stripped, or milked, to obtain a discharge.
   - (c. Fluid should be expressed until a pea-sized drop appears.
   - (d.) Patient may assist by holding a bottle of fixative beneath the breast so that the slide may be dropped in immediately.
   - (e.) The discharge is spread immediately on a slide and then dropped into the fixative bottle.
   - (f.) Specimen is identified with pertinent data, including from which breast it was obtained.
   - (g.) Specimen is sent without delay to the laboratory.

Clinical Implications

1. Abnormal results are helpful in identifying:
   - (a.) Benign breast conditions, such as mastitis and intraductal papilloma
   - (b.) Malignant breast conditions, such as papilloma intraductal cancer or intracystic infiltrating cancer

---

CLINICAL ALERT
Any discharge, regardless of color, should be examined. A bloody or blood-tinged discharge is especially significant.

Interfering Factors

Use of drugs that alter hormone balance, such as pheno-thiazines, digitalis, diuretics, and steroids, often result in a clear nipple discharge.

CYTOLOGIC STUDY OF URINE
(See also Chapter 2, *Urinalysis,* especially "Microscopic Analysis of Sediment.")

Normal Values

Negative. Epithelial and squamous cells are normally present in urine.

Explanation of Test

Cells from the epithelial lining of the urinary tract exfoliate readily into the urine. Urine cytology is most useful in the diagnosis of cancer and inflammatory diseases of the bladder, the renal pelvis, the ureters, and the urethra. This study is also valuable in detecting cytomegalic inclusion disease and in detecting bladder cancer in high-risk populations, such as workers exposed to aniline dyes, smokers, and patients previously treated for bladder cancer.

Procedure

1. Obtain a clean voided urine specimen of at least 180 cc. (adults) and 10 cc. (children).
2. Obtain a catheterized specimen, if possible, if cancer is suspected.
3. Deliver specimen immediately to the cytology laboratory. Urine should be as fresh as possible when it is examined.

Clinical Implications

1. Findings possibly indicative of *inflammatory conditions* of the *lower urinary tract:*

(a.) Epithelial hyperplasia
(b.) Atypical cells
(c.) Abundance of red blood cells
(d.) Leukocytes

Note: Inflammatory conditions could be due to any of the following:

Benign prostatic hyperplasia
Adenocarcinoma of the prostate
Kidney stones
Diverticula of bladder
Strictures
Malformations

2. Findings indicative of *cytomegalic inclusion disease:*
    (a.) Large intranuclear inclusions.

    Note: Cytomegalic inclusion disease is a viral infection that usually occurs in childhood but is also seen in cancer patients treated with chemotherapy and in transplant patients treated with immunosuppressives. The renal tubular epithelium is usually involved.

3. Findings possibly indicative of malakoplakia and granulomatous disease of the bladder of upper urinary tract:
    (a.) Histiocytes with multiple granules in an abundant, foamy cytoplasm.
    (b.) Michaelis-Gutmann bodies in malakoplakia

4. Cytologic findings possibly indicative of malignancy. If the specimen shows evidence of any of the changes associated with malignancy, cancer of the bladder, renal pelvis, ureters, kidney and urethra may be suspected. Metastatic tumor should be ruled out as well.

CYTOLOGIC STUDY OF CEREBROSPINAL FLUID (CSF)

Normal Values

1. Total Cell Count:
    Adult 0–10/cu. mm. (all mononuclear cells)
    Infant 0–20/cu. mm.

2. Negative for neoplasia
3. A variety of normal cells may be seen. Large lymphocytes are most common; small lymphocytes are also seen, as are elements of the monocyte-macrophage series.
4. The CSF of a healthy individual should be free of all pathogens.

Explanation of Test

Spinal fluid obtained by lumbar puncture is examined for the presence of abnormal cells and for an increase or decrease in the normally present cell population. Most of the usual laboratory procedures for study of CSF involve an examination of the white cells and a white blood cell count; chemical and microbiological studies are also done. In recent years, cell studies of the CSF have been used to identify neoplastic cells. These studies have been especially helpful in the diagnosis and treatment of the different phases of leukemia disorders. The nature of neoplasia is such that for tumor cells to exfoliate, they must actually invade the CSF circulation and enter such areas as the ventricle wall, the choroid plexus, or the subarachnoid space.

Procedure

1. A specimen of at least one to three ml. is obtained by lumbar puncture (see Chapter 4, p. 216).
2. Usually three tubes are collected.
3. The specimen is labeled with the patient's name, date, and type of specimen.
4. The sample is sent immediately to cytology laboratory for processing.

CLINICAL ALERT
The laboratory should be given adequate warning that a CSF specimen will be delivered. Time is a critical factor; cells begin to disintegrate if the sample is kept at room temperature for more than one hour.

Clinical Implications

1. Cerebrospinal fluid abnormalities may be helpful in the detection of:
   - (a.) Malignant gliomas that have invaded the ventricles or cortex of the brain. WBC $\leq$ 150/cu. mm. (The sample may be normal in 75% of patients.)
   - (b.) Ependymoma (neoplasm of differentiated ependymal cells) and medulloblastoma (a cerebellar tumor) in children
   - (c.) Seminoma and pineoblastoma (tumors of the pineal gland)
   - (d.) Secondary carcinomas:
     - (1.) Secondary carcinomas metastasizing to the CNS have multiple avenues to the subarachnoid space via the bloodstream.
     - (2.) The breast and lung are common sources of metastatic cells exfoliated in the CSF. Infiltration of acute leukemia is also quite common.
   - (e.) Central nervous system leukemia
   - (f.) Fungal Forms:
     - (1.) Congenital toxoplasmosis
       WBC 50–500/cu. mm. (Mostly monocytes present)
     - (2.) Coccidioidomycosis
       WBC 200/cu. mm.
   - (g.) Various forms of meningitis:
     - (1.) Cryptococcal meningitis
       WBC 800/cu. mm. (Lymphocytes are more abundant than polynuclear neutrophilic leukocytes)
     - (2.) Tuberculous meningitis
       WBC 25–1000/cu. mm. (mostly lymphocytes present)
     - (3.) Acute pyogenic meningitis
       WBC 25—10,000/cu. mm. (Mostly polynuclear neutrophilic leukocytes present)
   - (h.) Meningoencephalitis
     - (1.) Primary amebic meningoencephalitis
       WBC 400–21,000/cu. mm.

Red blood cells are also found.
Wright's stain may reveal amebas.

(i.) Hemosiderin-laden macrophages, as in subarachnoid hemorrhage.
(j.) Kipophages from CNS destructive processes
2. Characteristics of neoplastic cells:
(a.) Sometimes marked increase in size, most likely sarcoma and carcinomas
(b.) Exfoliated cells tend to be more polymorphic as the neoplasm becomes increasingly malignant.

Interfering Factors

The lumbar puncture can occasionally cause contamination of the specimen with squamous epithelial cells or spindly fibroblasts.

CYTOLOGIC STUDIES OF EFFUSIONS

Normal Values

Negative for abnormal cells
(Total cell counts and all cell types are reported.)

Background

Effusions are accumulations of fluids. They may be exudates, which generally accumulate as a result of inflammation, or transudates, which are fluids not associated with inflammation. Below is a comparison of these two effusions:

Exudate	*Transudate*
1. Accumulates in body cavities and tissues because of malignancy or inflammation	1. Accumulates in body cavities from impaired circulation of malignancy
2. Associated with an inflammatory process	2. Not associated with an inflammatory process
3. Viscous	3. Highly fluid

4. High content of protein, cells, and solid materials derived from cells
5. May have high WBC content
6. Clots spontaneously (because of high concentration of fibrinogen)
7. Malignant cells as well as bacteria may be detected
8. Specific gravity >1.018

4. Low content of protein, cells, or solid materials derived from cells
5. Has low WBC content
6. Will not clot
7. Malignant cells may be present
8. Specific gravity <1.018

Fluid contained in the pleural, pericardial, and peritoneal or abdominal cavities is a serous fluid. Accumulation of fluid in the peritoneal cavity is called ascites.

Explanation of Test

Cytologic studies of effusions—either exudates or transudates—are sometimes helpful in determining the cause of these abnormal collections of fluids. The effusions are found in the pericardial sac, the pleural cavities, and the abdominal cavities. *The chief problem in diagnosis is in differentiating malignant cells from reactive mesothelial cells.*

Procedure

Material for cytologic examination of effusions is obtained by either thoracentesis or paracentesis. Both of these procedures involve surgical puncture of a cavity for aspiration of a fluid. *Thoracentesis:*
1. Chest roentgenograms should be available at the patient's bedside so that the location of fluid may be determined.
2. Patient may be administered a sedative.
3. Chest is exposed. The physician inserts a long thoracentesis needle with a syringe attached.
4. At least 40 ml. of fluid is withdrawn. It is preferable to withdraw 300 to 1000 ml. of fluid.
5. The specimen is collected in a clean container and heparin is added. Alcohol should *not* be added.

6. Specimen should be labeled with patient's name, date, source of the fluid, and diagnosis.
7. The covered specimen should be sent immediately to the laboratory. (If the specimen cannot be sent at once, it may be refrigerated.)

Paracentesis (Abdominal)
1. Patient should be asked to void.
2. Patient is placed in Fowler's position.
3. A local anesthestic is given.
4. A #20 needle is introduced into the patient's abdomen and the fluid is withdrawn, 50 ml. at a time, until 300 to 1000 ml. is withdrawn.
5. Follow the same procedure as in #5, 6, and 7 of *thoracentesis*, above.

CLINICAL ALERT
Paracentesis may precipitate hepatic coma in a patient with chronic liver disease. Patient must be watched constantly for indications of shock: pallor, cyanosis, or dizziness. Emergency stimulants should be ready.

Clinical Implications

1. All effusions contain some mesothelial cells. (Mesothelial cells comprise the squamous layer of the epithelium covering the surface of all serous membranes.) The more chronic and irritating the condition, the more numerous and atypical are the mesothelial cells. Histiocytes and lymphocytes are common.
2. Evidence of abnormalities in serous fluids is characterized by:
    (a.) Degenerating RBC's, granular red cell fragments, and histiocytes containing blood. Presence of these structures means that injury to a vessel or vessels is part of the condition causing fluid to accumulate.
    (b.) Mucin, which is suggestive of adenocarcinoma.
    (c.) Large numbers of polymorphonuclear leukocytes,

which is indicative of an acute inflammatory process such as peritonitis.
- (d.) Prevalence of plasma cells which suggests the possibility of antibody formation.
- (e.) Numerous eosinophils which suggest parasitic infestation, Hodgkin's disease or a hypersensitive state.
- (f.) Presence of many reactive mesothelial cells together with hemosiderin histiocytes which may indicate:
     - (1.) Leaking aneurysm
     - (2.) Rheumatoid arthritis
     - (3.) Lupus erythematosus
- (g.) Malignant cells
3. Abnormal cells may be indicative of:
- (a.) Malignancy. The most important criterion of cancer is the arrangement of chromatin within the nuclei.
- (b.) Inflammatory conditions

Interfering Factors

Vigorous shaking and stirring of specimens will cause altered results.

Patient Preparation

Explain the purpose of test and procedure.

CHROMOSOME ANALYSIS

Normal Values

Women: 44 autosomes + 2X chromosomes; Karyotype: 46, XX

Men: 44 autosomes + 1X and 1Y chromosome; Karyotype: 46, XY

Background

Chromosome analysis is the study of the chromosomes, which are the cellular structures, containing the genes, the units of heredity. Two major factors are studied: 1) number of chromosomes, and 2) structure of chromosomes. Alteration in the total number of chromosomes or in their structure can result in a genetic disorder.

Most chromosome analyses are used as an aid in genetic counseling and diagnostic evaluation. This includes the study of chromosomes of fetal cells obtained by amniocentesis.

Studies are indicated in the following conditions:
1. Multiple malformation
2. Growth failure
3. Mental retardation
4. Ambiguous genital organs and hypogonadism
5. History of multiple miscarriages
6. Infertility
7. Primary amenorrhea or oligomenorrhea
8. Parents of children with known genetic disorders
9. Prospective mother over 35 years of age

Source of Specimen

Specimens used for chromosome analysis are generally taken from:
1. Leukocytes from peripheral blood
2. Bone marrow
3. Buccal or vaginal smear
4. Fibroblasts from skin or other tissues
5. Amniotic fluid

Of the sources, leukocytes are used most often because blood is the most easily obtained specimen.

Karyotyping

To evaluate chromosomes for anomalies in number of structure, a *karyotype* is prepared. A karyotype is an arrangement of pairs of chromosomes according to their size and structure, with the largest chromosomes placed first and the smallest placed last. The 23 pairs of chromosomes are arranged in seven groups—A through G. The sex chromosomes (two X's in normal females and an X plus a Y in a normal male) are usually placed apart from the autosomes but belong to the C group (X) and the E group (Y). (See Figure 10–1 for a karyotype of a male.)

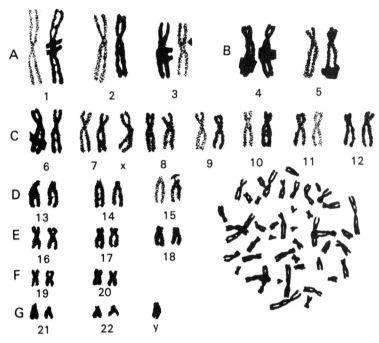

Fig. 10–1. A Human Karyotype. Pairs of homologous chromosomes are arranged in seven groups (A–G) according to total length. This figure shows a normal human male chromosome complement. (From Koss, Leopold G.: DIAGNOSTIC CYTOLOGY AND ITS HISTOPATHOLOGIC BASES. 3rd Ed., Philadelphia, J. B. Lippincott Co., 1979)

Individual chromosomes are distinguished by several characteristics:
1. Length
2. Location of the centromere position or the primary constriction
3. Arm ratios
4. Presence of secondary constrictions
5. Presence of satellites
6. Staining patterns

Nomenclature of the Karyotype

Placement of the letters and numbers of the karyotype has been agreed upon at international symposia. The following conventions are followed:

1. The first number is the total number of chromosomes.
2. The complement of sex chromosomes follows.
3. Then the chromosomes that are missing, extra, or abnormally formed are so indicated.

These principles are illustrated in the following examples:

Normal Female	46, XX
Normal Male	46,XY
Male with an additional No. 21 chromosome	47, XY, +21
Female with the short arm of No. 5 chromosome shorter than normal	46, XX, 5p−

Explanation of Test

1. Cells are cultured in the laboratory.
2. Time is allowed for the cells to undergo mitosis and to enter metaphase.
3. Further mitotic division is halted through chemical treatment of the cell culture.
4. Chromosomes are released when cell membrane is ruptured.
5. Chromosomes are placed on a glass slide, stained, and observed through a microscope.
6. Photomicrographs are taken of the chromosomes.
7. Individual chromosomes in the photo are cut apart and assembled to form the karyotype.
8. The patient's abnormalities are evaluated with respect to the karyotype.

Prenatal Chromosome Analysis

Certain genetic disorders, such as Down syndrome, can be detected in the early stages of a pregnancy (13th or 14th week) through chromosome analysis of fetal cells. A small amount of amniotic fluid is withdrawn through a needle inserted into the pregnant woman's lower abdominal wall. The fetal cells are analyzed as described above in "Explanation of Test." Results are available within two to three weeks. Only certain high risk Prospective mothers should have amniocentesis performed.

Clinical Implications

A. Chromosomal abnormalities involve whole chromosomes or parts of them. There may be too few or too many chromosomes; parts of a chromosome may be missing or it may be broken off and reattached to another chromosome. Common chromosomal disorders include:

  1. *Down syndrome* (formerly called Mongolism)
    Three types of cytogenetic abnormalities have been identified:

      (a.) *Trisomy 21.* This is the most common form of Down syndrome and is caused by an additional complete No. 21 chromosome. (There are three No. 21 chromosomes rather than a pair, giving a total chromosome count of 47.) This condition results in multiple defects with mental retardation, limb and facial anomalies, heart defects, and infertility in males. The disorder is due to failure of the two chromosomes of pair 21 to separate during sperm or egg development, resulting in an abnormal zygote with 47 chromosomes and a child with trisomy 21. Older women are much more likely to give birth to a child with Down syndrome. Risk increases progressively in women over age 35.

      (b.) *Translocation 21 trisomy.* This is rare and caused by extra chromosome 21 material attaching to chromosome 15. The same symptoms are produced as in standard trisomy 21. The actual chromosome count is the normal 46: however, persons with this form of Down syndrome have a longer No. 15 chromosome because the No. 21 chromosome is attached to it. This may be familial. When a parent, especially the mother, carries a chromosome 21 translocation, there is a substantial risk that her child will have Down syndrome.

(c.) *Mosaicism.* This is rare in Down syndrome. It is due to a mistake in the embryonic cell division and not a fault in the ovum or sperm formation. The affected individual has cells of different No. 21 chromosome counts dispersed throughout the body. The same symptoms as listed above are found, but the abnormalities are often less severe. This type of trisomy is not familial. Studies have shown that approximately 20 per cent of pregnancies will end in spontaneous abortion if mosaicism is present.

B. Sex chromosome abnormalities:

1. *Intersexuality.* In individuals with ambiguous genitalia, chromosome studies are helpful to establish the cellular sex of these persons. This information is important in guiding medical and surgical management.

2. *Turner syndrome.* The individual with only one X chromosome, missing either an X or a Y chromosome, has the Turner syndrome. This condition is associated with shortness of stature, infertility, heart disease and other manifestations.

3. *Klinefelter syndrome.* This is a major type of male hypogonadism and is caused by an extra X chromosome (karyotype is 47, XXY). Klinefelter syndrome can be detected by sex chromatin smears, since the second X chromosome forms a Barr body as in normal females, but it should be confirmed by chromosome analysis. (A discussion of Barr bodies and chromatin smears appears later in this chapter.)

C. Chromosome Analysis and Cancer

1. *Solid tumors.* Cells from many solid tumors can be characterized as having a broader range of chromosome count than found in normal tissue. However, there is little correlation between the type of chromosomal make-up and tumor histology.

2. *Leukemia.* A particular chromosomal aberration, the Philadelphia chromosome (Ph[1]), can be found in about 80 per cent of patients with chronic myelogenous leukemia. The Philadelphia chromosome is a deleted chromosome No. 22. It may be found in bone marrow cells even during remissions.

BARR BODY ANALYSIS; BUCCAL SMEARS FOR STAINING SEX CHROMATIN MASS

Normal Values

Barr body present: sex chromatin positive
Barr body absent: sex chromatin negative
Note: A Barr body occurs in 30 to 60 per cent of female somatic cells.

Explanation of Test

The Barr body is an inactive X chromosome, called sex chromatin which is contained in the nucleus of cells with two or more X chromosomes. Epithelial cells from a buccal smear or a vaginal smear may be stained with cresyl violet or other dyes and examined under the microscope. Techniques have also been developed to demonstrate the Barr body in cells from urine and amniotic fluid. The buccal smear however, is easily done and is an excellent screening method when a sex chromatin defect is suspected.

Analysis for the Barr body is done to detect sex chromosome abnormalities such as Turner syndrome and Klinefelter syndrome. It is important to remember that a sex determination is *not* being made when a chromatin test is done.

Procedure

1. Explain purpose of the test and the procedure to the patient.
2. Have patient rinse mouth well with mouthwash.
3. Using a metal spatula dipped in saline, scrape the buccal

mucosa. Discard the superficial layer of material. Scrape again firmly but gently, and spread the deeper layer of material on all slides. Prepare at least two slides from the same area.

4. Place the slides in a container containing a preservative.
5. Send specimen labeled with name, date, and site immediately to the laboratory.

Clinical Implications

1. Sex development abnormalities occur in:
    (a.) *Turner syndrome.* Negative for Barr body. Occurs in females who are sex chromatin negative and therefore have a karyotype of either 45, XO, or 46, XY, or 46, XX where one X chromosome is abnormal. Such females are characterized by amenorrhea and lack of secondary sexual maturation.
    (b.) *Klinefelter syndrome.* Positive for Barr body. Two Barr bodies may be found in the male with karyotype 48, XXXY or the karyotype 49, XXXYY. Three Barr bodies may be found in the male with karyotype 49, XXXXY. Such males have small testes, absent or decreased spermatogenesis, and show breast development and sparse body hair.
    (c.) Other sex chromosome abnormalities may be responsible for:
        (1.) Menstrual irregularities
        (2.) Infertility
        (3.) Mental retardation
        (4.) Growth abnormalities
        (5.) Retarded development of secondary sex characteristics
        (6.) Personality disorders
2. It is absolutely essential to remember that the sex chromatin tests cannot be used to determine the *true* genetic sex. The genetic sex depends upon the presence or absence of a Y chromosome, not upon the number of X chromosomes present. Buccal chromatin tests detect only the number of X chromosomes and only inferentially indicate the presence or absence of a Y chromosome.

REFERENCES

Brown, Walter V: TEXTBOOK OF CYTOGENETICS. St. Louis, The C. V. Mosby Company, 1972.

Brown, Walter V., and Bertke, Eldridge M: TEXTBOOK OF CYTOLOGY, 2nd Ed. St. Louis, The C. V. Mosby Company, 1974.

Fuhrmann, Walter, and Vogel, Friedrich: GENETIC COUNSELING. 2nd Ed. New York, Springer-Verlag, 1976.

Koss, Leopold G., DIAGNOSTIC CYTOLOGY AND ITS HISTOPATHOLOGIC BASES, 3rd Ed. Philadelphia, J.B. Lippincott Company, 1979.

Wallach, Jacques: INTERPRETATION OF DIAGNOSTIC TESTS—A HANDBOOK SYNOPSIS OF LABORATORY MEDICINE. 3rd Ed., Boston, Little, Brown and Company, 1978.

Zuher, M., and Naib, M.D., EXFOLIATIVE CYTOPATHOLOGY, 2nd Ed. Little, Brown and Co., 1976.

11 □□ COMMON ENDOSCOPIC STUDIES

INTRODUCTION

A group of diagnostic devices, known generically as "fiber-optic instruments," is used for direct visual examination of various internal body structures. Each of these instruments has a lighted mirror lens system attached to a flexible tube. In fiberoptics, light travels through an optic fiber by multiple reflections. Fiberoptic instruments are designed to redirect and transmit light around any number of twists and bends in the cavities and hollow organs of the body. The tube can be inserted into orifices and tracts of the body not easily accessible or directly visualized by other means. The insertion can be both for diagnosis of pathologic conditions and for therapy, such as in the removal of foreign objects. These examinations are done using local or general anesthetics. Biopsies are submitted for cytologic examination.

   This chapter will include discussions of the following procedures:

1. Mediastinoscopy—for examination and biopsy of lymph nodes in the mediastinum
2. Bronchoscopy—for visualization of the trachea and bronchi
3. Gastroscopy—for visual examination of the upper gastrointestinal tract
4. Colposcopy—for direct visualization of the vagina and cervix
5. Proctoscopy; sigmoidoscopy; proctosigmoidoscopy—for visualization of the rectum and sigmoid colon
6. Colonoscopy—for examination of the large intestine
7. Cystoscopy—for inspection of the bladder, urethra, orifices of the ureters, and prostate (in males)
8. Cystometry—This is not an endoscopic exam, but it is included because the procedure is often done in conjunction with cystoscopy. Cystometry is performed to study the pressure changes within the bladder during filling and voiding.

MEDIASTINOSCOPY

Normal Values

No evidence of disease; normal lymph glands.

Explanation of Test

This examination, which is performed under general anesthesia, involves the insertion of a lighted mirror lens instrument, similar to a bronchoscope, through an incision at the base of the neck. This procedure is done to biopsy the lymph nodes in the mediastinum. These nodes receive lymphatic drainage from the lungs, and biopsies may identify such diseases as carcinoma, granulomatous infection, and sarcoidosis. Mediastinoscopy has virtually replaced biopsy of the scalene fat pad for suspected nodes on the right side of the mediastinum. Mediastinoscopy is the routine method for establishing a tissue diagnosis of the stage of lung cancer. Nodes on the left side of the chest are usually biopsied through a limited left anterior thoracotomy (mediastinotomy) or occasionally, by scalene fat pad biopsy.

Procedure

1. Procedure is performed under general anesthesia in the surgical department.
2. The biopsy is done through a suprasternal incision.
3. Total procedure time is one and one-half hours.

Clinical Implications

1. Abnormal results in the examination aid in diagnosing:
    (a.) Sarcoidosis
    (b.) Tuberculosis
    (c.) Histoplasmosis
    (d.) Hodgkin's disease (this condition commonly involves the lymph nodes)
    (e.) Granulomatous infections
    (f.) Lung cancer
2. The procedure helps to demonstrate spread of lung tumors

Patient Preparation

1. Purpose of test and procedure should be explained to patient.
2. A legal permit must be signed prior to the examination.
3. Preoperative care is the same as for any patient who is going to have general anesthesia and surgery.
4. The patient must be NPO for 12 hours prior to test.

Patient Aftercare

Following the examination, care is the same as for any patient who has had surgery and a general anesthetic.

CLINICAL ALERT
1. Previous mediastinoscopy is a contraindication to another examination because adhesions make an adequate dissection of nodes extremely difficult and sometimes impossible.
2. The main complication of the procedure results from the general anesthesia.

BRONCHOSCOPY

Normal Values

Normal trachea, bronchi, and alveoli

Explanation of Test

This test permits visualization of the trachea and bronchi via a flexible bronchoscope. The procedure is used to diagnose tumors or granulomatous lesions, to biopsy, to take brushings for cytologic examinations, to improve drainage, and to remove foreign bodies. The exam is usually done under local anesthesia in the outpatient department or in the small operating room of a surgical suite.

Procedure

1. A local anesthetic is administered. The tongue, pharynx, and epiglottis are sprayed and swabbed with a local anesthetic.
2. The patient lies on his back with the neck hyperextended.
3. The flexible bronchoscope is inserted carefully through the mouth or nose into the pharynx and trachea.
4. The procedure is uncomfortable for most persons. When the bronchoscope is passed, the patient may feel that he cannot breathe or that he is suffocating.

Clinical Implications

Abnormalities that will be revealed include:
1. Abscesses
2. Bronchitis
3. Carcinoma
4. Tumors
5. Tuberculosis
6. Alveolitis
7. Site of hemorrhage

Patient Preparation

1. Explain purpose and procedure of the exam to the patient.
2. An informed consent form must be signed.
3. The patient must be NPO for four to six hours prior to the

procedure to reduce the risk of aspiration after reflexes are blocked.
4. Dentures and contact lenses must be removed prior to the exam.
5. Analgesics or tranquilizers/sedatives and atropine are ordered and administered one-half to one hour prior to bronchoscopy. The patient must be as relaxed as possible prior to and during the procedure.

Patient Aftercare

1. Be certain that the patient can swallow or cough before allowing foods or liquids.
2. Provide gargles to relieve a mild pharyngitis which may persist for 4 to 24 hours after exam.

CLINICAL ALERT
Observe for possible complications, including:
1. Cardiac arrhythmias
2. Hypoxemia
3. Laryngospasm
4. Bronchospasm
5. Pneumothorax
6. Respiratory failure
7. Bleeding following biopsy

GASTROSCOPY

Normal Values

Essentially normal upper GI tract.

Explanation of Test

This test allows the physician to visualize the lumen of the upper gastrointestinal tract via a fiberoptic instrument. This instrument is a tube that incorporates a lighted mirror-lens system. This method is valuable in determining the cause of upper gastrointestinal tract (UGI) bleeding, to confirm suspicious findings on x-rays, to establish a diagnosis in a symptomatic patient with a negative x-ray report, to biopsy

UGI lesions, and to diagnose hiatal hernia and esophagitis. It is also valuable in helping to determine if a gastric ulcer is benign or malignant. Note: "Endoscopy" is a general term denoting visual inspection of any body cavity with an endoscope. Endoscopic examination, therefore, may be ordered under any of the following terms: panendoscopy, esophagoscopy, gastroscopy, duodenoscopy, esophagostroscopy or esophagostroduodenoscopy.

Procedure

1. This examination is usually done in the outpatient department or surgical suite.
2. A topical anesthetic is applied to the throat in the form of a gargle.
3. Intravenous Valium is often given by the physician during the procedure. The Valium is injected slowly into a vein until the patient becomes relaxed and somewhat sleepy.
4. The endoscope is gently inserted into the esophagus and advanced slowly into the stomach and duodenum. Air is insufflated through the scope to distend the area being examined and to permit good visualization of the mucosa. Biopsies and brushings for cytology may be obtained during the examination. Photos may also be taken during the examination.
5. Feelings of pressure are felt, but there is no pain involved.
6. Immediately after completion of the examination, the patient will be asked to sit up and deep breathe, cough, and expectorate.
7. Examining time is about 15 minutes.

Clinical Implications

Abnormal results will indicate:
1. The site of hemorrhage
2. Hiatal hernia
3. Esophagitis
4. Neoplastic tissue
5. Gastric ulcers, benign or malignant

Patient Preparation

1. Explain the purpose of the test and the procedure.
2. Instruct patient that no food or water is to be ingested eight hours prior to the examination. In the hospital, this restriction is usually begun at midnight, prior to the examination. Give patient a written reminder of the fasting.
3. With outpatients, oral hygiene is to be done prior to coming to laboratory. With hospital patients, give assistance with oral care, if needed.
4. Patient is encouraged to urinate or defecate before the examination.
5. A tranquilizing medication may be given by injection 30 minutes prior to examination, if ordered.

Patient Aftercare

1. After the test is completed, no food or liquids are permitted for two hours.
2. Be certain that client is able to swallow before offering anything to drink.
3. Blood pressure, pulse, and respirations are checked every 30 minutes times four, especially if biopsies have been obtained during the examination.
4. A side-lying position in bed with the side rails up is to be maintained until the sedative has worn off, usually two hours.
5. The patient should experience no discomfort or side effects once the sedative has worn off.

COLPOSCOPY

Normal Values

Essentially normal vagina and cervix

Explanation of Test

Colposcopy is examination of the vagina and cervix with a colposcope, which is an instrument with a magnifying lens that is inserted into the vagina for visualization of the vagina and cervix. This examination is an aid in the diagnosis of benign and preclinical cancerous lesions of the cervix. It is now common to examine by colposcope all patients who have abnormal Papanicolaou (Pap) smears. With colposcopy, it is possible to do biopsies, and to take scrapings of cells under direct visualization.

The most common criteria for biopsy are leukoplakia vulvae and irregular blood vessels. (Leukoplakia vulvae is a precancerous condition characterized by grayish infiltrated patches on the vulvar mucosa.) The colposcope has a definite advantage in detecting atypical epithelium, which is designated in the literature as "basal cell activity." Atypical epithelium may be considered epithelium that cannot be called benign and yet does not fulfill all the criteria for a diagnosis of carcinoma *in situ*. Its detection is of value in cancer prophylaxis.

Patients receiving colposcopy may often be spared a conization (the removal of a cone of tissue from the cervix), which is a surgical procedure requiring hospitalization.

Procedure

1. The vagina and cervix are exposed with a speculum, as is usual in a gynecologic examination. No part of the colposcope is inserted into the vagina (see Figure 11–1). There is no discomfort when the speculum is inserted, just feelings of slight pressure.
2. A long cotton applicator stick is used to dry any cervical secretions.
3. The cervix and vagina are usually swabbed with acetic acid to improve contrast of the epithelial tissues.
4. Suspicious lesions are drawn on a diagram for the patient's record or photographs are made.
5. Biopsies of the lesions are done with a fine biopsy forceps. Some patients note discomfort at this time and others do not.
6. A small amount of vaginal bleeding for a few hours is not abnormal. A vaginal tampon may be inserted to absorb the flow.

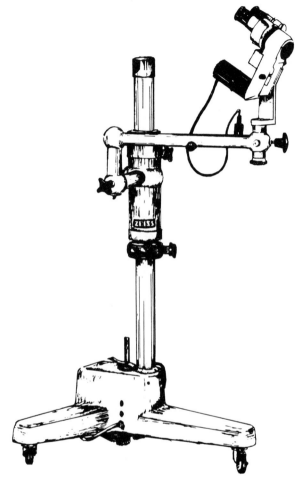

Fig. 11–1.   *The Colposcope. (Courtesy of Carl Zeiss, Inc., New York)*

Clinical Implications

A description is given of any abnormal lesions or unusual epithelial patterns:
1. Leukoplakia
2. Abnormal blood vessels

3. Atypical epithelium (Columnar epithelium may be replaced by squamous epithelium.)
4. Neoplastic tissue
5. Cancer *in situ*

Patient Preparation

1. Explain purpose of the examination and the procedure.
2. Inform patient that there will be a slight sensation of pressure when the speculum is inserted and that there may be a few hours of bleeding from the biopsy.

Patient Aftercare

Insert a vaginal tampon to absorb any bleeding.

PROCTOSCOPY; SIGMOIDOSCOPY; PROCTOSIGMOIDOSCOPY

Normal Values

Essentially a normal rectum and sigmoid

Explanation of Test

These tests involve the examination of a 31-cm. (or 12-inch) area of rectum and sigmoid with a proctoscope or sigmoidoscope. Both devices are essentially tubes incorporating a lighted mirror-lens system for illuminating the rectum and sigmoid. The main use of these studies is the detection and diagnosis of cancers. In cancer screening of people over 40, these exams should be routine. (Note: Men over 45 are the high-risk group for this form of malignancy.) These tests are also indicated in the evaluation of hemorrhoids, when blood is present in the stool, when bowel symptoms are present, and in unexplained anemia.

Procedure

1. Patient is placed in a knee-chest position for the exam, and the proctoscope or sigmoidoscope is carefully inserted.
2. The exam can be done with the patient in bed or on a special tilt table.
3. Usually the procedure takes three to five minutes.
4. There is no pain, but the patient may feel a very strong urge to defecate. This is a very natural reaction.

Clinical Implications

These tests may be ordered and may help to confirm any of the following conditions:
1. Ulcerative or granulomatous colitis
2. Inflammation of rectosigmoid area
3. Tumors of rectosigmoid area

Patient Preparation

1. Explain the purpose of the examination and the procedure to the patient.
2. The patient does not need to fast, but he may be placed on a light diet the evening before the test.
3. Laxatives may be given the night before the exam, and an enema or suppository may be administered an hour before the procedure. (In young, active patients, a small enema one hour before the scheduled exam is ample preparation.)

CLINICAL ALERT
1. Patients having acute rectal symptoms, particularly those with suspected ulcerative or granulomatous colitis, should be given the exam *without* any preparation—that is, without enemas, laxatives, or suppositories.
2. Perforation of the intestinal wall is an infrequent complication of these tests.
3. Do not give laxatives or enemas to pregnant women.

COLONOSCOPY

Normal Values

Normal large intestine

Explanation of Test

Colonoscopy is the examination of the large intestine with a fiberoptic instrument. This examination permits visualization of the colon by the use of a colonoscope, which is inserted through the anus to the ileocecal valve. The technique is valuable in differentiating inflammatory disease from neoplastic disease or in evaluating polypoid lesions beyond the reach of the sigmoidoscope. Polyps, foreign bodies, and specimens can be removed with the colonoscope, and photographs can be taken. Air, which passes through an accessory channel of the colonoscope, is used to distend the intestinal walls.

Clinical Implications

Abnormal results will indicate:
1. Polyps
2. Tumor
3. Areas of ulcerative colitis

Procedure

1. A clear liquid diet is usually ordered 72 hours prior to exam, and the patient must fast for eight hours before procedure.
2. Laxatives are ordered for one to three days before the test, and enemas are often ordered the night before.
3. The examination is done under analgesia or light anesthesia, using combinations of Talwin (pentazocine hydrochloride), Demerol (meperidine hydrochloride), Valium (diazepam), or Pentothal (thiopental sodium). The patient should be alert enough to inform the doctor of any gross complication during the examination.
4. Intravenous anticholinergics and glucagon are used when needed to relax local bowel spasms.

5. The patient is placed on his left side or Sim's position, and the rectum is dilated. Feelings of pressure are felt, but pain is usually not experienced.
6. The examination may take from one-half to two hours and is done by an endoscopist, who maneuvers the colonoscope through the twists and turns of the colon.

Patient Preparation

1. Explain purpose of the examination and the procedure to the patient.
2. Instruct the patient that he will be on a clear liquid diet 72 hours prior to test.
3. Administer medications and enemas, if ordered.
4. Explain that thorough cleansing of the bowel is very important and that this is the reason for the liquid diet and enema.
5. A legal consent form must be signed by patient.

Patient Aftercare

1. The patient should be NPO for two hours after the exam and on bedrest for six hours.
2. The stools should be observed for gross bleeding. Patient should be alert to abdominal pain because perforation and hemorrhage are possible complications.
3. Vital signs should be checked for six hours.
4. Flat plate x-ray of abdomen is done in the x-ray department (See chapter 9) late in the day following this procedure and again the following day.

CLINICAL ALERT
1. Contraindications for colonoscopy include:
   (a.) Perforating disease of the colon
   (b.) Peritonitis
   (c.) Acute conditions of the anus and rectum
   (d.) Recent abdominal surgery
   (e.) Recent myocardial infarction
2. Patients who have adhesions are not good candidates for this procedure.

CYSTOSCOPY

Normal Values

Normal structure and function of the bladder, urethra, orifices of the ureters, and prostate (in males)

Explanation of Test

This examination provides a view of the interior of the bladder, urethra, and prostatic urethra by means of the cystoscope, which is a tubular lighted telescopic lens. The procedure is done to observe bladder function and to detect deformation of the bladder, ureters, and prostate. The function of each kidney may be studied separately by means of catheterization of the ureters and collection of urine from each kidney.

The cystoscope is used not only for diagnostic but also for therapeutic purposes. Small stones and other foreign bodies may be removed from the urethra, ureter, and bladder. Biopsy specimens can be obtained, bladder stones can be crushed, and bladder tumors can be fulgurated.

Procedure

1. The examination is performed in a cystoscopy room which is part of the operating room suite of the hospital. It is also performed safely in the urologist's office.
2. The external genitalia are scrubbed and sprayed with an antiseptic solution such as Betadine (povidone-iodine).
3. The patient is placed in the lithotomy position with legs in stirrups.
4. A local anesthetic in the form of jelly is instilled into the urethra. In the male patient, the anesthetic is held in the urethra by a clamp applied near the end of the penis. For best results the local anesthetic is applied five to ten minutes before passage of the cystoscope.
5. The cystoscope is connected to an irrigation system.
6. The actual examination takes 15 minutes; however, the patient's time in the examining room is about one hour.

Clinical Implications

1. Cystoscopy is the most important and precise of all urologic diagnostic methods. This procedure may be indicated with the following conditions:
   - (a.) Unexplained hematuria
   - (b.) Recurrent urinary tract infection
   - (c.) Infection resistant to medical treatment
   - (d.) Unexplained urinary symptoms (*e.g.*, dysuria, frequency, urgency, hesitancy, intermittency, and straining)

Note: In an intravenous pyelogram (IVP) it is almost impossible to see the area from the neck of the bladder to the end of the urethra. Cystoscopy makes it possible to diagnose abnormalities in this area of the body.

2. Abnormal conditions that are revealed by this method include:
   - (a.) Prostatic hyperplasia
   - (b.) Cancer of the bladder
   - (c.) Bladder stone
   - (d.) Urethral stricture
   - (e.) Prostatitis
   - (f.) Vesical neck contracture

Patient Preparation

1. Explain the purpose and procedure of the test. Advise the patient that there is little pain or discomfort from cystoscopy. (Most persons will complain of more discomfort from a catheterization procedure.)
2. If cystoscopy is performed in the hospital, have the patient sign a legal consent form.
3. The patient is permitted a full liquid breakfast the morning of the examination, and liquids are permitted until the time of the exam.
4. Sedatives or analgesics are administered prior to examination. It is common practice to give Nembutal (pentobarbital sodium) three to four hours prior to cystoscopy. Patients who receive morphine sulfate for analgesia and scopolamine seem to experience less discomfort during the procedure.

Valium may also be given intravenously. Male patients up to 60 years of age experience more pain and discomfort than do older men. Female patients require less sedation because the urethra is shorter.

Patient Aftercare

1. For 24 hours following cystoscopy, the patient's capacity to void should be determined, as well as whether his bladder emptying is complete.
2. When the patient is able to void, fluids should be encouraged.
3. Any bleeding that occurs should stop, because clots will form.
4. Inability to void or to empty bladder completely may signify large clot formation.
5. Frequency of urination and some dysuria is anticipated following cystoscopy.
6. Antibiotics are usually given one day prior and three days following examination to prevent infection.
7. The urethra is such a vascular organ that any break in the tissues allows bacteria to enter directly into the bloodstream. Observe and report chills and fever (urethral chill) to the urologist.

CYSTOMETRY

Normal Values

Normal filling pattern; normal sensation of fullness at 100 to 450 ml., urge to void at 350 to 450 ml.; filling bladder pressure constant until capacity reached with contraction at capacity; normal thermal sensation when hot and cold sterile fluids are introduced into the blood.

Explanation of Test

This study of intravesical pressure changes during filling and emptying (voiding) of the bladder is an aid in evaluating bladder function and in determining whether bladder pathophysiology is due to neurologic, infectious, or obstructive disease. The primary purpose of cystometry is to determine if a detrusor (pushing down) reflex exists. These studies are indicated when there is evidence of neurologic disease: spina bifida, myelomeningocele, cord injury, extensive pelvis dissection, cordotomy, neurectomy or a specific neuropathy such as multiple sclerosis, cord tumor, diabetes, and tabes dorsalis. This examination is also useful in evaluating clients with known neurologic disease but with symptoms of dysuria, small or weak urinary stream, frequency, enuresis, overflow or stress incontinence, residual urine, or recurrent infection. This exam is often done in conjunction with cystoscopy, which is described earlier in the chapter.

Procedure

1. After the patient voids, a catheter is inserted and is then connected to the cystometer. (A cystometer is a device for studying the neuromuscular mechanism of the bladder by measuring capacity and pressure.) The bladder is then filled with water or a gas.
2. Observations are recorded during the cystometric examination about these sensations:
   - (a.) Heat and cold
   - (b.) Bladder fullness
   - (c.) Urge to void
   - (d.) Ability to inhibit voiding when contractions occur
3. The patient is asked to void, and the urine flow rate and voiding pressure are recorded.
4. The patient is asked to report sensations that are related to the neurologic stimulation of the bladder and sphincter muscles:
   - (a.) Flushing
   - (b.) Sweating
   - (c.) Pain
   - (d.) Nausea
   - (e.) Bladder fullness
   - (f.) Strong urge to void
5. During the examination cholinergic and anticholinergic drugs (*e.g.,* Banthine [methantheline bromide], atropine, and Urecholine [bethanechol chloride]) may be administered to determine their effects on bladder function. The following questions may be probed:

(a.) Is an atonic bladder capable of being stimulated by cholinergic parasympathomimetic drugs such as Urecholine, or are detrusor muscle fibers so decompensated that no response can be elicited?

(b.) Can overactive motor stimuli be altered sufficiently with cholinergic blocking parasympatholytic drugs such as atropine to allow a near-normal bladder volume that will produce an acceptable voiding pattern?

6. To determine the effect of these drugs, a cystometric study is performed as a control (see procedure for cystometry), followed by another tracing 20 to 30 minutes after injection of the drugs.

7. Examination time is one-half to one hour.

Clinical Implications

Abnormal flow rates and voiding pressure may indicate:

1. Lower urinary tract obstruction, as in bladder tumors
2. Neurogenic or cord bladder and absence of detrusor reflex, as in

   (a.) Spina bifida   (e.) Cordotomy
   (b.) Myelomeningocele   (f.) Neurectomy
   (c.) Cord injury
   (d.) Extensive pelvic dissection

3. Bladder dysfunction due to upper or lower motor neuron lesions, as in

   (a.) Spinal cord tumor
   (b.) Diabetes
   (c.) Tabes dorsalis

Patient Preparation

Explain purpose of examination and procedure to patient.

REFERENCES

Bolten, Karl and Jacques, William. "Introduction to Colposcopy", Abbott Laboratories, 1959.

Brunner, L. S., and Suddarth, D.: THE LIPPINCOTT MANUAL OF NURSING PRACTICE, 2nd Ed., Philadelphia, J. B. Lippincott Co., 1978.

Clarke, S. W. "Fiberoptic Bronchoscopy", NURS MIR, Nov. 27, 1979
    p. 47–49.

Glenn, James F., editor, DIAGNOSTIC UROLOGY, New York,
    Harper and Row, 1964..

Guidelines for the VINCE LOMBARDI COLON CLINIC, unpub-
    lished, Milwaukee County Hospital, Milwaukee, Wisconsin,
    1978.

Luckman, J., and Sorensen, K. C.: MEDICAL-SURGICAL
    NURSING. Philadelphia, W. B. Saunders Co., 1974.

Marice, Frank. "The Flexible Fiberoptic Bronchoscope", AM J
    NURS, October, 1973, p. 1776–1778.

Overholt, Bergein, E. "Colonoscopy", AMERICAN CANCER SOCI-
    ETY PROFESSIONAL EDUCATION PUBLICATION, 1975.

Savage, Edward D. "Correlation of Colposcopically Directed Biopsy
    and Conization with Histologic Diagnosis of Cervical Lesions."
    J REPRO MED, Vol. 15, December, 1975, p. 211.

12 □□ ULTRASOUND STUDIES

INTRODUCTION

Overview

Ultrasonography is a noninvasive procedure for visualizing soft tissue structures of the body by recording the reflection of ultrasonic waves directed into the tissues. This harmless diagnostic procedure, which requires very little patient preparation, is now being used in many branches of medicine for accurate diagnosis of certain pathologic conditions. It may be used diagnostically with the obstetric and gynecologic patient, the cardiac patient, and in abnormal conditions of the kidney, pancreas, gallbladder, lymph node, liver, spleen, thyroid, and peripheral blood vessels. Frequently, it is used in conjunction with radiography or radioisotope scans. The procedure is relatively quick (often requiring only a few minutes to an hour) and causes little discomfort.

Principles of the Technique

Ultrasound employs high frequency sound waves to examine the position, form, and function of anatomical structures within the body. Both superficial and deep structures may be visualized. This method can be used to examine moving structures (*e.g.*, the heart) and beautifully demonstrates fetal movements. Utilizing principles first employed in sonar, ultrasound involves transmission of a sound frequency higher than that detectable by the human ear.

The basic principles of ultrasound are the following:
1. An ultrasound beam is directed into the patient's body.
2. By vibration the beam is propagated through body tissue.
3. The body tissue, being composed of structures of different densities, reflects the sound waves in various ways.
4. Reflected sound waves are electronically processed and shown on imaging displays.
5. Recordings of the reflected sound waves may be made on Polaroid film or videotape.

Evidences of pathology are detectable because lesions are of different density and elasticity than the surrounding normal tissue. However, ultrasound cannot be used diagnostically with the air-filled lung or the gas-filled intestine because the ultrasound beam is almost totally reflected by air-containing organs. For this reason the ultrasound beam cannot be employed where air-filled lung or gas-filled intestine will come between the beam and the part of the body being studied.

Terminology

"Ultrasonography" is the term most frequently used for the procedure using ultrasound. "Echography" may be used interchangeably with "ultrasonography." "Echogram" or "sonogram" is the record made by ultrasonography (echography). The record may also be called the "scan." The technician examining the patient is the "ultrasonographer" and applies a device called a "transducer" to the surface of the patient's skin. Ultrasound waves are transmitted through the skin to deeper body structures. A lubricant applied to the skin to serve as a conductor of sound waves is called the "coupling agent."

Display Techniques

The complexities of the ultrasonic equipment used in ultrasound studies as well as the physical principles involved are beyond the scope of this book. However, it is helpful to have a general understanding of the types of equipment used and the techniques for displaying the image.

A cathode ray tube (CRT) displays the amplitude of the echoes and the time required for the reflection of the sound waves. Several different types of imaging displays are available:

1. A-mode display. This was the earliest type of display used. All other displays are derived from this. Time and amplitude are given.
2. B-mode display. This is a two-dimensional display that provides a cross–sectional image.
3. Real-time display. This is a high-speed scanner that allows for visualization of moving structures such as the living fetus, the heart, and blood vessels.

Recording Display Images

Images are displayed on a cathode ray tube. However, a permanent record of the patterns is needed so that the images can be carefully studied. Following are some of the methods used at present:

1. Photographs may be taken of A-mode or B-mode scans that are displayed on non-storage oscilloscopes.
2. A storage oscilloscope can provide a display image that may be seen while the scan is being produced.
3. Certain real-time imaging systems are equipped with sensitized paper that continuously moves in front of the display image, providing a continuous permanent record that may be checked at any time and filed as part of the patient's history.

4. Methods of recording the echoes of ultrasound include:
   - (a.) "A" mode (amplitude)
   - (b.) "B" mode (brightness)
   - (c.) "M" mode (motion)
   - (d.) Gray scale
   - (e.) Real time

Uses of Ultrasound

1. Obstetrical use of ultrasound is the most common application of this diagnostic modality. This is because fluid-filled uterus is an ideal environment from which to gain information with diagnostic ultrasound.
2. Ultrasound has been frequently used in diagnosis of brain disorders to determine shifts in the intracranial midline structures; however, this technique is used less often since the advent of computed tomography (CT) of the head. Ultrasound studies are still useful when CT and radionuclide studies are not available and in following young children with hydrocephalus.
3. Other uses of ultrasound include studies of the genitourinary system with promising results identified in the examination of the urinary bladder, scrotum, and prostate and in the diagnosis of renal masses.
4. A 98.8 per cent accuracy rate has been reported in use of ultrasound to detect aortic aneurysms.
5. Ultrasound is the method of choice in screening for suspected pancreatic disease. Included in this category are pancreatic tumors, pancreatitis, and pseudocytes.
6. Echograms of the thyroid have their greatest value when used in conjunction with palpation of the gland by an experienced clinician. It is useful in differentiating cysts from tumors.
7. Echograms of the eye aid ophthalmologists in removal of foreign bodies and allows the ophthalmologist to study the posterior parts of the eye, especially when the lens is opaque (cataracts or in vitreous hemorrhage). It is also helpful in evaluating retinal detachment.
8. Ultrasound studies of the gallbladder will detect disease as well as gallstones. Diseases of the gallbladder often are not

detected when conventional x-ray techniques are used because the distressed organ cannot concentrate the dye used in testing. Ultrasonography does not depend on organ function and thus can be used even in the presence of significant jaundice which would interfere with radiologic techniques dependent on organ function.

Procedure (General)

1. A gel or lubricant, such as mineral oil or glycerin, is applied to the skin over the area to be examined. The oil or gel acts as a conductor of the sound waves.
2. In certain cases, water is used as the conductor of sound waves. The patient is then either immersed in a water bath or a water bath is hung over the area to be scanned.
3. A transducer is handheld by an examiner, who watches a screen while moving this device over a specific area of the body. Often a "sweeping" or "brushing" motion is used.
4. The examination is performed by a technician called an ultrasonographer.
5. The physician then views the recorded images and takes scan pictures of the images.
6. The examination causes no physical discomfort. However, if the examining time is long, the patient could become very tired.
7. All tests take at least 35 to 45 minutes. This test time refers to the actual time the patient is in the examining department.
8. Some examinations require fasting and enemas.
9. Certain tests are best performed with a full bladder.
10. Each individual examining department will determine its own guidelines.

Contact Technique vs. Water Bath Technique

Since air provides a poor medium for transmission of ultrasound beams, another medium must be used to couple the ultrasonic energy from the probe into the patient. Two major kinds of coupling agents have been used: water and various kinds of oils and gels.

1. *Water bath.* Early scanning devices relied heavily on the immersion of the patient in a water bath. This method provided good detail or internal structure and good sound beam control, but it was cumbersome, and the condition of the patient often made immersion inadvisable. Several newer ultrasound devices have returned to the water bath as a coupling agent. This is especially true when visualizing small organs such as the eye or the thyroid.
2. *Contact method.* This technique utilizes oils, glycerin, and water soluble gels that are applied directly to the patient's skin. The transducer is swept across the skin with a brushing motion, with the probe always moving along a layer of the coupling material. Advantages of this technique are that it is easy to use, and the device is portable.

Advantages of Ultrasound Studies

1. Noninvasive procedure
2. Requires little, if any, patient preparation
3. Procedure is safe for both patient and examiner. (To date, the procedure has been shown to be safe even for the developing fetus.)
4. Examination can be repeated as many times as necessary without being injurious to patient. There is no harmful cumulative effect.
5. Studies can obviate the need for extended hospitalization.
6. Since ultrasound studies demonstrate structure rather than function, they may be useful with patients whose organ function is impaired.
7. Useful in detection and examination of moving parts, such as the heart.
8. Does not require the injection of contrast materials, isotopes, or ingestion of opaque materials.
9. Fasting is not required.
10. Examination time is generally short—from a few minutes to a half hour.

Disadvantages of Ultrasound Studies

1. An extremely skilled technician is required to operate the transducer. The scans must be read immediately and inter-

preted for adequacy. If the scans are unusable, the examination must be repeated.
2. Air-filled structures (*e.g.*, lungs) cannot be studied via ultrasonography.
3. Certain patients cannot be studied adequately unless specially prepared (*e.g.*, restless children, extremely obese patients).

Patients Difficult to Study

The following general categories of patients may provide some difficulties in ultrasound studies:
1. Postoperative patients. If possible, dressings should be removed and a sterile coupling agent and probe should be applied gently to the skin.
2. Patients with abdominal scars. The scar tissue causes attenuation of the ultrasound.
3. Children. Since the procedure requires the patient to remain very still, children may need to be sedated so that their movements do not cause artifacts.

CLINICAL ALERT
Inadequate contact between the skin and the probe is one of the principal causes of unusable scans. Sufficient quantities of coupling agent, such as oil, must be applied to the skin and frequently reapplied.

Interfering Factors

1. Barium has an adverse effect on the quality of abdominal studies, so echograms should be scheduled before barium studies are done.
2. If a patient has a large amount of gas in the bowel, the exam will be rescheduled because air (bowel gas) is a very strong reflector of sound and will cause inaccuracies.
3. Because a gel or lubricant on the skin is used as a conductor, the examination cannot be performed over an area of open wounds or dressings.

OBSTETRIC ECHOGRAM

Normal Values

Normal pattern image reported in a B-mode of fetal and placental position and size.

Explanation of Test

Ultrasound studies of the obstetric patient are valuable in (a) confirming pregnancy, (b) determining fetal age, (c) confirming multiple pregnancy, and (d) ascertaining whether fetal development is normal, through sequential studies.

The pregnant uterus is ideal for echographic evaluation because the amniotic fluid-filled uterus provides strong transmitting interfaces between the fluid, placenta, and fetus. Ultrasonography has become the method of choice in evaluating the fetus, thus eliminating the need for the potentially injurious x-ray studies previously used. Since ultrasonography as used in obstetrics is about 98 per cent accurate in detecting placental site, radionuclide studies of the pregnant patient have been abandoned.

Procedure

1. Patient lies in the supine position with her abdomen exposed.
2. A coupling agent (*e.g.*, mineral oil, olive oil, or special gels) is applied liberally to the skin.
3. The scanner is positioned either to the left or right of the patient.
4. Generally, standards established by the American Institute of Ultrasound in Medicine are used. This provides for some measure of agreement in the interpretation of the scans.
5. The examining time is about 30 minutes.

Clinical Implications

1. Pregnancy can be diagnosed as early as five weeks after the last missed menstrual period.

2. Fetal age can be determined through ultrasound cephalometry. (Such a study may be done from 14 weeks to term. Before 14 weeks' gestation, fetal age may be determined by crown-rump length measurements.)

3. A growth-retarded fetus can be determined by serial cephalometry coupled with estriol measurements.

4. The fetal position may be accurately noted. This information is particularly valuable in breech presentation or transverse lie, when normal vaginal delivery may not be possible.

5. The placenta may be easily identified. Conditions such as abruptio placentae (premature separation of the placenta) and placenta previa (placental development in the lower uterine segment, partially or completely covering the cervical os) can also be identified.

6. Various conditions associated with the larger-than-expected pregnant uterus can be differentiated: incorrect calculation of dates, multiple pregnancy, molar pregnancy, fibroids, or polyhydramnios.

7. Multiple pregnancies may be diagnosed after 13 to 14 weeks' gestation by demonstration of more than one fetal head.

8. Fetal cranial abnormalities such as anencephaly and hydrocephalus can be diagnosed. *In utero* diagnoses of congenital heart problems and polycystic renal disease are possible.

9. Fetal death can be determined by a series of sequential scans that show lack of total growth, including uterine growth, loss of fetal outline, and increased fetal intracranial echoes. Fetal death is suggested by bizarre echoes from the fetal thorax and skull, failure to grow, diminished growth, and overlapping of cranial bones.

Interfering Factors

1. Artifacts can be produced when the transducer is moved out of contact with the skin. This can be resolved by adding more coupling agent to the skin and repeating the scan.

2. Artifacts (reverberation) may be produced by echoes emanating from the same surface several times. This can be avoided by careful positioning of the transducer.

Patient Preparation

1. Instruct patient about the purpose(s) of the test and explain the procedure.
2. Give the patient three to four glasses (200 to 400 cc.) of water or liquids one hour prior to the exam. Instruct her not to void until the test is completed.
3. Inform the patient that the examination will be done when she has an urge to void but is not yet uncomfortable.
4. Assure the patient that the test is not painful and will not cause discomfort.
5. Advise patient that the studies can be repeated without harm to the mother. There is no known harm to the fetus, but the procedure is being studied carefully to determine whether there are any adverse side effects.
6. Explain that a liberal coating of coupling agent, such as mineral oil, must be applied to the skin so that there is no air between the skin and the probe (transducer) and so that the probe will pass easily across the skin.

CLINICAL ALERT
A full bladder may not be needed or desired in the patient who is in the late stages of pregnancy or is in active labor.

GYNECOLOGIC ECHOGRAM

Normal Values

Normal pattern image of bladder, uterus, and vagina.

Explanation of Test

Ultrasound studies of the gynecologic patient may be used to evaluate pelvic masses and to aid in the diagnosis of cysts and tumors. Information can be provided on the size, location, and structure of the masses. These examinations cannot give definitive diagnoses of pathology, but they can be used as an adjunct procedure when the diagnosis is not readily apparent. Ultrasound exams may be used to pinpoint the location of an IUD; x-ray studies will merely indicate that the device is in the pelvis. These studies are also used in treatment planning and follow-up radiation therapy of gynecologic cancer.

With this test, a full bladder is necessary. The distended bladder serves four purposes: (1) acts as a "window" for transmission of the ultrasound beam, (2) pushes the uterus away from the pubic symphysis, thus providing a less-obstructed view, (3) pushes the bowel out of the pelvis, and (4) may be used as a comparison in evaluating the internal characteristics of a mass under study.

Procedure

1. The patient lies on her back on the examining table during the test.
2. A coupling agent is applied to the area under study.
3. The active face of the transducer is placed in contact with the patient's skin and swept across the area being studied.
4. A contact B-scanner or real-time scanner is used.
5. The examination time is about 30 minutes.

Interfering Factors

1. Results are only fair (see Clinical Implications) and can only be used in conjunction with other studies.
2. Echograms are difficult to do in the pelvic area because of the gas-filled intestine and the bladder.

Clinical Implications

1. Ultrasound studies may raise the suspicion that a uterine fibroid exists; such studies, however, cannot confirm this diagnosis. It may also be difficult to differentiate a uterine fibroid from a solid adnexal tumor.
2. Adnexal masses smaller than three cm. in diameter may not be demonstrated by ultrasound studies. Larger masses studied with this technique can provide information on size and consistency.

3. Ovarian cysts will appear as smoothly outlined, well-defined masses. Cysts cannot be confirmed as either malignant or benign, but ultrasound studies can increase the suspicion that a particular mass is malignant.
4. Ultrasound studies can help to determine whether a pelvic mass is mobile.
5. Solid pelvic masses, such as fibroids and malignant tumors, may be differentiated from cystic masses, which will show sound patterns similar to the bladder.
6. Lesions may be shown to have metastasized.
7. Studies may aid in the planning of tumor radiation therapy.
8. Position of an intrauterine contraceptive device may be determined.

Patient Preparation

1. Instruct patient about the purpose of the test and the procedure to be followed.
2. Have patient drink three to four glasses of water or liquid one hour prior to the exam. Advise her not to void until the test is over.
3. Reassure her that there is no pain or discomfort involved.

KIDNEY ECHOGRAM

Normal Values

Normal pattern image indicating normal size and position of the kidney.

Explanation of Test

This noninvasive test, often done to differentiate renal masses, has become an accepted clinical procedure following intravenous pyelography (IVP). It is of value in monitoring the status of the transplanted kidney. Using the IVP, the exact location of the renal mass can be located before ultrasonic exams are performed. However, in the case of impaired renal function and iodine allergies which preclude the use of IVP, renal echograms are fairly reliable and easy to do and can be used alone to establish a diagnosis.

Procedure

1. The patient lies quietly in a prone position on an examining table. However, the right kidney may also be examined with the patient supine, employing the liver as an "acoustic window."
2. Warm oil is applied to the back.
3. For visualization of the upper poles of the kidney, the patient must inspire as deeply as possible.
4. The total study time varies from 45 to 120 minutes.

Clinical Implications

1. Abnormal pattern readings will reveal:
   (a.) Cysts   (c.) Hydronephrosis
   (b.) Solid masses   (d.) Obstruction of ureters
2. Studies can provide information on the size, site, and internal structure of a nonfunctioning kidney.
3. Studies can differentiate between bilateral hydronephrosis, polycystic kidneys, and the small end-stage kidneys of glomerulonephritis or pyelonephritis.
4. Ultrasound may be used to follow the kidney development in children with congenital hydronephrosis. This approach is safer than repeated IVP's.
5. Perirenal hematomas or abscesses may be discovered.
6. Solid lesions may be differentiated from cystic lesions.

Interfering Factors

Retained barium from x-rays will give poor results.

Patient Preparation

1. Instruct the patient about the purpose of the test and procedure.
2. Assure patient that there is no pain involved; the only dis-

comfort is that caused by lying quietly for a long period of time.
3. Explain that *no fasting is necessary.*

CLINICAL ALERT
1. Scans cannot be done over open wounds or dressings.
2. This examination must be performed before barium x-ray. If such scheduling is not possible, at least 24 hours must elapse after barium procedure before the renal echogram is done.
3. Biopsies are often done using ultrasound as a guideline. If a biopsy is done, a surgical permit must be signed by the patient.

PANCREAS ECHOGRAM

Normal Values

Normal pattern image on gray scale, B-scan imaging indicating normal size and position of pancreas. The normal gland is an echo-producing structure.

Background

The pancreas is an extremely inaccessible abdominal organ; various diagnostic procedures have been attempted to ascertain pathologic conditions of this organ. Ultrasound studies are probably the safest and most accurate procedures available. With gray scale ultrasound equipment, the normal pancreas can be visualized 75 per cent to 95 per cent of the time (Hagen-Ansert, 1978).

Explanation of Test

Ultrasound studies are done to establish a diagnosis of chronic pancreatitis, pseudocysts, and carcinoma. It is the method of choice for screening for suspected pancreatic disease and to monitor the response of pancreatic tumors to therapy. The results of these studies are used as a guide for percutaneous aspiration and biopsy. Liver and pancreatic ultrasound studies may be done at the same time. The pancreas may be visualized more easily and precisely by echogram than by any other method.

Procedure

1. The patient lies on his back on the examining table.
2. The skin is covered with a layer of mineral oil.
3. Patient must inspire deeply before the scans are taken.
4. Total time of the examination is one to one and one-half hours.

Patient Preparation

Explain the purpose of the test and the procedure.

Clinical Implications

1. Abnormal image patterns can identify the following conditions:
   (a.) Acute and chronic pancreatitis
   (b.) Possible sequelae of pancreatitis
   (c.) Pseudocysts
   (d.) Carcinoma of the pancreas
2. In the patient with pancreatitis, the borders of the pancreas are more distinct, and the fibrous tissues septae inside the gland become more apparent.

CLINICAL ALERT
If the patient with pancreatitis has an unusual amount of bowel gas, the scan will be repeated.

---

3. With ultrasound studies pseudocysts appear as well defined masses with echofree interiors. (A pseudocyst occurs when a portion of the pancreas is deprived of its normal route of drainage through the pancreatic duct. Enzymes which con-

tinue to be secreted form walled-off cysts with no mucosal lining.)
4. Pancreatic carcinoma may be identified as an irregular mass with scattered internal echoes and poorly defined borders. This condition may easily be confused with lymph node enlargement secondary to lymphoma.

Interfering Factors

1. Air, gas, or bone near the pancreas could interfere with visualization of the organ.
2. If the stomach, costal cartilage, or fat overlies the pancreas, visualization is impeded.
3. The obese patient presents an impediment to visualization because of the difficulty of ultrasound waves passing through layers of fat.
4. Movement of the organ can cause difficulties, but this is less of a problem if real time imaging techniques are used.
5. Barium from recent radiographic studies will cause problems in visualization.

GALLBLADDER AND BILIARY SYSTEM ECHOGRAM

Normal Values

Normal pattern image reported via the B-mode technique indicating normal size and position of the gallbladder and bile ducts.
    Normal gallbladder: 3 cm. wide; 7.5–10 cm. long

Explanation of Test

This test is used to differentiate hepatic disease from biliary obstruction. The gallbladder and sometimes the common bile and cystic duct can be identified using echography. This method is the procedure of choice when a patient with poor liver function has an elevated serum bilirubin and contrast x-rays cannot be performed.

Procedure

1. The patient lies on his back on the examining table.
2. If gallstones are suspected, the patient will have to stand up during the exam.

Clinical Implications

1. Abnormal pattern images will indicate:
    (a.) Enlarged gallbladder
    (b.) Obstruction of the common bile duct
    (c.) Dilatation of the biliary tree
    (d.) Stones in the gallbladder and common bile duct
    Note: Gallstones smaller than two to three mm. in diameter often cannot be visualized. These stones are often the most dangerous because they can obstruct the flow of bile by entering the bile ducts.
2. Stones usually cause dense echoes in the gallbladder area.
3. Inflammation of the gallbladder (cholecystitis) will be indicated by a slightly enlarged sonolucent structure with thickened walls.
4. At low and medium sensitivities a fluid-filled gallbladder may seem echo-free. Use of the gray scale may allow for easier localization of this organ.

Patient Preparation

1. Explain the purpose of the test and procedure.
2. Instruct patient not to eat solid food for 12 hours prior to exam. (This allows the greatest dilatation of the gallbladder.)
3. Water is permitted.
4. In some instances, enemas will be ordered prior to testing.

CLINICAL ALERT
When it is difficult to differentiate between an abnormal gallbladder and a normal gallbladder with good contractility, give patient a fatty meal and do another scan after 40 minutes to check contractility.

LYMPH NODE ECHOGRAM

Normal Values

Normal lymph nodes, which are smaller than a finger tip, are *not* visible with ultrasound. Only when the lymph nodes enlarge, as with tumor or infection, are they visible.

Explanation of Test

This test is ordered for a patient who has aortic or iliac lymph node enlargement and lymphoma is suspected. Localization of lymph node masses by this method prior to radiotherapy is very useful in planning treatment and may be used as a follow-up study to assess shrinkage of the mass. These studies are easy to do and fairly reliable with 28 per cent chance of error. Ultrasound studies of the lymph nodes are often done in conjunction with lymphangiography.

Procedure

1. The patient lies on his back during the test.
2. Scans in two planes—longitudinal and transverse—must be taken.
3. If scans are taken below the umbilicus, the patient should have a full bladder to push the bowel out of the pelvis.

Clinical Implications

1. Abnormal pattern readings indicate retroperitoneal adenopathy.
2. Lymph nodes that have enlarged will be more homogeneous than surrounding structures.

Patient Preparation

1. Instruct patient about the purpose of the test and procedure.
2. A 12-hour fast from solid food prior to the test is usually required.
3. Water is permitted.

Interfering Factors

With scans taken below the umbilicus, a gas-filled bowel may cause difficulty in visualizing the image.

LIVER ECHOGRAM

Normal Values

Normal pattern image indicating normal size, shape, and position of liver and normal relationship to adjacent anatomic structure.

Explanation of Test

This noninvasive diagnostic technique is used to determine the cystic, solid, or complex nature of a liver defect. Pleural effusion can be seen and the intrahepatic ducts and veins can also be visualized. This examination is an excellent guide in evaluating ascites and is used prior to biopsy. Liver echograms are also used with good results mainly to differentiate cysts and abscesses from tumors. Liver sonograms are extremely useful in conjunction with hepatic radioisotope studies. Unfortunately, liver echograms are not reliable in detecting metastasis.

Procedure

1. The patient lies on his back on the examining table.
2. Scans in several different planes are taken: supine longitudinal, supine transverse, and supine oblique.

Clinical Implications

1. Abnormal pattern readings will reveal:
    (a.) Biliary duct obstruction
    (b.) Cirrhosis
    (c.) Liver masses (intrahepatic, extrahepatic, or subhepatic)
    (d.) Necrotic tumors

(e.) Metastasis to liver

(f.) Cause of jaundice

2. Cystic masses, solid masses, and abscesses may be distinguished from one another (cystic lesions have an echo-free nature, while abscesses may contain internal echoes). Solid masses will have internal echoes and will alternate the sound beam more than cystic lesions or abscesses.

3. A cirrhotic liver is more echogenic (contains more echoes than the normal liver).

4. Serial scans can be used to determine the volume of the liver.

5. An adenocarcinoma will have a dense central echo pattern surrounded by a less echo-producing halo. The image pattern is thus called the "bulls eye" (Hagen-Ansert, 1978).

Patient Preparation

Instruct patient about the purpose of the test and the test procedure.

Interfering Factors

Images of the right lobe may be somewhat obscured by rib artifacts.

SPLEEN ECHOGRAM

Normal Values

Normal pattern image; concave sonolucent structure in left upper quadrant; highly echo-producing.

Explanation of Test

This test is useful when the spleen is enlarged, because it is then easily detectible. Ultrasound is often used when a splenectomy is contemplated, such as with thrombocytopenic purpura. These studies can be used to estimate spleen size and volume and may spare the patient discomfort from other kinds of diagnostic procedures. Ultrasound is often used in conjunction with a radioisotope scan, except in the case of pregnant women.

Procedure

1. The patient will be on his back or abdomen on examining table during the test.
2. Examining time is about 30 minutes.

Clinical Implications

1. Abnormal pattern readings will reveal an enlarged spleen, splenic metastasis, and cysts.
2. Although splenic metastases are rare, they will produce stronger than normal echoes.
3. Cysts within the spleen are identified because they give off no echoes.
4. In pregnant women who have experienced trauma to the spleen, a splenic hematoma may develop, causing distortion of the border of the spleen; hemorrhagic areas may be separated by a band of echoes.
5. The spleen is often large and echo-free in early sickle cell disease, but shrinks in size and is echo-producing in later stages of the disease.

Patient Preparation

1. Instruct patient about the purpose of the test and procedure.
2. Fasting from food for 12 hours prior to examination is usually necessary.
3. Water is permitted.

THYROID ECHOGRAM

Normal Values

Normal pattern image of thyroid; echoes will be uniformly reflected throughout the gland; boundaries are unevenly displayed. (The normal thyroid is moderately echogenic and will be surrounded by the trachea, carotid sheath, and anterior strap muscles.)

Explanation of Test

This ultrasound study is used to determine the size of the thyroid, to differentiate cysts from tumors, and to reveal the depth and dimension of thyroid goiters and nodules. The response of a mass in the thyroid to suppressive therapy can be monitored by successive examinations. Theoretically, this technique offers the possibility of a good estimation of thyroid weight—information that is important in radioiodine therapy for Graves' disease.

The examination is easy to do, is done prior to surgery, and gives 85 per cent accuracy. Often these studies are done in conjunction with radioactive iodine uptake tests. With pregnant patients, ultrasound studies are the method of choice; radioactive iodine is harmful to the developing fetus.

Procedure

1. The patient lies on his back on the examining table, with his neck hyperextended.
2. Oil is applied to the patient's neck.
3. A pillow is placed under the shoulder for the patient's comfort and to bring the transducer into better contact with the thyroid.
4. An alternate procedure involves separation of the neck surface from the transducer by a plastic bag filled with water. The water-filled bag is clipped on a stand and hung over the patient's neck. This water bath device allows for proper transmission of the ultrasound waves through the thyroid.

Clinical Implications

1. An abnormal pattern reading will present a cystic, complex, or solid echo pattern.
2. Solitary "cold nodules" identified on radioisotope scans of one to three cm. in size can be described as cystic or solid nodules by means of the ultrasound studies.

3. Cysts, which are generally benign, are usually echo-free with many echoes occurring distal to the posterior wall.
4. Solid tumors are usually malignant in the thyroid.
5. Thyroid adenoma will be demonstrated by a core of high-amplitude echoes with a halo of low-amplitude echoes.
6. Thyroid carcinomas appear to be lesions that are echo-poor with an irregular display of peripheral echoes.

Interfering Factors

1. Nodules less than one cm. in diameter may escape detection.
2. Cysts not originating in the thyroid may show the same ultrasound characteristics as thyroid cysts.
3. Lesions of more than four cm. in diameter frequently contain areas of cystic or hemorrhagic degeneration and give a mixed echogram that is difficult to correlate with specific disease.

Patient Preparation

1. Instruct patient about the purpose of the test and the test procedure.
2. The procedure usually takes about 30 minutes.

ABDOMINAL AORTA ECHOGRAM

Normal Values

Normal pattern image of contour and diameter of the aorta usually reported in B mode, gray scale or real time. The walls strongly reflect echoes, while the blood-filled lumen is echo-free.

Explanation of Test

Aortic echogram's greatest value is in the assessment of abdominal aortic aneurysms. Ultrasound is the least invasive diagnostic procedure available. The aorta is one of the easiest abdominal structures to visualize ultrasonically because of the marked change in acoustic impedance produced by the elasticity of its walls and its blood-filled interval structure. Echograms can evaluate the body tissues from below the xyphoid process to the aortic bifurcation. Ultrasound is an ideal method for serial examinations before and after surgery and in patients with small aneurysms. For the pregnant patient, ultrasound studies are the only diagnostic method used (usually not a clinical problem in pregnant women).

Procedure

1. The patient will lie on his back or side on the examining table, and may also be asked to sit up during the test.
2. The skin surface in the testing area will be lubricated with a gel to permit maximum contact between the transducer and body surface.
3. Length of examination time is 30 minutes.

Clinical Implications

The typical abnormal pattern readings will reveal aortic aneurysms with or without thrombus.

Interfering Factors

Retained barium from x-ray procedures will give poor results.

Patient Preparation

1. Instruct patient about the purpose of the test and procedure.
2. There is no pain or discomfort involved.

CLINICAL ALERT
This examination must be scheduled before barium x-ray procedures. If this cannot be arranged, at least 24 hours must elapse after barium tests before aortic echogram is done.

HEART ECHOGRAM (ECHOCARDIOGRAM)

Normal Values

Normal position, size, movement of heart valves and chamber walls recorded in "M" mode and real time.

Left ventricular dimensions: $\begin{cases} \text{Diastolic} \\ \text{Systolic} \end{cases}$ 3.7–5.6 cm.

Ejection fraction: $\begin{cases} \text{Thickness} \\ \text{Motion} \end{cases}$ 0.6–1.1 cm.

Interventricular septum	$\frac{2}{3}$ LVPW Motion
LV posterior wall thickness	0.6–1.1 cm.
Ratio: $\dfrac{\text{IVS}}{\text{LVPW}}$	<1.3
LV outflow tract width (early systolic)	2.0–3.5 cm.
Right ventricular dimensions	0.7–2.3 cm.
Change	0.0–0.6 cm.
Aortic root dimension	2.0–3.7 cm.
Left atrial size	1.9–4.0 cm.
Mitral valves: amplitude	1.5–2.5 cm.
Diastolic closing velocity (EF slope)	50–150 mm./sec.
Aortic cusp separation	1.6–2.6 cm.
Pre-ejection period	Q wave to aortic opening
Ejection time	Period of aortic opening
Mean V_{cf} (left ventricular velocity of fiber shortening)	1.22–1.73 circm./sec.
Peak V_{cf}	1.15–2.10 circm./sec.

Explanation of Test

This noninvasive technique of examining the heart can provide information about the position, size, and movements of the valves and chambers by means of reflected ultrasound. Echoes from pulsed high-frequency sound waves are used to locate and study the movements and dimensions of cardiac structures such as the valves and chamber walls. Because the heart is a blood-filled organ, sound can be transmitted through it readily to the opposite wall and to the heart-lung interface. It is commonly used to determine or rule out mitral stenosis or pericardial effusion, to furnish direction for further diagnostic study, and to follow cardiac patients over an extended period. One of the advantages of this diagnostic technique is that it is a noninvasive procedure which can be performed at the patient's bedside using mobile equipment, or it can be done in the laboratory.

Procedure

1. A specific diagnosis should accompany the request for the test (*e.g.*, R/O pericardial effusion or determine severity of mitral stenosis).
2. The patient is asked to lie on his back, and he may be asked to turn on his left side and sit up, leaning slightly forward.
3. There is no pain or discomfort involved. ECG leads are attached for a simultaneous electrocardiogram and ultrasonic record (see ECG Chapter 14).
4. Examination time is 15 to 30 minutes.

Clinical Implications

Abnormal values help to diagnose:
1. Mitral stenosis
2. Pericardial effusion
3. Subaortic stenosis
4. Tricuspid valve disease
5. Pulmonary embolism
6. Congenital heart disease

Patient Preparation

Explain the purpose of the test and procedure to the patient.

BRAIN ECHOGRAM (ECHOENCEPHALOGRAM)

Normal Values

Normal sized ventricles. Midline structure of the brain in normal position recorded in "A" mode and can be recorded in B-mode gray scale in infants and young children.

Explanation of Test

This ultrasound examination of the brain is done to determine the position of the midline structure of the brain, to detect a shift in the midline of the brain due to space occupying intracranial lesions, and to estimate the size of the ventricle. In infants and children up to two years of age, studies of the brain can be done through the open sutures and fontanels.

The study of the intracranial structure of the brain was one of the earliest applications of ultrasound. This diagnostic modality is used less, since the advent of computed tomography (CT) of the brain. It is useful, however, when CT scans and radioisotope studies are not available.

Procedure

1. The test is done with the patient either sitting up or lying down.
2. A gel is applied to the scalp.
3. Three to four projections are made.

Clinical Implications

Abnormal pattern images will indicate:
1. Shift in midline structure
2. Ventricles of abnormal size
    (a.) Hydrocephalus
    (b.) Anancephalus
    (c.) Dilated ventricles
    (d.) Posterior fossa abnormalities

Patient Preparation

Explain the purpose of the test and the procedure.

Interfering Factors

Long or thick hair interferes with scanning contact and can result in inadequate examination in the B-mode gray scale.

REFERENCES

Hagen-Ansert, Sandra L.: TEXTBOOK OF DIAGNOSTIC UL-TRASONOGRAPHY. Saint Louis, The C. V. Mosby Company, 1978.

Hassani, Sam N. (in collaboration with R. L. Bard): ULTRASOUND IN GYNECOLOGY AND OBSTETRICS. New York, Springer-Verlag, 1978.

Shirley, Isabel M., et al.: A USER'S GUIDE TO DIAGNOSTIC UL-TRASOUND. Baltimore, University Park Press (distributor); Kent, England, Pitman Medical Publishing Company Ltd., 1978.

Thompson, Horace E., and Bernstine, Richard L.: DIAGNOSTIC ULTRASOUND IN CLINICAL OBSTETRICS AND GYNECOLOGY. New York, John Wiley & Sons, 1978.

13 □□ PULMONARY FUNCTION STUDIES; BLOOD GASES ANALYSES

INTRODUCTION

Pulmonary Physiology

Patients with pulmonary disease usually complain of difficulty in breathing. During breathing, the lung-thorax system acts as a bellows that provides fresh air to the alveoli for adequate gas exchange. Like springs, the lung tissue possesses the property of elasticity. When the inspiratory muscles contract, the thorax and lungs expand, and when the muscles relax and the force is removed, the thorax and lungs recoil to their resting position.

Use of Tests

Pulmonary function tests are designed to determine the presence, nature and extent of pulmonary dysfunction caused by either obstructive or restrictive disease. The primary function of the lung is to oxygenate mixed venous blood and to remove carbon dioxide from this blood. These two functions depend upon the integrity of the airway, the vascular system, and the alveoli. The results of pulmonary function studies are used for both medical and surgical diagnostic reasons. The tests may reveal abnormalities in the airways, alveoli, and pulmonary vascular bed early in the course of disease when physical examinations and x-rays are still normal. Although these tests indicate how function has been altered by disease, they cannot determine either the etiology or the pathology causing the abnormality. For example, tests may indicate the existence of an abnormality in the pulmonary vascular bed, but they cannot differentiate involvement by scleroderma from that of a pulmonary embolism.

Indications for Tests

1. Early detection of pulmonary or cardiac pulmonary disease
2. Differential diagnosis of all patients with dyspnea
3. Evaluation of patients before surgical procedures
4. Determination of the risk of using certain diagnostic procedures
5. Detection of early respiratory failure
6. To follow course of disease in patients known to have bronchopulmonary disease
7. Periodic examination of workers in industries in which a dust or fume hazard exists
8. Epidemiologic studies of population to provide clues to the causes of pulmonary diseases

Classification of Pulmonary Diseases

1. "Restrictive" Diseases:
   Characterized by interference with elastic behavior of lungs, causing them to be stiff; actual reduction in the volume of air that can be inspired
   Examples:
   (a.) Pulmonary fibrosis
   (b.) Pneumonia
   (c.) Replacement of lung tissue by tumor, infiltration, fluid, fibrosis, consolidation

(d.) Surgical removal of lung tissue

(e.) Fibrothorax

(f.) Conditions restricting expansion of chest (*e.g.,* kyphoscoliosis)

2. "Obstructive" Diseases

Characterized by need for unusual effort to produce airflow; respiratory muscles must work with difficulty to overcome resistive forces during breathing. Patient experiences prolongation and impairment of airflow during expiration.

Examples:

(a.) Bronchitis

(b.) Emphysema

(c.) Bronchospasm

(d.) Edema of bronchial mucosa

(e.) Bronchial secretions

Most pulmonary function tests evaluate the status of the airways, vascular system, and alveoli in an indirect, overlapping way. The patient's age, height, weight and sex are recorded prior to testing because they are the basis for the determination of predicted values.

Classification of Tests

Pulmonary function tests are generally divided into three categories:

1. Conventional Pulmonary Function Tests

Usually includes spirometry (or flow-volume loops), static lung volumes, diffusing capacity determinations and arterial blood gas studies at rest.

2. Specialized Pulmonary Function Tests

Includes such procedures as closing volume, isoflow volume, body plethysmography, CO_2 response, maximum voluntary ventilation, metacholine challenge, respiratory stress testing, and exercise arterial blood gas studies.

3. Preoperative Pulmonary Screening

Generally includes only the spirometry (before and after bronchodilator administration if indicated).

SPIROMETRY

Lung capacities, volumes, and flow rates are clinically measured by various devices. The *spirometer* (Fig. 13–1) is the instrument most often used for these determinations.

A spirometer consists of a bell suspended in a container of water. The bell rises and falls in response to the breathing of the patient, who inhales and exhales into a tube connected to the spirometer. The proportional movements of the bell are recorded, either on a kymograph (a rotating drum on which a tracing is made with a stylus) or on an electrical potentiometer. Values obtained are compared via computer with the predicted values for a particular age, sex, and height.

Spirometry is designed to determine the effectiveness of the various forces involved in the movement of the lungs and chest wall. The values obtained will provide quantitative information

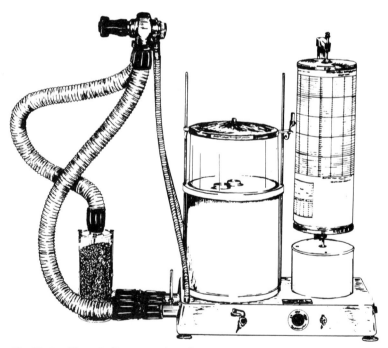

Fig. 13–1. *The Collins Stead-Wells Spirometer (Courtesy Warren E. Collins, Inc., Braintree, Massachusetts).*

about 1) degree of obstruction to airflow, 2) restriction of the amount of air which can be inspired.

Screening Spirometry

Screening spirometry is a clinical procedure that takes 15 to 20 minutes to perform and reveals the following values:
1. Forced vital capacity (FVC)
2. Forced expiratory volumes FEV_1, FEV_3 (*i.e.*, the volumes exhaled during the first and third seconds of forced vital capacity)
3. Air flow rates (*e.g.*, forced expiratory flow FEF 200–1200, FEF 25–75)

Note: Spirometry plus lung volumes will take 40 minutes to complete and includes measurement of spirometry plus functional residual capacity, residual volume, expiratory reserve volume, and total lung capacity.

Procedure

1. The patient is fitted with a mouthpiece that is connected to the spirometer.
2. A nose clip is used so that only mouth breathing is possible.
3. The patient is either sitting down or standing up.
4. Patient is asked to inhale maximally, breathe-hold momentarily, and then exhale forcibly and completely.
5. The patient is allowed to rest for a few minutes, and the above step is repeated twice.
6. The procedure takes 15 to 20 minutes to perform.
7. The best tracing from the spirometer is used to provide spirometric measurements of FVC, FEV_1, $FEF_{200-1200}$ and FEF_{25-75}.

PULMONARY FUNCTION TESTING

Lung Volumes

Lung volumes can be considered as basic subdivisions of the lung (not anatomic subdivisions), and may be subdivided as follows:

1. Total lung capacity (TLC)
2. Tidal Volume (V_T)
3. Inspiratory capacity (IC)
4. Functional residual capacity (FRC)
5. Expiratory reserve volume (ERV)
6. Vital capacity (VC)
7. Residual volume (RV)

Combinations of two or more volumes are termed capacities. There are two basic methods for the determination of lung volumes:

1. The multiple breath nitrogen washout technique (open circuit)
2. The helium dilution technique (closed circuit)

Both methods employ the use of a gas (oxygen or helium, respectively) to either wash out or dilute the air left in the lung at end tidal expiration.

These volumes and capacities are shown graphically in Figure 13–2. Also shown are values found in the normal adult

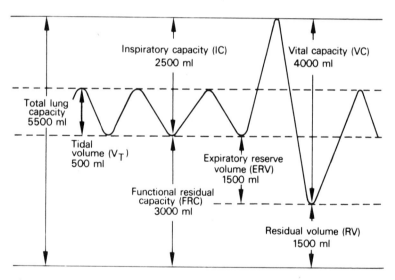

Fig. 13–2.   *Subdivisions of lung volume in the normal adult. (From Geschickter, Charles F.: THE LUNG IN HEALTH AND DISEASE. Philadelphia, J. B. Lippincott Co., 1973.)*

male. Measurement of these values by means of such devices as the spirometer can provide information about the severity of airway obstruction and can serve as an index of dynamic function.

Flow Rates

Flow rates provide information about the severity of airway obstruction and serve as an index of dynamic function. The lung volume at which the flow rates are measured is a most important value. Lung capacities, volumes, and flow rates are measured with a spirometer. A breathing system into and out of this device allows for the addition or removal of accurate amounts of gas. The electrical recording of the amounts of gas breathed in and out form the *spirogram*. The values obtained and the predicted values for age, sex, height, and weight are compared by a computer.

Diffusion

The measurement of lung diffusion gives information about the amount of functioning capillaries in contact with functioning alveoli and these measurements are of value in the diagnosis of pulmonary vascular disease.

Arterial Blood Gases

The measurment of arterial blood gases integrates the whole of respiratory function and allows evaluation of an important factor not obtained from routine pulmonary function tests: that is, the degree of ventilation matched to perfusion. The measurement of the alveolar to arterial oxygen gradient $(A\text{-}aD_{O_2})$ gives information about the cause of hypoxemia. When an unexplained decrease in vital capacity is observed, measurement of lung compliance is not considered a screening procedure because the patient must swallow an esophageal balloon and special expertise is required to perform the study.

LIST OF SYMBOLS AND ABBREVIATIONS*

Pulmonary function studies and blood gas analyses measure gas mixtures and their components, blood and its constituents, and various factors affecting these quantities. The symbolic expression of these quantities was standardized at a conference held in 1950 by American physiologists. The list of symbols and abbreviations given here is based on those standards.

Once you have mastered the meaning of the major symbols and the secondary symbols, you should be able to interpret any combination of these symbols. This list will introduce you to general principles and then will apply them to measurements included in the chapter.

General Principles

Gas Volumes. *Large capital letters* denote primary symbols for gases:

V = Gas volume

$\dot{V}$ = Gas volume per unit time (The dot over the symbol indicates the factor per unit time.)

P = Gas pressure or partial pressure of a gas in a gas mixture or in blood

F = Fractional concentration in gas

Small capital letters that are set as subscripts to large capital letters indicate the type of gas measured:

A = Alveolar gas

D = Dead space gas

E = Expired gas

I = Inspired gas

T = Tidal gas

Chemical symbols for gases may be set as subscripts to the small capital letters listed above:

O = Oxygen

CO = Carbon monoxide

CO_2 = Carbon dioxide

N_2 = Nitrogen

*Adapted from Pace, William R., Jr.: PULMONARY PHYSIOLOGY IN CLINICAL PRACTICE, 2nd Ed., Philadelphia, F. A. Davis Company, 1970.

Combinations of Symbols. Following are some of the ways these symbols may be combined in the measurement of gases:

V_T = Tidal volume
V_E = Volume of expired gas
$P_{A_{CO_2}}$ = Partial pressure of carbon dioxide in alveolar gas

Blood Gas Symbols. *Large capital letters* are used as primary symbols for blood:

C   = Concentration of a gas in blood
S   = Per cent saturation of H_gb with CO or O_2
Q   = Volume of blood
Q   = Volume of blood per unit time

To indicate whether blood is capillary, venous, or arterial, *lower case letters* are used as subscripts:

v   = Venous blood
a   = Arterial blood
c   = Capillary blood
s   = Shunted blood

Combinations of Symbols. Blood gas symbols may be combined in the following ways:

P_{O_2} = Oxygen tension or partial pressure of oxygen
$P_{V_{O_2}}$ = Venous oxygen tension or partial pressure of oxygen in venous blood
$P_{a_{O_2}}$ = Arterial oxygen tension or partial pressure of oxygen in arterial blood
$P_{A_{O_2}}$ = Alveolar oxygen tension or partial pressure of oxygen in the alveoli
P_{CO_2} = Partial pressure of carbon dioxide
$P_{a_{CO_2}}$ = Partial pressure of carbon dioxide in arterial blood
$P_{V_{CO_2}}$ = Partial pressure of carbon dioxide in venous blood
S_{O_2} = Oxygen saturation
$S_{a_{O_2}}$ = Percent saturation of oxygen in arterial blood
$S_{V_{O_2}}$ = Percent saturation of oxygen in venous blood
T_{CO_2} = Total carbon dioxide content

Lung Volume Symbols. The following list indicates symbols used in measuring lung volumes as well as the units used in expressing these measurements.

FVC   = *F*orced *V*ital *C*apacity-Maximal amount of air

	that can be exhaled forcibly and completely following a maximal inspiration (units:liters)
FEV	= *F*orced *E*xpiratory *V*olume in 1 second-Volume of air expired during the first second of the FVC maneuver (units:liters)
FEV_3	= *F*orced *E*xpiratory *V*olume in 3 seconds-Volume of air expired during the first three seconds of the FVC maneuver (units:liters)
$FEF_{200-1200}$	= *F*orced *E*xpiratory *F*low between 200 and 1200 milliliters-Flow of expired air measured after the first 200 milliliters and during the next 1000 milliliters of the FVC maneuver (units: liters per second)
FEF_{25-75}	= *F*orced *E*xpiratory *F*low between 25 and 75 per cent-Flow of expired air measured between 25 and 75 per cent of the FVC maneuver (units:liters per second)
PEFR	= *P*eak *E*xpiratory *F*low *R*ate-Maximum flow of expired air attained during an FVC maneuver (units:liters per second or liters per minute)
PIFR	= *P*eak *I*nspiratory *F*low *R*ate-Maximum flow of inspired air achieved during a forced maximal inspiration (units:liters per second or liters per minute)
$V \, max_{25}$	= Maximum flow at 25 per cent-Maximum flow of expired air at 25 per cent of lung volume achieved during an FEV maneuver (units: liters per second or liters per minute)
$V \, max_{50}$	= Maximum flow at 50 per cent-Maximum flow of expired air at 50 per cent of lung volume achieved during an FEV maneuver (units: liters per second or liters per minute)
$V \, max_{75}$	= Maximum flow at 75 per cent-Maximum flow of expired air at 75 per cent of lung volume achieved during an FEV maneuver (units: liters per second or liters per minute)
FRC	= *F*unctional *R*esidual *C*apacity-Volume of gas contained in the lung at the end of a normal expiration (units:liters)
IC	= *I*nspiratory *C*apacity-Maximum amount of air

that can be inspired from end tidal expiration (units:liters)

ERV = *E*xpiratory *R*eserve Volume-Maximum amount of air that can be expired from end tidal expiration (units:liters)

RV = *R*esidual Volume-Volume of gas left in the lung following a maximal expiration (units: liters)

VC = *V*ital *C*apacity-Maximum volume of air that can be expired following a maximum inspiration (units:liters)

TLC = *T*otal *L*ung *C*apacity-Volume of gas contained in the lungs following a maximal inspiration (units:liters)

DL_{CO} = Carbon monoxide diffusing capacity of the lung-Rate of diffusion of carbon monoxide across the alveolar/capillary membrane (*i.e.*, rate of gas transfer across the alveolar/capillary membrane. (units:ml/min./torr)

CV = *C*losing Volume-Volume at which the lower lung zones cease to ventilate, presumably as a result of airway closure (units:percent of VC)

MVV = *M*aximum *V*oluntary *V*entilation-Maximum number of liters of air a patient can breathe per minute by a voluntary effort (units:liters per minute)

$V_{ISO}\dot{V}$ = Volume of isoflow-Volume in which flow was the same with air and with helium during an FVC maneuver.

Miscellaneous Symbols. Following is an assortment of symbols you may encounter throughout the chapter:

A = Age in years

W = Weight in pounds

H = Height in inches

torr = A unit of pressure equal to 1/760 of normal atmospheric pressure or to the pressure necessary to support a column of mercury one mm. high at 0°C and standard gravity

f = Frequency of breathing

C   = Compliance
He   = Helium
Hg   = Mercury
D   = Diffusing capacity
$D_{L_{CO}}$ = Carbon monoxide diffusing capacity of the lung (ml./min./torr)
$D_{L_{O_2}}$ = Oxygen diffusing capacity of the lung (ml./min./torr)
A-a D_{O_2} Ratio = Alveolar to arterial oxygen ratio
BSA   = Body surface area (unit:meters^2)
H_2CO_3 = Carbonic acid
HCO_3 = Bicarbonate
TGV   = Thoracic Gas Volume (also expressed as V_{TG})
R_{aw} = Airway resistance
F-V   = Flow volume
pH   = Negative logarithm of the hydrogen ion concentration, used as a positive number to indicate acidity or alkalinity inspired

TESTS

Functional Residual Capacity (FRC)

Normal Values
     Approximately 2400–3000 ml.
     Predicted values are based on age, height, weight, and sex. The observed value should be 75 to 125 per cent of the predicted value.

Explanation of Test. This test is used to evaluate both restrictive and obstructive defects of the lung. Changes in the elastic properties of the lungs are reflected in the FRC. This test measures the volume of gas contained in the lungs at the end of a normal quiet expiration and is mathematically equal to the sum of the expiratory reserve volume and the residual volume (FRC = ERV + RV). Calculation of the functional residual capacity is based on the fact that 81 per cent of the air in the lung is nitrogen. The nitrogen (N_2) is "washed" out from the lungs by having the patient breathe 100 per cent oxygen (O_2) and then measuring the volume of nitrogen collected.

Procedure

1. The patient is fitted with noseclips and asked to breathe through the mouthpiece on the lung volume apparatus.
2. Depending on instrument, patient either:
   - (a.) Breathes 100% O_2 until the alveolar nitrogen reaches 1% or seven minutes elapses (which ever comes first) or
   - (b.) Rebreathes a 10–12% helium/room-air-concentration until equilibrium is reached
3. Results are recorded on a spirogram.
4. At the end of the test, the following values are computed. The choice of the formula depends on the method being used.

$$FRC = \frac{\% \, N_2 \, \text{Final} \times \text{Expired Volume}}{\% \, N_2 \, \text{Atmospheric}}$$

$$FRC = \frac{\% \, \text{He initial} - \% \, \text{He Final}}{\% \, \text{He Final}} \times \text{Initial Volume}$$

Clinical Implications

1. A value less than 75 per cent is indicative of restrictive disease.
2. Restrictive defects are characterized by normal or decreased FRC.
3. A value of greater than 125 per cent demonstrates air trapping, which is consistent with obstructive airway disease.
4. An increase in the FRC represents hyperinflation, which may result from emphysematous changes, asthmatic or fibrotic obstruction of the bronchioles, compensation for surgical removal of lung tissue, or a thoracic cage deformity (Ruppel, 1979).

Patient Preparation

1. Instruct patient about purpose of the test and the procedure.
2. Obtain the patient's weight and height and record this information prior to doing the test.

Total Lung Capacity (TLC)

Normal Values
Approximately 5500 ml.
Predicted values are based on age, height, and sex.

Explanation of Test. This test is mainly used to evaluate obstructive defects of the lungs. It measures the volume of gas contained in the lungs at the end of a maximal inspiration. Mathematically, it is the sum of the vital capacity (VC) and the residual volume (RV) or the sum of the primary lung volumes (see Fig. 13–2). This value is determined indirectly from other tests.

Procedure
1. There is no procedure to perform.
2. It is a mathematical formula: TLC = VC (Vital capacity) + RV (Residual Volume)

Clinical Implications
1. An obstructive defect is characterized by an *elevated* total lung capacity. However, a normal or *increased* total lung capacity does not mean that ventilation or the surface area for diffusion is normal.
2. The TLC may be normal or *increased* in broncheolar obstruction with hyperinflation and in emphysema.
3. The TLC is *decreased* in edema, atelectasis, neoplasms, pulmonary congestion, pneumothorax or thoracic restriction.

Vital Capacity (VC)

Normal Values
About 4000–4800 ml. in the normal male
Predicted values are based on age, sex, and height.

Explanation of Test. This measurement is used to identify defects which can be due to lung or chest wall restriction. It measures the largest volume of gas that can be expelled from the lungs after the lungs are first filled to the maximum extent and then emptied to the maximum extent. The vital capacity is the mathematical sum of the inspiratory capacity and the expiratory reserve volume (see Fig. 13–2).

Procedure
1. Have the patient inhale as deeply as possible and then exhale completely, with no forced or rapid effort.
2. The inhalation and exhalation is done into a spirometer and the results are recorded on a spirogram.
3. No time limit is set.

Clinical Implications
1. A "reduced" vital capacity is considered to be less than 80 per cent of the predicted value.
2. Causes of decreased vital capacities can be related to depression of the respiratory center in the brain, neuromuscular diseases, pleural effusion, pneumothorax, pregnancy, ascites, and limitations of thoracic movement due to pain (Ruppel, 1979).

Interfering Factors
1. Vital capacity increases with physical fitness and height.
2. Vital capacity decreases with age.
3. Vital capacity is generally smaller in females than in males for the same age and height.

Patient Preparation.   Instruct patient about the purpose and procedure of the test.

Residual Volume (RV)

Normal Values
Approximately 1200–1500 ml.
Predicted values are based on age, sex, and height.

Explanation of Test.   This test is used to evaluate obstructive defects of the lungs. It is a measurement of the volume of gas remaining in the lungs after a maximal exhalation. Because the lungs cannot be completely emptied and since all the gas cannot be expelled by maximal expiratory effort, it is the only volume that cannot be measured directly from the spirometer. This value is calculated mathematically: Residual volume equals the functional residual capacity minus the expiratory reserve volume: (RV = FRC − ERV) (see Fig. 13–2).

Procedure.   The RV is determined indirectly from other tests. There is no procedure.

Clinical Implications
1. An increase in the residual volume indicates that in spite of a maximal expiratory effort, the lungs still contain an abnormally large amount of gas. This type of change occurs in young asthmatics and is usually reversible.
2. Increases of the residual volume are also characteristic of emphysema, chronic air trapping, and chronic bronchial obstruction.
3. The residual volume and the functional residual capacity usually increase together, although this is not always true.
4. The residual volume sometimes decreases in diseases that occlude many alveoli (Ruppel, 1979).

Patient Preparation.   Instruct patient about the purpose and procedure of the test.

Expiratory Reserve Volume (ERV)

Normal Values
Approximately 1200–1500 ml.
Predicted values are based on age and height.

Explanation of Test.   This test measures the largest volume of gas that can be exhaled following normal resting expiration. This measurement is used to identify lung or chest wall restriction. The ERV can be estimated mathematically by subtracting the inspiratory capacity from the vital capacity. The expiratory reserve volume comprises approximately 25 per cent of the vital capacity and can vary greatly in subjects of comparable age and height.

Procedure
1. Record the patient's age and height.
2. Have the patient breathe normally for several breaths and then exhale maximally into a spirometer from end tidal expiratory level.
3. The results are recorded on a spirogram.

Clinical Implications
1. A decreased ERV implies a chest wall restriction due to nonpulmonary causes.
2. Decreased values are associated with elevated diaphragms as seen in massive obesity, ascites or pregnancy. These decreased values also occur in conjunction with massive enlargement of the heart, pleural effusion, kyphoscoliosis, and thoracoplasty.

Patient Preparation.   Instruct the patient about the purpose and procedure of the test

Forced Vital Capacity (FVC) and Forced Expiratory Volume (FEV)

Normal Values.   Approximately 4800 ml. The value can also be given in liters per second or an FVC:VC ratio. A normal timed vital capacity is at least 81 and 95 per cent of the forced vital capacity at one and three seconds. The total vital capacity should be exhaled in six seconds.
   81–83% exhaled in 1 second
   90–94% exhaled in 2 seconds
   95–97% exhaled in 3 seconds
Predicted values for a patient of a specific age and height may be determined by use of a nomogram (See Figure 13–3).

Explanation of Test.   This test is used to evaluate the severity of airway obstruction. The maximum amount of air that can rapidly be exhaled after a maximum deep inspiration is recorded. Three separate exhalations are measured and the highest volume is recorded as the forced vital capacity. The recording is given in liters or as the FVC:VC ratio. The volumes exhaled within one and three seconds are referred

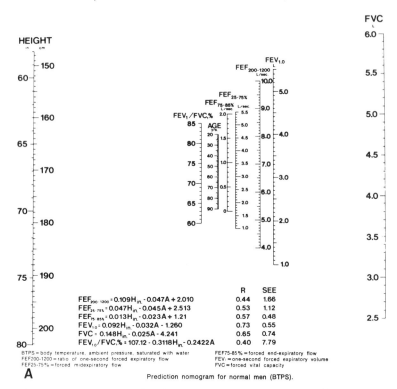

Fig. 13–3. *Nomogram for determining various expiratory flow rates in normal males (A), and normal females (B). The values are determined by laying a ruler across the height scale and age scale (corresponding to patient's height and age) and then reading the values where the ruler crosses the other scales. (From Burton, George G., Gee, Glen N., and Hodgkin, John E.: RESPIRATORY CARE: A GUIDE TO CLINICAL PRACTICE. Philadelphia, J. B. Lippincott Co., 1977.)*

to as the forced expiratory volumes $FEV_{1.0}$ and $FEV_{3.0}$ or timed vital capacities. These measurements are useful in the evaluation of a patient's response to bronchodilators.

Procedure. The patient is asked to breathe normally, inspire maximally and then exhale as forcefully and as rapidly as possible into the spirometer.

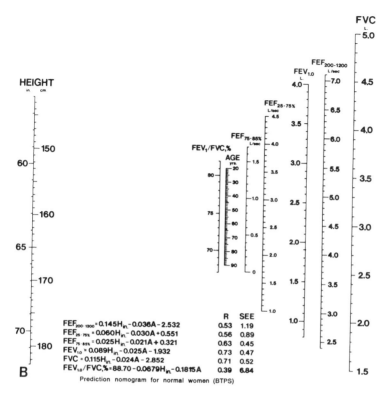

Fig. 13–3B

Clinical Implications
1. Obstructive lung disease is a cause of reduced volume and flow rates.
2. Decreased values occur in chronic lung diseases which cause trapping of air such as emphysema, pulmonary fibrosis and asthma.
3. In restrictive lung disease, the FVC is reduced; however, the flow rates can be normal or elevated.

Patient Preparation. Instruct patient about the purpose and procedure of the test.

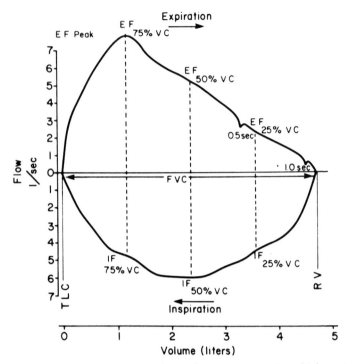

Fig. 13–4. *Flow-volume loop. Flow-volume spirogram in which an FEV and an FIV maneuver are recorded in succession. Flow rate is plotted on the vertical axis and volume on the horizontal axis. Peak flows for inspiration and expiration can be read directly, as can the FVC. (From Guenter, Clarence A., Welch, Martin H., and Hogg, James C.: CLINICAL ASPECTS OF RESPIRATORY PHYSIOLOGY, Philadelphia, J. B. Lippincott Co., 1978.)*

Flow Volume Loops (F-V Loops)

Normal Values. Normal curves or loops are characteristic of absence of lung disease.

Explanation of Test. This test is designed to provide both a graphic analysis and quantitative measurement of flow rates at any lung volume. It is used to evaluate the dynamics of both large and small airways and is quite helpful in the diagnosis of small airway disease. Values obtained in this determination include the FVC, FEV, FEF$_{25-75}$, PEIR, PIFR, V$_{max25}$, V$_{max50}$, and V$_{max75}$. See Figure 13–4 for an example of a flow-volume loop.

Procedure. The procedure is the same as for spirometry except for the addition of a maximal forced inspiration at the end of the forced expiratory maneuver.

Clinical Implications
1. Characteristic: Abnormal flow volume loops are indicative of:
   (a.) Obstructive lung disease
       (1.) Small airway obstructive disease, as in emphysema and asthma.
       (2.) Large airway obstructive disease such as tumors of trachea and bronchioles.
   (b.) Restrictive diseases when the disease is far advanced.

Patient Preparation. Explain the purpose and procedure of the test.

Carbon Monoxide Diffusing Capacity of the Lung (DL$_{CO}$)

Normal Values
Approximately 25 ml./min./torr

75% of predicted value based on patient's height, age and hematocrit

Note: "A" = Age in years; "BSA" = Body surface area in meters.

Male DL$_{CO}$ = 15.5 (BSA) − 0.238 (A) + 6.8

Female DL$_{CO}$ = 15.5 (BSA) − 0.117 (A) + 0.5

Background. Carbon monoxide combines with hemoglobin about 210 times more readily than does oxygen. If there is a normal amount of hemoglobin in the blood, the only other significant limiting factor to carbon monoxide uptake is the state of the alveolar capillary membranes. Normally there is no carbon monoxide in the blood to affect the test.

Explanation of Test.   This test is used to diagnose pulmonary vascular disease and is used to evaluate the amount of functioning pulmonary capillary bed in contact with functioning alveoli. During the measurement of this value, alveolar volume (VA) is also determined. D_L measures the diffusing capacity of the lungs for carbon monoxide (CO). The DL_{O_2} (oxygen diffusing capacity of the lung) is obtained by multiplying DL_{co} by 1.23. $DL_{O_2} = DL_{co} \times 1.23$

Procedure
1. Record age and height.
2. Two techniques are used by laboratories:
    (a.) *Single-Breath or Breathing-Holding technique*
        With this method the patient is asked to take a deep breath from a bag containing a mixture of neon, carbon monoxide, and air. The patient holds his breath for ten seconds and exhales.
    (b.) *Steady-State Technique*
        The patient is asked to take 12 breaths from a bag containing 0.1 to 0.6 per cent carbon monoxide and then exhale. This method requires an arterial blood sample.

Clinical Implications
1. *Decreased values* are associated with:
    (a.) Multiple pulmonary emboli
    (b.) Emphysema
    (c.) Anemia
    (d.) Lung restriction
    (e.) Pulmonary fibroses
        (1.) Sarcoidosis
        (2.) Scleroderma
        (3.) Systemic lupus erythematosus
        (4.) Asbestosis
2. The value is relatively normal in chronic bronchitis.

Interfering Factors.   Exercise, polycythemia, and anemia will increase the value.

Patient Preparation.   Instruct patient about the purpose and procedure of the test.

Peak Inspiratory Flow Rate (PIFR)

Normal Values
An average value of at least 300 liters per minute
Predicted values based on age, sex, and height

Explanation of Test. This measurement of flow rate is used to identify reduced breathing on inspiration and is totally dependent on the effort the patient makes in inspiration. PIFR is the maximum flow of air achieved during a forced maximal inspiration.

Procedure
1. The peak inspiratory flow rate is obtained from the flow volume loop procedure using the spirometer with an X-Y recorder.
2. The patient is asked to inspire maximally, exhale forcibly and completely, and then inspire forcibly and completely.

Clinical Implications
1. The value is reduced in neuromusclar disorders, weakness, poor effort and extrathoracic airway obstruction (*i.e.*, substernal thyroid, tracheal stenosis, and laryngeal paralysis).
2. The PIFR will be less than the peak expiratory flow rate in the above conditions.

Interfering Factors. Poor patient effort

Patient Preparation. Instruct patient about the purpose and procedure of the test.

Peak Expiratory Flow Rate (PEFR)

Normal Values
An average of at least 300 liters per minute
Predicated values are based on age, sex, and height.

Explanation of Test. This measurement of lung volume flow rate is used as an index of large airway function. It is the maximum flow of expired air attained during a forced vital capacity (FVC) maneuver.

Procedure

1. The peak expiratory flow rate is obtained from the flow volume loop procedure using the spirometer with an X-Y recorder.
2. The patient is asked to inspire maximally, exhale forcibly and completely, and then inspire forcibly and completely.

Clinical Implications

1. The value is normally decreased in obstructive disease such as emphysema when air is trapped.
2. The value is usually normal in restrictive lung disease, except in severe restriction, when it is reduced.

Patient Preparation.   Instruct patient about the purpose and procedure of the test.

Inspiratory Capacity (IC)

Normal Values

Approximately 2500 to 3600 ml.
Predicted values are based on age and height.

Explanation of Test.   This test measures the largest volume of air that can be inhaled in one deep breath after a normal expiration or that can be inhaled from the end tidal expiratory level. This measurement is used to identify lung or chest wall restriction. This measurement mathematically equals the tidal volume plus the inspiratory reserve volume. This value is not commonly measured because many diseases do not affect inspiratory capacity.

Procedure

1. Record age and height of patient.
2. The patient is asked to breathe normally into a spirometer for several breaths and then to inhale deeply or maximally expanding the lungs as much as possible from end tidal expiration. Normal breathing is then resumed.
3. Step Two is usually repeated two or more times and the largest inspired volume is selected.

Clinical Implications. Changes in the inspiratory capacity usually parallel increases or decreases in the vital capacity.

Patient Preparation. Instruct the patient about the purpose and procedure of the test.

Maximum Voluntary Ventilation (MVV)

Normal Values. Approximately 170 l./min.
  Based on age, height, and sex; and a healthy person may vary by as much as 25–35 per cent of mean group values.
  Mean Group Values:
1. MVV (in men) = 3.39 (H) − 1.26 (A) − 21.4
2. MVV (in women) = 138 − 0.77 (A)
(H = height in inches; A = age in years)

Explanation of Test. This test measures several physiological phenomenona occurring at the same time (*e.g.*, thoracic cage compliance, lung compliance, airway resistance, and muscle force available). It is a determination of the liters of air that a person can breathe per minute by a voluntary effort.

Procedure
1. Patient breathes into a spirometer as deeply and rapidly as possible for 10 to 15 seconds. (Generally the frequency is 40–70 breaths per minute and tidal volume is 50% of VC).
2. Actual value is then extrapolated from the 10 to 15 second time interval, to a one-minute time period.

Clinical Implications
1. Obstructive defects, chronic obstructive pulmonary disease (COPD), abnormal neuromuscular control, and poor patient effort are causes of reduced values.
2. In restrictive disease, the value will usually be normal.

Patient Preparation
1. Instruct patient about the purpose and procedure of the test.
2. Obtain and record patient's age and height.

Closing Volume (CV)

Normal Values. Average is about 10 to 20 per cent of vital capacity. Values are derived from mathematical regression equations and are based on age and sex.
Mean Group Values:
1. CV (in men) = 0.562 + 0.357 (A) + 4.15
2. CV (in women) = 2.812 + 0.293 (A) + 4.90
(A) = age in years

Explanation of Test. In the healthy person, the concentration of nitrogen diluted with 100 per cent oxygen rapidly increases near the end of expiration. This rise is due to closure of the small airways in the lower alveoli. The point at which this closure occurs is termed "closing volume."

This measurement is used as an index of pathological changes occuring within the small airways (those airways less than 2 mm. in diameter). The conventional pulmonary function tests are not sensitive enough to make this determination. The principle of the determination relies on the fact that the upper lung zones contain a proportionately larger residual volume of gas than the lower lung zones and that there is a gradient of intrapleural pressure from the top of the lung to the bottom of the lung.

Procedure
1. The patient is asked to exhale completely, inhale 100 per cent oxygen, hold the breath for a couple of seconds, and then exhale completely at the rate of approximately one-half liter per second.
2. During the exhalation, the percent of alveolar nitrogen is monitored with a nitrogen meter. A sudden increase in nitrogen represents the closing volume.

Clinical Implications. The value is increased in diseases in which the airway is decreased, in pulmonary edema, in chronic smokers, and in old patients.

Interfering Factors. Increases with age

Patient Preparation. Instruct patient about the purpose and procedure of the test.

Volume of Isoflow ($V_{ISO}\dot{V}$)

Normal Values. values cover a wide range based on age and sex.

$V_{ISO}\dot{V} = 0.450 \text{ (A)} + 4.69$

(A = age in years)

Explanation of Test. This test is designed to detect pathological changes occurring in the small airways and may be more sensitive than conventional pulmonary function tests. Small airways contribute only 10 per cent to total pulmonary resistance, therefore, considerable change can occur without detectable alteration in flow rates or lung volumes.

Procedure
1. Patient is fitted with noseclips and allowed to breathe into a mouthpiece connected to a spirometer which is interfaced with an X-Y recorder.
2. Patient is then instructed to perform a flow-volume loop maneuver.
3. Next, the patient is asked to breathe an 80 per cent helium and 20 per cent oxygen gas mix for several breaths and then perform another flow-volume loop maneuver.
4. From the tracings obtained in steps 2 and 3, the volume of isoflow is measured.

Clinical Implications
1. An *increased* volume of isoflow is consistent with the diagnosis of mild airway obstruction (*i.e.*, small airways disease).
2. A *decreased* volume of isoflow is normal.

Patient Preparation. Explain the purpose and procedure of the test.

Body Plethysmography

Normal Values

Based on height in inches (H) and weight in pounds (W)

TGV = approximately 2400 ml.

TGV = 0.081 (H) − 2.94 (W) in men

TGV = 0.135 (H) − 0.008 (W) − 4.74 in women
C = 0.2 l./cm. H_2O
RAW = 0.6 to 2.4 cm. H_2O/l./sec.

Explanation of Test. This test is designed to measure thoracic gas volume compliance and airway resistance. Thoracic gas volume (TGV) equals all of the air contained within the thorax whether or not it is in ventilatory communication with the rest of the lung. Compliance (C) is an indication of the elasticity of the lung, and airway resistance (RAW) is a measurement of resistance to airflow in the tracheobronchial tree.

Procedure

1. Patient is seated in the body box, fitted with nose clips and breathes through a mouthpiece connected to a transducer.
2. The box door is secured and the test is not begun for a couple of minutes, while the box pressure is allowed to stabilize.
3. The patient is instructed to perform a panting maneuver while holding his cheeks rigid and glottis open. The technician makes a recording of box pressure and mouth pressure on the oscilloscope. This recording provides the necessary data for mathematical derivation of TGV.
4. Next, the patient is instructed to breathe rapidly and shallowly. The technician makes a recording of box pressure changes versus flow on the oscilloscope and this provides the necessary data for mathematical derivation of RAW.
5. For the compliance determination, a balloon catheter must be passed into the patient's esophagus through the nose. The balloon is then inflated with a couple of cc.'s of air, and the patient is instructed to breathe normally. The technician makes a recording of intraesophageal pressure changes during normal respiration and this provides the necessary data for the mathematical derivation of C.

Clinical Implications

1. An *increased* thoracic gas volume (TGV) demonstrates air trapping which is consistent with obstructive pulmonary disease.
2. An *increased* airway resistance (RAW) demonstrates an

increased resistance to airflow thru the traechobronchial tree which is seen in asthma, emphysema, bronchitis and other forms of obstruction. RAW is useful in distinguishing between a restrictive ventilatory defect versus an obstructive ventilatory defect as the former does not increase the resistance to airflow.

3. An *increase* in Compliance (C) (*i.e.*, more distensible) is seen in obstructive diseases.
4. A *decrease* in Compliance (C) (*i.e.*, lung is more stiff) is seen in fibrotic diseases, restrictive diseases, pneunonia, congestion, atelectasis.

Patient Preparation
1. The height, weight and sex are recorded.
2. Explain the purpose and procedure of the test.

Patient Aftercare. Allow patient to rest quietly after test is completed.

Methacholine Challenge

Normal Values
Negative response.

Explanation of Test. Occasionally the diagnosis of asthma cannot be made with certainty from the history, physical examination, and conventional pulmonary function tests. Therefore, a test for bronchial asthma is needed, that is, methacholine challenge. The asthmatic patient is more sensitive to the bronchoconstrictive effects of cholinergic agents (*e.g.*, methacholine chloride) than the normal patient.

Clinical Implications. A positive response to methacholine is consistent with a diagnosis of asthma.

Procedure
1. Patient is instructed to perform an FVC maneuver and the FEV is measured.
2. Patient is now asked to take an inhalation of 3.12 mg. of methacholine chloride per millileter via a nebulizer, wait

five minutes, and repeat the FVC maneuver. A 20 per cent reduction in the FEV is a positive response.

3. If there is no response, the dilution of methacholine chloride is progressively increased (6.25 mg./ml., 12.5 mg./ml., 12.5 mg./ml. and 25 mg./ml.) and patient repeats step #2. However, once a 20 per cent reduction is observed at any dilution ration, this represents a positive response, and the test is terminated.

4. If a patient goes through all four dilution ratios without a 20 per cent reduction in the FEV, this is a negative test.

Patient Preparation
1. Explain the purpose and procedure of the test.

Carbon Dioxide (CO_2) Response

Normal Values. Breathing 2 per cent carbon dioxide (CO_2) should result in a three-fold increase in minute volume when compared to minute volume when breathing room air (0.03% CO_2).

Explanation of Test. This test is designed to evaluate the respiratory response to increasing levels of inspired carbon dioxide concentration. As levels of carbon dioxide increase in alveolar air, so does arterial carbon dioxide. The central chemo-receptors respond by initiating impulses to the respiratory control centers, and this in turn causes an increase in the rate and depth of breathing in the healthy person.

Procedure
1. The patient's minute volume is determined while breathing room air. This is done by allowing patient to breathe for several minutes into an instrument which records frequency (f) of breathing and tidal volume (V_T). The minute volume is then calculated for one minute by computing the value of F $\times$ V_T.

2. Next, the patient is instructed to breathe a gas mixture of two per cent carbon dioxide and balanced room air for five minutes. During the last two minutes frequency of breathing (f) and tidal volume (V_T) are recorded.

3. Next, the patient breathes a gas mixture of four per cent carbon dioxide, balanced room air, and the above procedure is repeated. This is also done with six per cent carbon dioxide and sometimes even eight per cent carbon dioxide and room air.
4. Finally a graph is constructed which plots changes in minute volume against increasing inspired carbon dioxide concentrations.

Clinical Implications. Unresponsiveness to increasing inspired carbon dioxide (CO_2) concentrations suggests a disturbance in the normal physiological pathway of ventilatory changes to hypercapnia.

BLOOD GASES

INTRODUCTION

Reasons for obtaining blood gases:
1. Assessment of adequacy of oxygenation
2. Assessment of adequacy of ventilation
3. Assessment of the acid/base status by measuring the respiratory and nonrespiratory components

Reasons for using *arterial* blood rather than *venous* blood to measure blood gases:
1. Arterial blood is a good way to sample a mixture of blood that has come from various parts of the body.
   (a.) Venous blood in an extremity gives information mostly about that extremity. The metabolism in the extremity can differ from the metabolism in the body as a whole. This difference is accentuated:
      (1.) In shock, when the extremity is cold or underperfused
      (2.) With local exercise of extremity, as opening and closing the fist
      (3.) In local infection of the extremity
   (b.) Blood from a central venous catheter (CVP) usually is an incomplete mix of venous blood from various parts of the body. For a sample of completely mixed blood, a sample would have to be obtained from the right ventricle or pulmonary artery and even then

information is not obtained about how well the lungs are oxygenating the blood.

2. Arterial blood gives the added information of how well the lungs are oxygenating the blood.

   (a.) If it is known that arterial oxygen concentration is normal (indicating that the lungs are functioning normally), but the mixed venous oxygen concentration is low, it can be inferred that the heart and circulation are failing.

   (b.) Oxygen measurements of CVP blood can tell if the tissues are getting oxygenated, but it does not separate the contribution of the heart from the lungs. If CVP blood has a low oxygen concentration, it means either:

      (1.) That the lungs have not oxygenated the arterial blood well so that venous blood has a low concentration.

      (2.) That the heart is not circulating the blood well. In this case, the tissues of the body must take more than the usual amount of oxygen from each cardiac cycle because the blood is flowing slowly. This produces a low venous O_2 concentration.

Note: The site of arterial puncture must satisfy three requirements:

1. Available collateral blood flow
2. Superficial or easily accessible
3. Periarterial tissues (should be non-sensitive)

The radial artery satisfies the criteria listed above.

Procedure for Obtaining Arterial Blood Sample

1. Place patient in either a sitting or supine position.
2. Elevate the wrist (with a small pillow) and ask patient to extend fingers donwnward (this will flex the wrist and move the radial artery closer to the surface).
3. Palpate the artery and rotate patient's hand back and forth until a good strong pulse is felt.
4. Swab the area liberally with an antiseptic agent such as Betadine.
5. Optional: Anesthetize the area with a small amount of one

per cent Xylocaine (approximately ¼ cc. or less). This allows a second attempt without undue pain if the first attempt is a failure.

6. Using a 20 or 21-gauge needle, make the puncture and then attach the prehepranized 12 cc. syringe once the artery has been entered.

7. Pull the plunger on the syringe (being careful not to accidentally pull the needle out of the artery) and collect a three to five ml. sample.

8. Withdraw needle and place a 4″ × 4″ absorbant bandage over the puncture site and maintain pressure with two fingers for a minimum of two minutes.

9. Meanwhile any air bubbles in the blood sample should be expelled as quickly as possible; the syringe should then be capped and gently rotated to mix heparin with blood.

10. If the sample is not going to be analyzed for 15 to 20 minutes, place in an ice water container until such time it can be analyzed.

ALVEOLAR TO ARTERIAL OXYGEN GRADIENT (A-aD$_{O_2}$ RATIO)

Normal Values

9 torr or less in a patient breathing room air

Explanation of Test

This test gives an approximation of the oxygen in the alveoli and arteries. It is used to identify the cause of hypoxemia and intrapulmonary shunting: (1) ventilated alveolus but no perfusion, (2) unventilated alveolus with perfusion or (3) collapse of both alveolus and capillaries.

Procedure

An arterial blood sample is obtained.
    The following mathematical formula is solved.

$$A\text{-}aDO_2 = P_A - P_{a_{O_2}}$$
$$P_{a_{O_2}} = \text{Arterial oxygen tension}$$

$P_{A_{O_2}}$ = Alveolar oxygen tension
D   = difference

Clinical Implications

1. Increased values may be due to:
   (a.) Mucus plugs
   (b.) Bronchospasm
   (c.) Airway collapse as seen in:
      (1.) Asthma
      (2.) Bronchitis
      (3.) Emphysema
2. Hypoxemia, due to an increased A-a_{O_2} difference is also caused by:
   (a.) Atrial septal defects
   (b.) Pneumothorax
   (c.) Atelectasis
   (d.) Emboli
   (e.) Edema

PARTIAL PRESSURE OF CARBON DIOXIDE (P_{CO_2})

Normal Values

$P_{a_{CO_2}}$ (arterial blood) 35–45 torr
$P_{v_{CO_2}}$ (venous blood) 41–51 torr
Carried in blood in two ways: 10% carried in plasma
                              90% carried in RBC's

Explanation of Test

This test is a measurement of the pressure or tension exerted by dissolved carbon dioxide in the blood and is proportional to the partial pressure of carbon dioxide in the alveolar air. The test is commonly used to detect a respiratory abnormality and to determine the alkalinity or acidity of the blood. in order to maintain CO_2 within normal limits, the rate and depth of respiration vary automatically with changes in metabolism. It is an index of alveolar ventilation.

Carbon dioxide tension in the blood and cerebrospinal fluid is the major chemical factor regulating alveolar ventilation. When the CO_2 of arterial blood rises from 40 torr to 45 torr, it causes a three-fold increase in alveolar ventilation. A CO_2 of 63 torr in arterial blood increases alveolar ventilation ten-fold. When the carbon dioxide concentration of breathed air exceeds five per cent, the lungs can no longer be ventilated fast enough to prevent a dangerous rise of CO_2 concentration in tissue fluids. Any further increase in CO_2 begins to depress the respiratory center, causing a progressive decline in respiratory activity rather than an increase.

Procedure

1. Obtain an arterial blood sample.
2. Do not expose sample to air.
3. A small amount of blood is then introduced into a blood gas analyzing machine (*e.g.*, Radiometer, Corning, IL) and the carbon dioxide tension is measured via a silver-silver chloride electrode (Severinghaus electrode).

Clinical Implications

1. A rise in CO_2 is usually associated with hypoventilation; a decrease, with hyperventilation. Reduction in CO_2 through its effect on plasma bicarbonate concentration decreases renal bicarbonate reabsorption.
2. The causes of *decreased* P$_{co_2}$ include:
   - (a.) Hypoxia
   - (b.) Nervousness
   - (c.) Anxiety
   - (d.) Pulmonary emboli
   - (e.) Pregnancy
   - (f.) Other cause of hyperventilation
3. The causes of *increased* P$_{co_2}$ include:
   - (a.) Obstructive lung disease
      - (1.) Chronic bronchitis
      - (2.) Emphysema
   - (b.) Reduced function of respiratory center
      - (1.) Over reaction
      - (2.) Head trauma
      - (3.) Anesthesia

(c.) Other more rare causes of hypoventilation, such as Pickwickian syndrome

---

CLINICAL ALERT

Increased P_{CO_2} may occur even with normal lungs if the respiratory center is depressed. Always check laboratory reports for abnormal values. In interpreting laboratory reports remember that P_{CO_2} is a gas and is regulated by the lungs, not the kidneys.

OXYGEN SATURATION (S_{O_2})

Normal Values

Arterial blood saturation ($S_{a_{O_2}}$) = 95% or higher
Mixed venous blood saturation ($S_{V_{O_2}}$) = 75%

Explanation of Test

This measurement is a ratio of the actual oxygen content of the hemoglobin compared to the potential maximum oxygen-carrying capacity of the hemoglobin. The percentage of oxygen saturation is a measure of the relationship between oxygen and hemoglobin. The percentage of saturation does not indicate the oxygen content of arterial blood. The maximum amount of oxygen that can be combined with hemoglobin is called the oxygen capacity. The combined measurements of oxygen saturation, partial pressure of oxygen, and of hemoglobin will indicate the amount of oxygen available to the tissue (tissue oxygenation).

Procedure

1. Obtain an arterial blood sample. Two methods for determining oxygen saturation are used:
   (a.) The blood sample is introduced into the oximeter, which is a photoelectric device for determining the oxygen saturation of the blood. The value is measured directly with an oximeter (*i.e.*, spectrophotometry)

(b.) Oxygen saturation is calculated from the oxygen content and oxygen capacity determinations

$$\text{Percentage Saturation} = \frac{100 \times O_2 \text{ Content Volume \%}}{O_2 \text{ Capacity Volume \%}}$$

That is

$$\text{Percentage Saturation} = 100 \times \frac{\text{Vol. of } O_2 \text{ actually combined with Hemoglobin}}{\text{Vol. of } O_2 \text{ with which Hemoglobin is capable of combination}}$$

The oxygen content of blood sample is measured before and after exposure to atmosphere.

OXYGEN (O₂) CONTENT

Normal Values

Arterial blood: 15–22 Vol %
Venous blood: 11–16 Vol %
Vol % = Volume Percentage = ml./100 ml. of blood

Explanation of Test

The actual amount of oxygen in the blood is termed the "oxygen content." Blood can contain less oxygen than it is capable of carrying. About 98 per cent of all oxygen delivered to the tissues is transported in chemical combination with hemoglobin. One gram of hemoglobin can carry or is capable of combining with 1.34 ml. of oxygen, whereas 100 ml. of blood plasma can only carry up to 0.3 ml. of oxygen. This measurement is determined mathematically by multiplying the number of grams of hemoglobin in 100 ml. of blood by 1.34 times the partial pressure of oxygen in the blood.

Clinical Implications

Decreased arterial blood oxygen associated with increased arterial blood CO_2 can be due to:

1. Chronic obstructive lung disease
2. Patients with respiratory complications postoperatively
3. Flail chest
4. Kyphoscoliosis
5. Neuromuscular impairment
6. Obesity hypoventilation

Procedure

1. An arterial or venous blood sample is obtained.
2. Mathematical Formula: O_2 content $= S_{a_{O_2}} \times H_g b \times 1.34 + P_{a_{O_2}} \times 0.003$

PARTIAL PRESSURE OF OXYGEN (P_{O_2})

Normal Values

$P_{a_{O_2}}$ 80 torr or greater: Arterial sample
$P_{V_{O_2}}$ 30–40 torr: Venous or peripheral blood sample

Background

Oxygen is carried in the blood in two forms: (1) dissolved, and (2) in combination with hemoglobin. Most of the oxygen in the blood is carried by hemoglobin. It is the partial pressure of a gas that determines the force it exerts in attempting to diffuse through the pulmonary membrane. The partial pressure reflects the amount of oxygen passing from the pulmonary alveoli into the blood and is directly influenced by the amount of oxygen being inhaled.

Explanation of Test

This is a measure of the pressure exerted by the amount of oxygen dissolved in the plasma. It is a test that measures the effectiveness of the lungs to oxygenate the blood. The severity of impairment of the ability of the lungs to diffuse oxygen across the alveolar membrane into the circulating blood is indicated by the level of partial pressure of oxygen.

Procedure

1. An arterial blood sample is obtained.
2. A small amount of blood is then introduced into a blood gas analyzing machine and the oxygen tension is measured via a polarographic electrode (Clark electrode).

Clinical Implications

1. *Increased* levels are associated with
    (a.) Polycythemia
    (b.) Hyperventilation in an arterial blood sample
    (c.) Increased F_IO_2
2. *Decreased* levels are associated with:
    (a.) Anemias
    (b.) Cardiac decompensation
    (c.) Insufficient atmospheric oxygen
    (d.) Intracardiac shunts
    (e.) Chronic obstructive disease
    (f.) Restrictive pulmonary disease
    (g.) Hypoventilation due to neuromuscular disease
3. *Decreased* arterial PO_2 with normal or decreased arterial blood P_{co_2} tension is associated with:
    (a.) Diffuse interstitial pulmonary infiltration
    (b.) Pulmonary edema
    (c.) Pulmonary embolism
    (d.) Postoperative extracorporeal circulation

CARBON DIOXIDE (CO_2) CONTENT OR TOTAL CARBON DIOXIDE (T_{co_2})

Normal Values

24–30 mEq/l.

Background

In normal blood plasma, more than 95 per cent of the total CO_2 content is contributed by bicarbonate (HCO_3), *which is regulated by the kidneys.* The other five per cent of carbon dioxide is contributed by the dissolved CO_2 gas and carbonic acid (H_2CO_3). Dissolved CO_2 gas, which is regulated by the lungs, therefore contributes little to the total CO_2 content. Total CO_2 content gives little information about the lungs.

Bicarbonate in the extracellular spaces exists first as carbon dioxide, then as carbonic acid, and thereafter, much of it is changed to sodium bicarbonate by the buffers of the plasma and red cells.

Explanation of Test

This test is a general measure of the alkalinity or acidity of the venous, arterial, or capillary blood. This test measures carbon dioxide from:
1. Dissolved carbon dioxide (CO_2)
2. Total carbonic acid (H_2CO_3)
3. Bicarbonate (HCO_3)
4. Carbamino carbon dioxide

Total carbon dioxide = $HCO_3 + .03 \times P_{CO_2}$

Procedure

1. A venous or arterial blood sample of six ml. is collected in a heparinized syringe.
2. If the collected blood sample cannot be studied immediately, the syringe should be placed in an iced container.

Clinical Implications

(See also Table 13–1)
1. *Elevated* carbon dioxide content levels occur in:
   - (a.) Severe vomiting
   - (b.) Emphysema
   - (c.) Aldosteronism
   - (d.) Use of mercurial diuretics
2. *Decreased* carbon dioxide content levels occur in:
   - (a.) Severe diarrhea
   - (b.) Starvation
   - (c.) Acute renal failure
   - (d.) Salicylate toxicity
   - (e.) Diabetic acidosis
   - (f.) Use of chlorothiazide diuretics

Note: In diabetic acidosis the supply of ketoacids exceeds the demands of the cell. Blood plasma acids rise. Blood plasma bicarbonate decreases because it is used in neutralizing these acids.

CLINICAL ALERT
A double use of the term carbon dioxide (CO_2) is one of the main reasons why understanding acid-base problems may be difficult. Use the terms CO_2 *content* and CO_2 *gas* to avoid confusion. Remember the following:
1. CO_2 *content* is mainly bicarbonate and a base. It is a solution and is regulated by the kidneys.
2. CO_2 *gas* is mainly acid. It is regulated by the lungs.

Interfering Factors

1. Drugs which may cause *increased or decreased* levels include:
   (a.) Nitrofurantoin
   (b.) Salicylates
2. Drugs which may cause *decreased* levels include:
   (a.) Dimercaprol (BAL)
   (b.) Lipomul oil injection
   (c.) Methicillin

BLOOD pH

Normal Values

Arterial blood: 7.35–7.45
Venous blood: 7.31–7.41

Background

The pH is the negative logarithm of the hydrogen ion concentration in the blood. The sources of hydrogen ions are (1) volatile acids, which can vary between a liquid and a gaseous state and (2) nonvolatile acids that cannot be volatilized and are fixed (*e.g.*, dietary acids, lactic acids, and ketoacids).

TABLE 13–1. FOUR BASIC FORMS OF ACID/BASE IMBALANCE AND THEIR COMPENSATORY MECHANISMS

Forms of Acid-Base Imbalance	Cause	Occurrence	Compensatory Mechanism
1. Respiratory Acidemia	Primary increase in P_{CO_2} and a decreased pH	*Depression of respiratory centers:* (a.) Drug overdose (b.) Barbiturate toxicity (c.) Use of anesthetics *Interference with mechanical function of thoracic cage* (a.) Deformity of thoracic cage (b.) Kyphoscoliosis *Airway Obstruction* (a.) Extrathoracic tumors (b.) Asthma (c.) Bronchitis (d.) Emphysema *Circulatory Disorders* (a.) Congestive heart failure (b.) Shock	Renal reabsorption of the bicarbonate ion. Examples: (a.) Uncompensated respiratory acidemia (acute ventilatory failure) *Values:* pH = 7.26; P_{CO_2}= 56 Bicarbonate= 24 (b.) compensated respiratory acidemia (chronic respiratory failure) *Values:* pH = 7.36; P_{CO_2} = 63 Bicarbonate = 34
2. Respiratory Alkalemia	Primary decrease in P_{CO_2} and increased pH	*Hyperventilation* (a.) hysteria *Lack of oxygen* *Toxic stimulation of the respiratory centers:* (a.) high fever (b.) cerebral hemorrhage (c.) excessive artificial respiration (d.) salicylates	Glomerular filtration of the bicarbonate ion. Examples: (a.) Uncompensated respiratory alkalemia (acute alveolar hyperventilation) *Values* pH = 7.52; P_{CO_2} = 28 Bicarbonate = 22 (b.) Compensated respiratory alkalemia (chronic alveolar hyperventilation) *Values* pH = 7.43; P_{CO_2} = 24 Bicarbonate = 15

TABLE 13–1. FOUR BASIC FORMS OF ACID/BASE IMBALANCE AND THEIR
COMPENSATORY MECHANISMS (*Continued*)

Forms of Acid-Base Imbalance	Cause	Occurrence	Compensatory Mechanism
3. Nonrespiratory Acidemia or Metabolic Acidemia	Increase in hydrogen ions with a secondary decrease in bicarbonate	*Acid Addition* (a.) renal failure (b.) diabetic keto-acidosis (c.) lactic acidosis (d.) anaerobic metabolism *Hypoxia* *Base subtraction* (a.) diarrhea (b.) renal tubular acidosis	Hyperventilation through stimulation of central chemoreceptors. Examples: (a.) uncompensated nonrespiratory acidemia (acute) *Values* pH = 7.20, P_{CO_2} = 38 Bicarbonate = 15 (b.) compensated respiratory acidemia (chronic) *Values* pH = 7.20, P_{CO_2} = 25 Bicarbonate = 15
4. Nonrespiratory Alkalemia or Metabolic Alkalemia	Increase in bicarbonate secondary to a decrease in hydrogen ions	*Acid subtraction* (a.) Loss of gastic juice (b.) vomiting *Potassium or chloride depletion* *Base addition* (a.) excessive bicarbonate or lactate administration	Hypoventilation. Examples: (a.) uncompensated nonrespiratory alkalemia (acute) *Values* pH = 7.56, P_{CO_2} = 44 Bicarbonate = 38 (b.) compensated respiratory alkalemia (chronic) *Values* pH = 7.44, P_{CO_2} = 55 Bicarbonate = 38

NOTE: 1. Although these four basic imbalances occur individually, more frequently a combination of two or more is observed. These disturbances may have an antagonistic or a synergestic effect upon each other.
2. Compensation is most efficient in respiratory and nonrespiratory acidemia.

Explanation of Test

This is a measurement of the chemical balance in the body and is a ratio of acids to bases. A determination of the blood pH is one of the best ways to tell if the body is too acid or too alkaline. Low pH numbers (<7.35) indicate an acid state and higher pH numbers (>7.45) indicate an alkaline state. This balance is extremely intricate and must be kept within the very slight margin of 7.35 to 7.45 pH (alkaline) in the extracellular fluid. (Recall that 1.00-7.00 represents acidity; 7.00 is neutrality; and 7.00-14.00 represents alkalinity.) pH limits compatible with life are 6.9 to 7.8.

The respiratory response to changes in blood pH is almost instantaneous. Acidosis (CO_2 retained, pH falls) stimulates ventilation; alkalosis, (CO_2 blown off, pH rises) depresses ventilation. The respiratory center in the medulla appears to respond to a pH intermediate between those of the blood and cerebrospinal fluid (7.35–7.40)

Procedure

1. An arterial blood sample is obtained.
2. Two methods of determining the pH are used; the direct method and the indirect method.
   - (a.) *Direct method:* A small amount of blood is introduced into a blood gas machine and the pH is measured.
   - (b.) *Indirect method:* The Henderson Hyasselbalch equation is solved.
$$pH = {_p}k' + \log \frac{(HCO_3) \text{ major blood base}}{(H_2CO_3) \text{ major blood acid}}$$

Clinical Implications

1. Generally speaking, the pH is *decreased* in acidemia because of increased formation of acids. pH is *increased* in alkalemia because of a loss of acids.
2. When attempting to interpret an acid/base abnormality one must: (a) check the pH to see if there is an alkalemia or an acidemia, (b) check P_{CO_2} to see if there is a respiratory abnormality, and (c) check bicarbonate (HCO_3) or base excess to see if there is a metabolic abnormality.
3. See Table 13–1 for a more complete explanation of the changes occurring in respiratory and metabolic acidemia and respiratory and metabolic alkalemia.

CLINICAL ALERT
Observing the rate and depth of respiration may give a clue to blood pH:
1. Acidosis usually *increases* respirations.
2. Alkalosis usually *decreases* respirations.

Interfering Factors

1. Drugs that may cause *increased* levels include:
   - (a.) Potassium oxalate
   - (b.) Sodium bicarbonate
   - (c.) Sodium oxalate
2. Drugs that may cause *decreased* levels include:
   - (a.) Acetazolamide
   - (b.) Ammonium chloride
   - (c.) Ammonium oxalate
   - (d.) Calcium chloride
   - (e.) EDTA
   - (f.) Methyl alcohol
   - (g.) Paraldehyde
   - (h.) Salicylates
   - (i.) Sodium citrate

BASE EXCESS/DEFICIT

Normal Values (±3 mEq./l.)

Positive value indicates a base excess (*i.e.*, nonvolatile acid deficit)

Negative value indicates a base deficit (*i.e.*, nonvolatile acid excess)

Explanation of Test

This determination is an attempt to quantify the patient's total base excess or deficit so that clinical treatment of acid base disturbances (specifically those that are nonrespiratory in nature) can be initiated. It is also referred to as the whole blood buffer base and is the sum of the concentration of buffer anions (in mEq./l.) contained in whole blood. These buffer anions are the bicarbonate (HCO_3^-) ion in plasma, red blood cells and the hemoglobin, plasma proteins and phosphates in plasma and red blood cells.

Total quantity of buffer anions is 45 to 50 mEq. per l. or about twice that of bicarbonate which is 24 to 28 mEq. per l. Thus the quantity of bicarbonate ions accounts for only about half of the total buffering capacity of the blood. Therefore, the base excess/deficit measurement provides a more complete picture of the buffering taking place and is a critical index of non-respiratory changes in acid/base balance versus respiratory changes.

Procedure

Calculation is made from the measurements of pH, $P_{a_{CO_2}}$ and hematocrit. These values are plated on a nomogram and the base excess/deficit is read.

Clinical Implications

1. Negative value (below 3 mEq./l.) reflects a nonrespiratory or metabolic disturbance. It indicates a nonvolatile acid *accumulation* due to
   (a.) Dietary intake of organic and inorganic acids
   (b.) Lactic acid
   (c.) Ketoacidosis
2. Positive value (above 3 mEq./l.) reflects a nonvolatile acid deficit.

REFERENCES

Berkow, Robert (ed.): THE MERCK MANUAL OF DIAGNOSIS AND THERAPY, 13th Ed. Rahway, N.J., Merck Sharp & Dohme Research Laboratories, 1977.

Boren, H., Kory, R., Snyder, J.: "The Veterans Administration–Army Cooperative Study of Pulmonary Function: II–The Lung Volume and Its Subdivisions in Normal Men;" Amer. J. Med., *41*(1):96–114, 1966.

Borrows, Benjamin, Kasik, John, E., Niden, Albert H., and Barclay, William, R.: "Clinical Usefulness of the Single-Breath Pulmonary Diffusing Capacity Test. Amer. Rev. Resp. Dis., 84:789–806, 1961.

Brust, S. A., and Ross, B. B.: "Predicted Values for Closing Volumes using a Modified Single Breath Nitrogen Test." Amer. Rev. Resp. Dis., 107:744, 1973.

Cherniack, Reuben M.: PULMONARY FUNCTION TESTING. Philadelphia, W. B. Saunders Company, 1977.

Fraser, Robert G., and Paré, J. A. Peter: ORGAN PHYSIOLOGY: STRUCTURE AND FUNCTION OF THE LUNG. 2nd Ed. Philadelphia, W. B. Saunders Company, 1977.

Geschickter, Charles F.: THE LUNG IN HEALTH AND DISEASE. Philadelphia, J. B. Lippincott Company, 1973.

Gilb, Arthur F., Molony, Patrick A., Klein, Edward and Aronstam, Peter S.: "Sensitivity of Volume of Isoflow in the Detection of Mild Airway Obstruction." Amer. Rev. Resp. Dis., 112:401–405, 1975.

Goldman, H. O., and Becklake, M. R.: "Respiratory Function Tests. Normal Values at Median Altitudes and the Prediction of Normal Results." Amer. Rev. Tuber. Pul. Dis., 79:457, 1979.

Pace, William R., Jr.: PULMONARY PHYSIOLOGY IN CLINICAL PRACTICE. 2nd Ed. Philadelphia, F. A. Davis Company, 1970.

Petty, Thomas L.: PULMONARY DIAGNOSTIC TECHNIQUES. Philadelphia, Lea & Febiger, 1975.

Ruppel, Gregg: MANUAL OF PULMONARY FUNCTION TESTING. 2nd Ed. St. Louis, The C. V. Mosby Company, 1979.

Shapiro, Barry A., Harrison, Ronald A., and Walton, John, R.: CLINICAL APPLICATION OF BLOOD GASES. 2nd Ed., Year Book Medical Publishers, Inc., Chicago, London, 1977.

Slonim, N. Balfour, and Hamilton, Lyle H.: RESPIRATORY PHYSIOLOGY. 3rd Ed. St. Louis, The C. V. Mosby Company, 1976.

14 □□ SPECIAL TESTS OF CARDIOVASCULAR AND CENTRAL NERVOUS SYSTEM FUNCTION

INTRODUCTION

These special tests of the cardiovascular and central nervous systems have been selected to appear in this chapter because of their great importance in diagnosing alterations in the functions of these two vital systems.

ELECTROENCEPHALOGRAPHY (EEG)

Normal Values

Normal symmetrical pattern of alpha, beta, and delta wave

676

Explanation of Test

This test measures and records electrical impulses in the brain. Electrodes are placed outside the cranial vault to record the electrical manifestations of brain activity. It is used to diagnose epilepsy and as an aid in identifying brain tumors, abscesses and subdural hematomas; cerebrovascular diseases, such as cerebral infarcts and intracranial hemorrhage; and cerebral diseases, such as advanced cases of multiple sclerosis, narcolepsy and acute delirium.

It is common practice to use the EEG pattern to define cerebral death. A record which is flat is usually the result of cerebral hypoxia or ischemia, and the brain is largely necrotic. When this occurs, there is no change of neurologic recovery and the patient may be considered dead, despite the preservation of cardiovascular functions supported by mechanical respiration.

Procedure

1. The test is usually scheduled early in the day.
2. It is usually done in a small room adjacent to, but separate from, the EEG machine; this prevents the machine from picking up extraneous electric signals, giving the patient the privacy needed for quiet and relaxation.
3. The technician will place electrodes in the form of small discs on the scalp, fastening them with ointment electrical conduction paste, or by use of a cap or headband. The electrodes, numbering from 16 to 25, are arranged in one of several patterns, or montages, on the scalp.
4. Patient will be seated in an easy chair or will be requested to lie on a bed or couch.
5. Instructions are given to keep eyes closed, to relax, and to rest.
6. A flashing light may be used over the face at frequencies of 1 to 20 times per second with the eyes opened or closed. The light is used to activate the EEG. This technique often causes abnormal discharge. Hyperventilation may also be used to activate the EEG.
7. Near the end of the examination, the patient may be asked to breathe deeply, 20 times a minute through the mouth for three minutes. This hyperventilation may cause dizziness

or numbness in hands or feet, but it is nothing to be alarmed about. Rapid shallow breathing contributes to alkalosis with vasoconstriction which may activate a seizure pattern.

8. Some patients may be given a mild sedative prior to the test to promote rest and sleep. Sleep is especially helpful in bringing out abnormalities, especially temporal lobe epilepsy.

9. The technician will remove the discs after the test and the ointment or paste will be removed from the scalp.

10. Total examining time is 30 to 45 minutes.

Clinical Implications

1. Abnormal pattern readings will reveal generalized seizures (*e.g.*, grand mal and *petit mal* epilepsy) provided the EEG is recorded during the seizure. If a patient suspected of having epilepsy shows a normal EEG, the test may have to be repeated.

   (a.) The EEG is also abnormal during lesser types of seizure activity (*e.g.*, focal or psychomotor, infantile myoclonic, and Jacksonian seizure).

   (b.) Between seizures, as many as 20 per cent of patients with petit mal epilepsy and 40 per cent with grand mal epilepsy show a normal pattern.

   (c.) The diagnosis of epilepsy can be made only by correlating the clinical history with the EEG abnormality, if one exists.

2. An EEG may often be normal in the presence of cerebral pathology.

   (a.) However, 100 per cent of brain abscess and 90 per cent of glioblastomas cause EEG abnormalities.

   (b.) EEG changes due to cerebrovascular accidents (CVA's) depend on the size and location of the infarcts or hemorrhage.

   (c.) Following a head injury, a series of EEG's may be helpful in identifying the prospect of epilepsy, a result of the trauma.

3. The EEG is abnormal in almost all diseases in which there is an impairment of consciousness.

   (a.) The more profound the change in consciousness, the more abnormal the EEG pattern.

Interfering Factors

1. Sedative drugs and mild hypoglycemia may affect the normal EEG.
2. Oily hair or hair spray interferes with the placement of leads and a true tracing
3. Drugs which interfere with the test include:
   - (a.) Barbiturates
   - (b.) Anticonvulsants
   - (c.) Tranquilizers

   These drugs should not be administered before the test. Check with doctor or pharmacist.
4. Artifacts may appear even in technically well done EEG's. Eye movements and body movements cause changes in the wave pattern and must be noted so that they may not be mistaken for brain waves.

Patient Preparation

1. Explain the purpose and procedure of the test. Some people are very fearful of the test, even though it involves no pain or discomfort. Emphasize that it is not a test of thinking or intelligence. No electrical impulses pass from the machine to the patient, and the test has no relation to any type of shock treatment.
2. Check with physician or pharmacist about medications which should not be given prior to testing.
3. Food may be taken, but no coffee, tea, or cola is permitted within eight hours before the test. Emphasize that food should be eaten to prevent hypoglycemia.
4. Smoking is usually allowed.
5. Hair should be shampooed the evening before the test so that leads will remain firmly in place.
6. An adult patient should retire late and arise early before the EEG so that he will have as little sleep as possible (4–5 hours preferred) and be tired enough to fall asleep at the time of the test.
7. A young child should be put to bed two hours later than his regular time and awakened at his usual time the next morning. If the child has an afternoon appointment, he should not nap during the morning.

Patient Aftercare

1. If anti-convulsant drugs have been withheld prior to testing, administer them as soon as test is completed.
2. Hair should be shampooed after testing to remove oil or ointment if used to fasten discs.

OPHTHALMODYNAMOMETRY

Normal Values

Very little difference in the pressure readings of both eyes.

Explanation of Test

This procedure, using an ophthalmoscope, measures arterial systolic and diastolic blood pressures in the main retinal branch or branches of the ophthalmic artery. It is helpful in evaluating internal transient ischemia attacks and cerebral infarctions. It is indicated in the evaluation of cerebrovascular insufficiency due to carotid artery stenosis or occlusion.

Procedure

1. The ophthalmoscope, the instrument that measures the pressure, is pressed gradually against the eye. A blood pressure cuff is also applied to an arm and a brachial blood pressure determined.
2. The examination is not painful.
3. Mydriatic eye drops are instilled if the patient does not have glaucoma.
4. The test cannot be performed unless the patient cooperates.
5. The test takes only a few minutes.

Clinical Implications

1. A marked decrease in the retinal arterial pressure with the brachial arterial pressure remaining normal when the client moves from a supine position to the upright position is important evidence of carotid occlusive disease.

2. A difference of 15 to 20 per cent is almost always a sign of internal carotid artery occlusion or stenosis.
3. Acute carotid thrombosis can usually be detected and differentiated from thrombosis or embolism of the middle cerebral artery.

Patient Preparation

Explain the purpose and procedure of the test.

ELECTROCARDIOGRAPHY (ECG or EKG)
(With brief description of vector cardiogram)

Normal Values

Normal deflections on an ECG graphic record (Fig. 14–1) See also Table 14–1.

1. A *normal P wave* represents the electrical activity associated with the original impulse from the SA node and its subsequent spread through the atria. If P waves are present and of normal size, shape, and deflection, it can be assumed that the stimulus began in the SA node; if these waves are absent or altered, it implies that the impulse originated outside the SA node.
2. A *normal PR interval* is the period from the start of the P wave to the beginning of the QRS complex. It represents the time taken for the original impulse to reach the ventricles and initiate ventricular contraction (depolarization). During this period (which normally does not exceed 0.2 seconds) the impulse has traversed the atria and the AV node. If the PR interval is prolonged beyond 0.2 seconds, it may be assumed that a conduction delay exists in the AV node. In some cases the PR interval is unusually short (less than 0.1 seconds) which implies that the current reached the ventricle through a shorter than normal pathway as in the Wolff-Parkinson-White syndrome.
3. A *normal QRS complex* consists of waves that represent the contraction or depolarization of the ventricular muscle. They consist of an initial downward deflection (Q wave), a

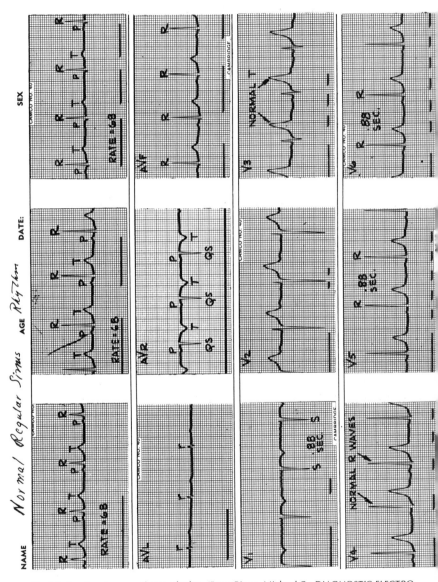

Fig. 14–1. *Regular normal sinus rhythm. (From Ritota, Michael C.: DIAGNOSTIC ELECTRO-CARDIOGRAPHY. 2nd Ed., Philadelphia, J. B. Lippincott Co., 1977.)*

large upward deflection (R wave) and a second downward wave (S wave). Together this complex reflects the time necessary for the impulse to spread through the bundle of His and its branches to complete ventricular activation. When the duration of this impulse (normally less than 0.12 seconds) is increased, it is evidence that the ventricles have been stimulated in a delayed, abnormal manner, as in a bundle branch block.

4. A *normal ST segment* is an interval representing the period between the completion of depolarization and repolarization (recovery) of the ventricular muscles. The segment may be elevated or depressed if there is ischemia or injury to the muscle.

5. A *normal T* wave represents the recovery phase after contraction. If repolarization or recovery period is abnormal, usually because of tissue injury or ischemia, the T wave may be inverted.

Explanation of Test

An electrocardiogram (ECG) is a recording of the electrical impulses of the heart. This test is an important indicator of how well the heart is functioning. The ECG is used mainly to diagnose coronary artery disease, myocardial infarction, abnormal rhythms, electrolyte imbalance, pericardial effusion, and pericarditis.

Each normal heart beat begins with an electrical impulse that originates in a specialized area of the right atrium called the sinoatrial (SA) node. This island of tissue serves as a battery for the heart and normally discharges an electrical force 60 to 100 times a minute in rhythmic fashion. Because the SA node controls the rate of the heart beat, it is designated as the *pacemaker*. (All areas of the myocardium have the potential ability to serve in this capacity, but they assume this role only under abnormal circumstances.) The original impulse is transmitted through the heart in an orderly path. When it reaches the ventricular muscles, contraction occurs. After contracting, the muscles rest and recover while the ventricles fill with blood. The next impulse normally arrives when filling is complete and ventricular contraction again occurs. The combined periods of contraction (depolarization) and recovery (repolarization) constitute the cardiac cycle.

TABLE 14–1. NORMAL MEASUREMENTS AND RANGES OF COMPONENTS OF P-Q-R-S-T-U CYCLE*·†

	P Wave		P-R Interval	Q Wave Q% of R	
	Amplitude	Width			
	Maximum	Maximum	0.12-0.20 sec.	Width	Depth
	2.5 mm.	0.10 sec.		Less Than 0.04 sec.	Q/R Ratio
L₁					15% of R wave
L₂					20% of R wave
L₃				Up to 0.08 sec.	25% of R wave
ᴀVR				Up to 0.08 sec.	
ᴀVL				Less than 0.04 sec.	25% of R wave
ᴀVF				↓	
V₁				Up to 0.08 sec.	
V₂				↓	
V₃				Less than 0.04 sec.	
V₄					
V₅					
V₆	↓	↓	↓	↓	↓

*For practical purposes, these are the upper and lower limits of the normal ECG. However, there are "gray zones" and variation from these limits may not necessarily imply abnormality.

†From Ritota, Michael C.: DIAGNOSTIC ELECTROCARDIOGRAPHY. 2nd Ed., Philadelphia, J. B. Lippincott Co., 1977.

TABLE 14–1. NORMAL MEASUREMENTS AND RANGES OF COMPONENTS OF P-Q-R-S-T-U CYCLE (*Continued*)

QRS Interval	R Wave Amplitude	S-T Segment	T Wave	U Wave Amplitude	Width
0.10 sec.	Maximum to Minimum	1 mm.	1-5 mm.	1.5 mm.	0.24 sec.
	5-16 mm.	Above or Below			
		1 mm. Elevation			
	↓	↓	↓		
	Less than + 4 mm.		except in this lead (T is neg.)		
	5-13 mm. Transverse Heart	1 mm. Elevation			
	5-21 mm. Vertical Heart		↓		
	5-27 mm.	1-2 mm. Depression / 2 mm. to 4 mm. Elevation	13 mm.		
↓	↓	↓	↓	↓	↓

An ECG is a graphic record of the electrical impulses that are generated by contraction (depolarization) and recovery (repolarization) of the myocardium. The body fluid is an excellent conductor of electrical current. When the depolarization process sweeps in a wave across the cells of the myocardium, the electrical current generated is conducted to the body's surface where it is detected by special electrodes placed on the patient's limbs and chest.

An electrocardiogram tracing also shows the voltage of the waves and the time duration of both waves and intervals. By studying the amplitude and time duration of the waves and intervals, disorders of impulse formation and conduction can be diagnosed.

Principle of ECG

1. The conduction system of the heart produces small differences in electrical potential (a thousandth of a volt) as it stimulates the heart to contract.
2. The electrical activity of the heart can be recorded and measured.
3. The electrical forces from the heart are transmitted outward and reach the surface of the body, where they can be detected by electrodes attached to the chest wall and the extremities.
4. Deflections in the ECG recorder are caused by the ebb and flow of the electrical forces from the heart.
5. The resulting waves are amplified for greater visibility before being displayed on the oscilloscope or being printed on moving graph paper. This recording provides a continuous picture of the electrical activity during the cycle.

Recording the Electrical Impulses

1. Because the electrical forces extend in several directions at the same time, a comprehensive view can be obtained only if the flow of current in different planes is recorded.
2. Twelve leads are used simultaneously:
    (a.) Limb leads: I, II, III, AVF, AVL, AVR. These view the frontal plane of the heart.

(b.) Chest leads: V, V_2, V_3, V_4, V_5, and V_6. These record a horizontal view of the heart's electrical activity.

Electrocardiogram vs. Vectorcardiogram

The vectorcardiogram, like the electrocardiogram, records the electrical forces of the heart. The major difference between these methods is in the way in which these forces are displayed. A vectorcardiogram records a *three-dimensional* display of the heart's electrical activity, whereas the electrocardiogram shows activity in a *single plane.*

The three planes of the vectorcardiogram are as follows:
1. Frontal plane (combines the Y and X axes)
2. Sagittal plane (combines the Y and Z axes)
3. Horizontal plane (combines the X and Z axes)

Briefly, the two records of the heart's electrical activity may be compared as follows:

Electrocardiogram	*Vectorcardiogram*
Records electrical forces as deflections on a scale	Depicts electrical forces as vector loops, thereby showing the *direction* of electrical activity
Recorded in the frontal and horizontal planes of the body	Recorded on the frontal, horizontal, and sagittal planes of the body
	The term "vector" is used to indicate the direction of electrical activity.

Clinical Implications of ECG

1. The ECG *does not* depict the actual mechanical state of the heart or function of the valves.
2. An ECG may be quite normal in the presence of heart disease unless the pathologic process disturbs the electrical forces.
3. Final conclusions from an ECG should be done only with a full knowledge of the clinical status of the patient.
4. Abnormalities of an ECG are categorized into 5 general

areas: (1) heart rate, (2) heart rhythm, (3) axis or position of the heart, (4) hypertrophy, and (5) infarction. Certain specific abnormalities in these areas are typical of:

(a.) Pathological rhythms
(b.) Conduction system diseases
(c.) Myocardial ischemia
(d.) Myocardial infarction
(e.) Hypertrophy of the heart
(f.) Pulmonary infarction
(g.) Aortic stenosis
(h.) Electrolyte changes in potassium and calcium
(i.) Pericarditis
(j.) Effects of drugs (*e.g.*, digitalis and quinidine)

Clinical Implications of Vectorcardiogram

1. The vectorcardiogram is more sensitive than the ECG in the diagnosis of myocardial infarction, but it is probably not more specific.
2. Vectorcardiography is more specific than the ECG in the assessment of hypertrophy or dilatation of the ventricles of the heart in children.

Procedure

Note: The following steps apply to both the ECG and the vectorcardiogram.

1. The patient is placed in a supine position on a table, bed or couch, but the recording can also be done during exercise or the patient can be ambulatory and a halter device is used for a continuous 24 hour recording.
2. The skin is prepared (which can include shaving if there is excess hair) by the application of contact paste or prejelled discs.
3. Electrodes are placed on the four extremities (or their roots), on the groin and shoulder areas, and on the chest. The right leg is usually ground.
4. The operator then records the ECG through machine setting.

5. The test may take only a few minutes or it may take as long as 24 hours, if a continuous recording has been ordered.

Patient Preparation

Explain purpose and procedure of test, emphasizing that it is painless and that there is no current flow to the patient.

PHONOCARDIOGRAPHY

Normal Values

Normal heart sounds

Explanation of Test

This test graphically records the occurrence, timing, and length of sounds of the heart cycle. Heart murmurs can be both visualized and accurately timed. Sounds which originate in the heart and large vessels are recorded from the body's surface and correspond to what is heard through a stethoscope. This diagnostic technique involves the electronic detection, amplification, and recording of cardiac sounds onto specially designed phonocardiograph paper. For recording purposes, a specially designed microphone is placed upon the patient's chest. This device picks up the low-frequency cardiac vibrations for amplification and recording. The phonocardiograph is recorded simultaneously with carotid pulse, ECG, and respiration.

Phonocardiography provides information about underlying hemodynamics that is not obtainable through physical examination. It also provides a permanent objective record of events with which subsequent comparison may be made. It is useful in detecting abnormalities in valvular function and can be used in conjunction with other cardiovascular monitoring techniques to assess specific portions of the cardiac cycle such as systolic ejection time and pre-ejection time. It is a valuable teaching aid.

Procedure

1. The test should be done in a quiet room.
2. The patient is placed on a table in a supine position with pillows under his head.
3. Electrocardiographic leads are placed on all four extremities and standard lead two (2) is recorded throughout the procedure. A neck cuff for the indirect carotid pulse is secured in place and inflated to 15–20 mm. of mercury. Microphones for sound recording are placed over the pulmonary area and apex.
4. The patient is instructed to inhale deeply and to allow most of the air to escape from his lungs. Then he is instructed to suspend his breathing for a few seconds at this point in expiration, without tensing his muscles. Then the patient is asked to breathe quietly through his mouth and a recording is made.
5. The pulmonary area microphone then is removed and placed over the aortic area and a recording made during held expiration.
6. Next, the neck cuff is removed and the patient's upper body is lowered to one pillow. The upper microphone is then placed over the left sternal border in the fourth intercostal space, and a jugular pulse recording is made during held expiration.
7. The patient is turned on his left side and another recording is made.
8. Total examining time is about 30 minutes.

Clinical Implications

1. Phonocardiography can be used to augment, but not replace, auscultation.
2. The method can be used as an aid in diagnosis and differentiation of such valvular diseases as valvular pulmonary stenosis and valvular aortic stenosis.
3. Certain murmurs can be more accurately diagnosed with a stethoscope used by a skilled clinician.
4. Some cardiologists find it helpful to use phonocardiography so as to have a permanent record of the patient's heart

sounds before and after cardiac surgery. The phonocardiograms are useful in evaluating the patient's progress.

Patient Preparation

1. Explain the purpose and procedure of the test.
2. Reassure patient that no pain or discomfort is involved.

ELECTROMYOGRAPHY (EMG)

Normal Values

1. Normal nerve conduction
2. Normal muscle action potential:
   - (a.) on insertion
   - (b.) at rest
   - (c.) during minimum voluntary muscle contraction
   - (d.) during maximum voluntary muscle contraction

Explanation of Test

These studies, done to detect neuromuscular abnormalities, measure nerve conduction and electrical properties of skeletal muscle. Skin surface electrodes or monopolar electrodes are used to measure and record muscle nerve impulses: A needle electrode is inserted into the muscle to pick up the electrical activity. Normal muscle is electrically silent when at rest, but when muscles are voluntarily or electrically stimulated or contracted, action potentials of the muscle are greatly amplified and then can be viewed on a cathode ray oscilloscope (CRO). Sound equivalents of electrical activity are heard over a loudspeaker or recorded on a tape recorder. The tape can be played later and restudied as often as necessary.

These tests are useful in evaluating patients with symptoms of abnormal sensation or weakness (myasthenia gravis, myotonia) in lower motor neuron disease and peripheral nerve injuries.

Procedure

1. A history and physical (including reflexes and sensations) are done by the testing physician.
2. Test is done in a copper-lined room to screen out interference.
3. Patient lies on his back on a hard table, usually in a hospital gown.
4. Three electrodes are taped to the involved areas. The muscles and nerves the examiner checks are dependent on the patient's signs and symptoms, history and physical (certain nerves ennervate specific muscles).
5. Instructions are given to relax (the examiner may massage muscles to get patient to relax) and to contract certain muscles (*e.g.,* to point toes, when directed).
6. The test consists of two parts. The first test is done to determine *nerve conduction:*
   - (a.) Bipolar electrode is placed in a specific area and electrical current is passed through the individual. This will cause pain directly proportional to time involved.
   - (b.) Amplitude wave is read on an oscilloscope.
   - (c.) Electrical current leaves no mark but can cause considerable pain.
7. The second test is done to determine *muscle potential.*
   - (a.) A monopolar electrode (½–3″ very small diameter needle) is inserted and a pricking sensation may be felt as the needle pierces the skin. The needle is advanced into the muscle by increments. The examiner may move the needle around without removing it to see if readings change as well as reinserting the needle in another muscle area.
   - (b.) The electrode causes no pain unless the end of the needle is near a terminal nerve; then it can cause considerable pain. Ten or more insertions may be made.
   - (c.) Examiner watches the oscilloscope for a normal wave and listens to a loudspeaker for normal quiet sound at rest. A "machine-gun" popping sound is normally heard when the patient is asked to contract the muscles.

(d.) If the patient complains of pain, the examiner removes the needle because pain yields false results.

(e.) Total examining time is 45 to 60 minutes if testing is confined to single extremity—up to 2½ hours for more than one extremity. There is no completely "routine" EMG. The length of the test depends on the clinical problem.

Clinical Implications

1. Abnormal pattern readings can reveal
   (a.) early peripheral nerve degeneration
   (b.) regeneration
   (c.) presence, extent and prognosis of lower motor neuron disease.
2. Defects in nerves, neuro-muscular function, and muscle can be differentiated.
3. The EMG may be used in diagnosis of such disorders as anterior poliomyelitis and amyotrophic lateral sclerosis, in which there is involvement of the anterior horn cells.
4. EMG may be ordered in patients with suspected demyelinization of the peripheral neuron system, such as in diabetes mellitus and alcoholism.
5. In patients with muscular dystrophy, EMG may be used to differentiate neuropathy from myopathy.
6. In patients with suspected nerve injury, the EMG may be used to determine presence or absence of nerve injury, the extent of the injury and the location of any lesions.

Interfering Factors

1. Conduction can vary with age; conduction is normally decreased in the elderly.
2. Pain can yield false results.
3. Electrical activity from extraneous persons and objects can yield false results.

Patient Preparation

1. Instruct patient about the purpose and procedure of the test.
2. Sedation or analgesia may be ordered.

Patient Aftercare

1. If patient has experienced pain or is in pain, provide relief.
2. Provide restful, relaxing activities. Patient may be exhausted if examination time is lengthy.

CLINICAL ALERT
1. Enzyme levels which reflect muscle activity (SGOT, LDH, CPK) must be determined prior to testing because EMG will cause misleading elevation of these enzymes for up to ten days.
2. It is rare, but hematomas may form at needle insertion sites. Notify physician if this occurs.

CARDIAC CATHETERIZATION AND ANGIOGRAPHY (ANGIOCARDIOGRAPHY; CORONARY ARTERIOGRAPHY)

Normal Values

Normal heart and coronary arteries
Normal pressure and cardiac output
Normal percentage of oxygen saturation

Explanation of Test

This is a method of studying and diagnosing defects in the chambers of the heart, its valves and its vessels by inserting arterial and venous catheters carrying contrast material into the right and left sides of the heart. As the catheters are advanced, fluoroscopy and rapidly taken x-ray pictures projected on TV monitors show the action of the heart under study. The injected dye or contrast medium provides definition of the cardiac structures. Each coronary artery is filmed as well. An oscilliscope near the television monitor shows the patient's heart rate, rhythm and pressures.

Coronary arteriograms are highly useful in diagnosing heart disease, determining the extent of damage, diagnosing congenital abnormalities, identifying cardiac structure and function prior to surgery, measuring pressures within heart chambers and great vessels, determining cardiac output (using dye dilation, thermodilutin, and Fick method), and obtaining blood samples directly from heart to measure oxygen content of blood and oxygen saturation.

Cardiac catheterization with angiography is indicated in patients with angina, with incapacitating chest pain after healing has occurred following a myocardial infarction, syncope, valvular and ischemic disease; in patients with cholesteremia and familial heart disease who are experiencing chest pain; in patients with abnormal resting ECG's; in patients who have had cardiac revascularization with recurring symptoms; in young patients with a history of coronary insufficiency and ventricular aneurysm; and in patients with coronary neurosis who can be assured that their arteries are normal.

It is a serious examination and highly accurate as a diagnostic technique.

Procedure

1. The test is usually done in a darkened room.
2. To decrease fear of the procedure, the patient is continuously told what is being done.
3. The patient lies on an x-ray table; ECG leads are attached to the chest. During the procedure, the patient will be turned from side to side and may be asked to exercise (optional) to evaluate heart changes of any kind during activity.
4. The catheterization procedure is done under sterile conditions. Skin is prepared with an antiseptic solution. A local anesthetic is injected prior to the making of small incisions for the insertion of catheter into an artery and vein. (Incisions are not always made.) Catheters are gently pushed into the heart and great vessels.
5. The patient can watch all procedures on a screen of brightened heart image with "instant replay."
6. After x-rays have been taken at all angles, the catheters are removed and the skin incisions (if any) are closed with a few stitches. A sterile pressure bandage is applied. The procedure takes about one hour, or a little longer if the patient must exercise.

Clinical Implications

1. Abnormal results:
    - (a.) Advancing catheters will reveal altered intracardiac pressures
    - (b.) Injecting dye will reveal altered ventricular contractibility
    - (c.) Analyzing blood oxygen will confirm cardiac or arterial irregularities
2. Abnormal pressures are indicative of:
    - (a.) Valve stenosis
    - (b.) Left ventricular failure
    - (c.) Heart blockages
    - (d.) Rheumatic fever
3. Abnormal blood oxygen samples are indicative of:
    - (a.) Congenital or acquired shunting of blood
    - (b.) Septal defects
    - (c.) Leakage or abnormal sequential circulation of blood through heart
4. When dye is injected into ventricles, abnormal size, bulging, ejections, fractions, aneurysms of heart, leaks, stenosis, blockage and altered contractibility of heart can be detected.
5. When dye is injected into coronary arteries, abnormal circulation through coronary circulation can be detected.

Patient Preparation

1. Explain the purpose and procedure of the test. A legal permit must be signed prior to examination.
2. Usually a bland meal is eaten the evening before examination, but nothing can be consumed for at least three hours prior to testing.
3. Analgesics, sedatives, or tranquilizers are administered prior to examination.
4. Have patient void before going to the catheterization laboratory.
5. Allow the patient to wear dentures.
6. Patient should be aware that he will be asked to breathe deeply and cough during the test, and that he will experience certain sensations that are common to the procedure:
    - (a.) A slight shock (like hitting the "funny bone") is felt

when the artery is entered, and a tiny bump in the neck is experienced as the catheter is inserted and pushed through the artery into the chest. Neither of these sensations is too uncomfortable.

(b.) When dye is injected, a pumping sensation (with palpitations and warm flashes) lasts 30 to 60 seconds. The dye injection causes skin vessels to vasodilate, and warm systemic blood rises to skin surface, returning again as the heat fades.

(c.) Nausea, vomiting, and cough are minor side effects that some patients may experience.

Patient Aftercare

1. Bed rest is maintained for several hours after the test.
2. Check vital signs and dressing for swelling or bleeding.
3. Antibiotics may be administered before or after the examination to prevent infection.
4. Encourage fluids after testing.
5. Keep affected extremity extended (not elevated) and immobilized with sandbag to decrease discomfort and bleeding and apply ice to site, if ordered. Analgesics, if ordered, can be administered for pain at insertion sites.
6. Sutures, if used, are removed in seven days.

CLINICAL ALERT
1. This procedure is contraindicated in patients with gross cardiomegaly.
2. Complications which can occur include:
   (a.) Arrythmias
   (b.) Allergic dye reactions (evidenced by urticaria, pruritus, and conjunctivitis)
   (c.) Thrombophlebitis of cutdown vein
   (d.) Infection at cutdown site
   (e.) Pneumothorax
   (f.) Hemopericardium
   (g.) Embolism
   (h.) Tears in liver, especially in infants and children (results from poor technique)
3. Notify attending physician if there is any increased bleeding or a drastic fall or increase in blood pressure.

4. When angiography is performed, the following equipment should always be available for complications:
   (a.) Resuscitation equipment
   (b.) DC fibrillator
   (c.) External pacemaker
   (d.) Electrocardiographic monitor
   (e.) Cardiac drugs (epinephrine, norepinephrine, isoproterenol)

STRESS/EXERCISE TESTING
(GRADED EXERCISE TOLERANCE TEST)

Normal Values

Negative when a patient has no significant symptoms; arrythmias, or other ECG abnormalities

Explanation of the Test

This test measures the efficiency of the heart during a dynamic exercise stress period on a motor driven treadmill. It is valuable in diagnosing coronary artery disease.

When the patient is exercised at a given rate, the time it takes to reach a predetermined stress level is determined. The test is ended when the heart rate or blood pressure reaches a preset level. The systolic blood pressure normally increases with exercise, and the diastolic normally remains essentially unchanged.

Periodic stress testing is also recommended for any healthy person over the age of 35 and for an individual who is considering starting an exercise program.

Procedure

There are many different types of stress tests in use today. Most of them include the following steps:
1. Recording electrodes are placed on the patient's chest (see description of electrocardiogram) and attached to a monitor. A blood pressure recording device is also used.

2. While the patient walks on a motor-driven treadmill, a computerized electrocardiogram and heart monitoring device will record the performance. The patient walks at progressive speeds and elevations in an effort to increase heart rate and workload.
3. The ECG, heart rate, and blood pressure are recorded at rest. The patient is asked to report any symptom such as chest pain that is experienced during the test.
4. The patient is stressed in stages. Each stage consists of a predetermined level of the treadmill, in miles per hour, and in elevation of the treadmill, in per cent grade.
5. The ECG, heart rate, and blood pressure are constantly monitored for any signs of abnormality and any unusual symptoms such as dizziness, shortness of breath, chest pain, and severe cramping in the legs.
6. Usually a three-minute and ten-minute recovery stage are recorded. This is done with the patient seated. The test will be terminated if there are ECG abnormalities, fatigue and weakness, abnormal blood pressure changes, or intolerable symptoms.
7. Total exam time is about 30 minutes.

Clinical Implications

1. A stress test is positive when a patient has specific electrocardiographic changes with or without angina.
2. A stress test is abnormal when a patient complains of chest discomfort or if arrythmias are present.

Interfering Factors

A test is considered incomplete when the patient is unable to complete the test and falls short of the predetermined heart rate

Patient Preparation

1. Explain the purpose and procedure of the test.
2. Arrange to have patient wear comfortable walking shoes for the test. Bedroom slippers are not suitable.

CLINICAL ALERT

Stress exercise tests can be risky to patients who have had chest pain of recent onset and attacks of angina several times a day. The test should not be given to such a patient at that time, but may be rescheduled in four to six weeks.

DOPPLER ULTRASOUND FLOW STUDIES

Normal Values

Normal and equal arterial and venous blood flow. Ankle, brachial, and wrist segmental pressures in extremities should all be equal. Ankle/brachial index of one (or .95 or greater) normal.

Explanation of Test

The Doppler ultrasound flow studies are noninvasive diagnostic techniques that are used to determine the presence of deep and arterial venous obstruction; the right side is compared with the left and vice versa. The instrument used in these studies is the Doppler ultrasonic velocity detector, which incorporates piezoelectric crystals in a hand-held probe. A beam of ultrasound is sent through an acoustical gel on the skin. The reflected ultrasound produces an electrical impulse that is then converted into an audible signal.

With the Doppler probe, the technician can differentiate between various arterial and venous blood flows. The distinctive sounds of the flows can be characterized as normal, obstructed, or incompetent.

An assessment of cerebral blood flow is based upon an indirect measurement of carotid artery flow. Deep veins are tested for obstruction by measuring the amount of fluid in a limb. The amount of fluid is then changed by deep inspiration, by using the Valsalva manuever, or by using extrinsic pressure in the normal limb. The resting pressures in the peripheral vessels are determined.

Patients with suspected pulmonary emboli and with a positive lung scan are candidates for the venous vascular studies. The tests may also be requested for patients who have signs of thrombophlebitis and swollen extremities of unknown etiology. Other indications for arterial flow studies include absence of pulses, claudication, gangrene, chest pain, and following vascularization surgery, a patient who has signs of ischemia or sudden absence of distal pulses.

Procedure for Doppler Peripheral Blood Flow (Study of Extremity)

1. Patient is asked to lie down on an examining table.
2. Pressure cuffs are applied at various levels in the extremities.
3. The Doppler probe is used much the same as the stethoscope is used.
4. A mercury-rilled circle gauge is placed over the fingers and toes to determine the quality of the distal circulation.
5. Examining time is approximately 30 minutes.

Procedure for Doppler Carotid Flow (Studies of Neck)

1. The brachial blood pressure is measured.
2. Patient lies down on the examining table.
3. The Doppler flow meter (transducer) is pressed to the neck and face to obtain the maximum signal and to note direction of blood flow. Measurements are taken from the bifurcation of the carotid up to supraorbital artery of the pulses and blood flow. Pressure with the examiner's fingers temporarily compresses the temporal and carotid arteries during the exam.
4. There is no pain or discomfort.
5. Examining time is five to ten minutes.

Clinical Implications

1. A disparity of greater than 30 mm of mercury between levels is indicative of obstruction. The greater the difference, the more severe the obstruction.

2. In the obstructed extremity, respiratory or pressure maneuvers will not alter the base line impedance.
3. Mild ischemia: .85–.94
   Moderate ischemia: .50–.84
   Severe ischemia: .26–.49
   Limb Salvage: .25 and below
   The ankle/brachial index is employed in the lower extremities to determine the degree of ischemia.
4. Abnormal carotid studies give an idea of the level and degree of obstruction and the degree and level of arteriosclerosis.

Interfering Factors

1. Some vessels do not lend themselves to pressure measurements. Some will give widely divergent inconsistent readings, and others will not be compressible, as in the knee, ankle, and foot.
2. Diabetics develop a medial artery disease that reduces the elasticity of the vessel and eventually prohibits its compression.
3. A tense and nervous patient will have a higher pressure, and this condition can result in an inaccurate pressure reading. In this instance, the muscles are tensed and can alter the position of the Doppler probe.
4. Nicotine constricts the peripheral vessels. If the patient has smoked just prior to the test, and he already has poor circulation, it may be more difficult to locate these vessels with the Doppler probe.
5. Walking and related activities increase the demand for blood. In the presence of proximal arterial obstruction, there will be a drop in the arterial pressure at the ankle.

Patient Preparation

1. Explain the purpose and procedure of the test.
2. Emphasize that it is a noninvasive procedure.
3. Assure patient that there is no pain or discomfort involved. The patient should know that no needles or catheters are introduced into the body.

4. Be sure that the patient has been inactive and not smoking for 20 minutes prior to testing.
5. Try to keep the patient relaxed and comfortable.

CLINICAL ALERT
1. Noninvasive studies should always be scheduled prior to angiography or renography.
2. The vascular technician needs to know whether an arterial evaluation is requested and what the indications are for the test.

MYELOGRAPHY

Normal Values

Normal lumbar or cervical myelogram

Explanation of Test

Myelography is a radiographic study in which contrast material is introduced into the spinal subarachnoid space so that the spinal cord and nerve roots may be outlined and any distortion of the dura mater may be detected. This test is done to detect neoplasms, ruptured intravertebral disks. or other intraspinal pathology. This method of fluoroscopic and x-ray examination of the spinal subarachnoid space using a radiopaque substance is indicated when compression of spinal or of posteria fossa neural structures or nerve roots is suspected. The test is usually requested when surgical treatment for a ruptured vertebrae disk appears to be required.

5 to 15 ml. of an iodized oil (Pantopaque) which is heavier than cerebrospinal fluid is injected into the subarachnoid space in the lumbar region, or for special purposes, sometimes into the cisterna magna. The lumbar myelogram is the most widely used technique because it is safer and simpler to perform than other punctures. This method decreases the potential danger of herniation and brainstem compression. Oil is maneuvered up and down the spinal cord by tilting the patient on a table under

fluoroscopic control; x-ray films are then taken. The oil is removed after examination is completed. In some neurological practices, air contrast or water-soluble radiopaque materials are used instead of oil to visualize masses within the spinal cord. If an air contrast study is done, tomography is essential to improve visualization. Tomography will permit blurring above and below a preselected layer of tissues of predetermined thickness.

Disadvantages of air contrast studies include poor visualization and difficulty in controlling gas once it is introduced. Disadvantages of the oil contrast studies are irritation of tissues and poor absorption of the oil by subarachnoid space. This oily substance is still visible on x-ray up to one year following examination.

Procedure

1. The test is usually done in the x-ray department.
2. The lumbar area is shaved, if necessary.
3. The patient is positioned on his side as for lumbar puncture at the beginning of the examination.
4. The procedure is the same as for lumbar puncture (see Chapter 4, p. 217) until the added procedure of injection of the contrast substance and fluoroscopic x-ray films. Note: In children the puncture level is much lower than in adults to avoid the risk of puncturing the spinal cord.
5. With gas myelography, air or oxygen may be injected into the subarachnoid space so that the spinal cord may be outlined. In certain situations, gas myelography is needed for a differential diagnosis of lesions of the cervical cord. It may also be an alternative method in patients who are allergic to iodide materials.
6. The table is tilted during the procedure and the patient is turned onto the abdomen with the needle in place. A shoulder and foot brace help to maintain correct position. Some patients will express a fear of falling off the table. However, they are securely fastened to the table.
7. When the x-ray films are completed, the contrast material is aspirated and the needle is removed. The puncture site is then cleansed and covered with a small sterile dressing.

Clinical Implications

Abnormal results will reveal distortion of the outline of the subarachnoid space indicating:
1. Ruptured intervertebral disk
2. Compression of spinal cord
3. Exact level of intravertebral tumors
4. Obstruction of spinal cord
5. Avulsion of nerve roots

Patient Preparation

1. A legal consent form must be signed by the patient before the test may be administered.
2. Explain the purpose and procedure of the test.
3. Explain to patient that the examination table may be tilted during the test but that he is securely fastened and will not fall off.
4. Advise patient that fasting from food and liquids is usually required for approximately four to six hours prior to the test. If the test is scheduled in the afternoon, a light breakfast may be permitted.

Patient Aftercare

1. Bedrest is necessary for several hours after the test. Usually the patient will lie flat in bed in a prone position for two to four hours, then on his back for two to four hours.
2. Fluid intake is encouraged to hasten absorption of any retained contrast media, to replace CSF, and to reduce development of headache.
3. Check for bladder distention and the ability to void adequately.
4. Check vital signs every four hours for at least 24 hour post exam.

CLINICAL ALERTS
1. Observe patient for possible complications which include headache, fever, seizure, paralysis, arachnoiditis (inflammation of the coverings of the spinal cord), drowsiness, stupor, stiffness of

neck, convulsions and a sterile meningitis reaction (severe headache and symptoms of arachnoiditis).

2. Manipulation of cerebrospinal fluid pressure may cause an acute exacerbation of symptoms which may require immediate surgical intervention.

3. This test is to be avoided unless there is strong and sufficient reason to suspect a lesion. Multiple sclerosis, for example, may be worsened by the procedure.

4. If all of the contrast material has not been recovered by the physician, the head is elevated to prevent the substance from flowing into the brain.

REFERENCES

Armstrong, Michael L.: ELECTROCARDIOGRAMS—A SYSTEMATIC METHOD OF READING THEM, 4th Ed. A John Wright & Sons Ltd. Publication. Distributed by Yearbook Medical Publishers, Inc., Chicago, 1978.

Benchimol, A.: NONINVASIVE TECHNIQUES IN CARDIOLOGY FOR THE NURSE AND TECHNICIAN. New York, A Wiley Medical Publication, John Wiley & Sons, 1978.

Conn, Howard R., and Conn, Rex B., Jr. (eds.): CURRENT DIAGNOSIS, 5th Ed. Philadelphia, W. B. Saunders Company, 1977.

Fowler, Noble O.: CARDIAC DIAGNOSIS AND TREATMENT, 2nd Ed. Hagerstown, Medical Department, Harper & Row, Publishers, 1976.

Guinto, Faustino C., Jr., Radcliffe, William B., and Himadi, George M.: Radiologic Studies of the Spine and Myelography. In PRACTICE OF MEDICINE, Vol. II, Laboratory Methods/Diagnostic Procedures. Hagerstown, Harper & Row, 1978, Chapter 50.

Manchester, Joel H., and Shelburne, James C.: Angiocardiography. In PRACTICE OF MEDICINE, Vol II, Laboratory Methods/Diagnostic Procedures. Hagerstown, Harper & Row, 1978, Chapter 41.

Parisi, Alfred F., and Tow, Donald E.: NONINVASIVE APPROACHES TO CARDIOVASCULAR DIAGNOSIS. New York, Appleton-Century-Crofts, 1979.

Race, George J. (section ed.): PRACTICE OF MEDICINE, Vol. II, Laboratory Methods/Diagnostic Procedures. Hagerstown, Harper & Row, Publishers, 1978.

Remler, Michael P.: Electroencephalography. In PRACTICE OF MEDICINE, Vol. II. Laboratory Methods/Diagnostic Procedures. Hagerstown, Harper & Row, 1978, Chapter 48.

Stoner, Emery K.: Electromyography and Nerve Conduction Studies. In PRACTICE OF MEDICINE, Vol. II, Laboratory Methods/Diagnostic Procedures. Hagerstown, Harper & Row, 1978, Chapter 51.

Walker, H. K., Hall, W. D., and Hurst, J. W. (eds.): CLINICAL METHODS—THE HISTORY, *Physical and Laboratory Examinations*, Vol. 1. Boston/London, Butterworths, 1976.

A ☐ ☐ DRUGS AFFECTING RESULTS OF BLOOD STUDIES, ELECTROLYTES, BLOOD GASES ANALYSES, AND ISOTOPE STUDIES

*Substances with an asterisk in this table reportedly influence the laboratory test, but further study is needed to determine the exact effect and mechanism of action.

Substance Determined	Drugs Causing Increased Values or False Positives	Drugs Causing Decreased Values or False Negatives
Acid Phosphatase	Androgens (in female) Clofibrate	Alcohol Fluorides Oxalates Phosphates
Alkaline Phosphates	Acetohexamide Albumin Allopurinol Aluminum nicotinate Amitriptyline Anabolic/androgenic agents Azathioprine Bromsulphalein Carbamazepine Cephaloridine Chlorpropamide Clindamycin Colchicine Ergosterol Estrogens Erythromycin (Ilosone) Flurazepam (confirmation needed) Gold Salts N-hydroxyacetamide Imipramine	Fluorides Oxalates Phosphates Placebo* Propranolol Vitamin D

†Based on data in Martin, Eric W.: HAZARDS OF MEDICATION. 2nd Ed., Philadelphia, J. B. Lippincott Company, 1978.

Substance Determined	Drugs Causing Increased Values or False Positives	Drugs Causing Decreased Values or False Negatives

Alkaline Phosphates (cont.)	Indomethacin (rare)
	Isoniazid
	Lincomycin
	Methyldopa
	Methyltestosterone
	Mithramycin
	Nicotinic acid (large doses 3–6 g/day)
	Nitrofurantoin
	Novobiocin
	Oxacillin
	Oxyphenisatin
	Papaverine (reversible)
	P.A.S.
	Penicillamine
	Petrofane
	Phenothiazines
	Phenylbutazone
	Placebo*
	Procainamide
	Progestin-estrogen combination (oral contraceptives)
	Propranolol
	Rifampin
	Sulfonamides
	  Sulfamethoxazole
	  Sulfisoxazole
	Tetracycline
	Thiothixene
	Tolazamide
	Tolbutamide	

Amino Acids	ACTH Ampicillin Bismuth 11-oxysteroids Sulfonamides Uric Acid	Epinephrine Insulin

Ammonia	Acetazolamide (Diamox)
	Ammonium salts
	  Ammonium chloride in cough preparations
	Asparagine
	Barbiturates
	Colistimethate sodium (Colistin sulfate)
	Diuretics (oral)
	  Chlorthalidone (Hygroton)
	  Clopamide
	  Ethacrynic acid (Edecrin)
	  Furosemide (Lasix)
		Acetohydroxamic acid (AHA) urease inhibitor
		Arginine
		Diphenhydramine (Benadryl)
		Glutamate sodium
		Glutamic acid
		Lactobacillus acidophilus (Lactinex)
		Monoamine oxidase inhibitors
		  Iproniazid
		Neomycin (Mycifradin)
		Potassium salts

Substance Determined	Drugs Causing Increased Values or False Positives	Drugs Causing Decreased Values or False Negatives

Ammonia (cont.)	Glucose
	Glutamine
	Heparin
	Isoniazid (INH)
	Lipomul (oil injection)
	Methicillin
	  (Dimocillin, Staphcillin)
	Morphine
	Oral resins
	Polymyxin B
	Thiazide diuretics
	  Chlorothiazide (Diuril)
	Tetracycline
	  large doses produce
	  hepatic damage with ele-
	  vated ammonia levels (+)
	Urea
		Sodium salts
		Tetracycline
		  reduces ammonia produc-
		  tion by gut bacteria (−)

Amylase	ACTH
	Aminosalicylic acid (PAS)
	Bethanechol
	Chlorides
	*Codeine
	Corticosteroids
	Cyproheptadine
	Diatrizoate Sodium
	Diuretics (oral)
	  Chlorthalidone
	  Furosemide
	Ethanol (gross intake)
	Histamine
	Hypaque
	Indomethacin
	Isoniazid
	Lipemia
	*Meperidine
	Methylcholine
	*Morphine
	Oxyphenbutazone
	Pancreatic Extracts
	Pentazocine
	Phenylbutazone
	Salicylates
	Salicylazosulfapyridine
	Sulfamethizole
	Tetracycline
	Thiazide diuretics
	  Chlorothiazide
	  Hydrochlorothiazide
		Citrates
		Diuretics (oral)
		  Ethacrynic acid
		Fluorides
		Oxalates

Barbiturates	Antipyrine Theophylline (large doses)	

Substance Determined	Drugs Causing Increased Values or False Positives	Drugs Causing Decreased Values or False Negatives
Bicarbonate	Aldosterone Viomycin	Metformin Phenformin Triamterene

Bilirubin (& Icteric Index)	Acetaminophen (overdose)
	Acetazolamide
	Acetohexamide
	Allopurinol
	Aluminum nicotinate (rare)
	Aminosalicylic acid (PAS)
	Amphotericin B
	Amitriptyline
	Anabolic/androgenic
	  Steroids (reversible)
	   (conjugated)
	  Fluoxymesterone
	  Methandrostenolone
	  Methandriol
	  Norethandrolone
	  Norethisterone
	  Norethynodrel
	  Oxymetholone
	  Stanozolol
	Aspidium (unconjugated)
	Azathioprine
	Barbiturates
	Carbamazepine
	Carotin
	Chlordiazepoxide
	Chlorpropamide
	Chloroquine
	Clindamycin
	Desipramine
	Dextran
	Diazepam
	Diphenylhydantoin (rare)
	Erythromycin
	Ethacrynic acid
	Ethambutol
	Ethionamide
	Ethoxazene
	Flurazepam
	Fluorouracil
	Gentamicin
	Gold therapy (rare)
	Halothane (rare)
	Idoxuridine
	Imipramine
	Indandione anticoagulants
	Indomethacin
	Isoniazid
		Barbiturates
		Caffeine
		Chlorine
		Citrate
		Dicophane
		Ethanol (pregnant woman
		  near delivery)
		Placebos*
		Protein
		Salicylates (large amounts)
		Sulfisoxazole and penicillin
		Urea

Substance Determined	Drugs Causing Increased Values or False Positives	Drugs Causing Decreased Values or False Negatives
Bilirubin (& Icteric Index) (cont.)	Lincomycin	
	Lipochrome	
	Menadiol sodium diphosphate (large doses)	
	Menadione	
	Menadione sodium bisulfite	
	Mercaptopurine	
	Methimazole	
	Methotrexate	
	Methyldopa	
	Mithramycin	
	Monoamine oxidase inhibitors	
	Nicotinic acid (large doses)	
	Nitrofurans	
	Nitrofurantoin	
	Furazolidone	
	Novobiocin	
	Oxacillin	
	Oxyphenisatin (in Dialose Plus)	
	Papaverine	
	Penicillin & sulfisoxazole combination	
	Phenacetin (rare)	
	Phenazopyridine	
	Phenothiazines	
	Methotrimeprazine (unconjugated)	
	Phenylbutazone	
	Phytonadione (high dose)	
	Piprobroman	
	Placebos*	
	Primaquine	
	Procainamide	
	Procarbazine	
	Progestin-estrogen combination (oral contraceptives)	
	Norquen	
	Propylthiouracil	
	Protriptyline	
	Pyrazinamide	
	Quinacrine	
	Radiopaque contrast media sodium, calcium ipodates competition for excretion	
	Rifampin (unconjugated)	
	Sulfonamides	
	Gantanol	
	Gantrisin	
	Sulfamethizole	

Substance Determined	Drugs Causing Increased Values or False Positives	Drugs Causing Decreased Values or False Negatives
Bilirubin (& Icteric Index) (cont.)	Tetracyclines Tolbutamide Troleandomycin Trifluperidol Vitamin A Vitamin K, K₁ (large doses in newborn) Xanthophyll	
Blood Urea Nitrogen (B.U.N.)	Acetohexamide Acetone Alkaline antacids Amphotericin B Antimony compounds Arginine Arsenicals Ascorbic acid Bacitracin Blood, whole Capreomycin (reversible) Cephaloridine (high doses) Chloral hydrate Chloramphenicol Chlorobutanol Chlorthalidone Colistimethate sodium Creatinine Doxapram Ethacrynic acid Fluid therapy Fluorides Furosemide Gentamicin Guanethidine Guanachlor Hydroxyurea Indomethacin Kanamycin Lipomul (oil injection) Lithium carbonate Mercury compounds Methicillin Methyldopa Methysergide Mithramycin Morphine Nalidixic acid Neomycin Nitrofurantoin Pargyline Polymyxin B Propranolol Radiopaque contrast media	Dextrose infusions Phenothiazines Fluphenazine Thymol

Substance Determined	Drugs Causing Increased Values or False Positives	Drugs Causing Decreased Values or False Negatives
Blood Urea Nitrogen (B.U.N.) (cont.)	Salicylates Spectinomycin Streptokinase-streptodornase Sulfonamides Tetracyclines (Doxycycline does not give significant increase) Thiazide diuretics Triamterene Vancomycin	
Bromsulphalein (B.S.P.) Retention	Acetohexamide Aluminum nicotinate Amidone Anabolic/androgenic steroids Fluoxymesterone Methandriol Methandrostenolone Norethandrostenolone Norethisterone Norethynodrel Antifungal agents Aspidium (if absorbed) Barbiturates (stop drug 24 hours before the test) Capreomycin sulfate Carbamazepine (Tegretol) Cardiotonic glycosides Chlorpropamide cholestatic jaundice Chlortetracycline (Aureomycin) Choleretics Florantyrone (Zanchol) Clofibrate (Atromid-S) hepatic damage; chole-static jaundice Clomiphene citrate (Clomid) Dehydrocholic acid (Decholin) interferes with hepatic uptake or biliary excretion of B.S.P. Diphenylhydantoin (Dilantin) Estrogens intrahepatic cholestatic jaundice; depress hepatic secretory transport Ethambutol Ethoxazene (Serenium)	Albuminuria Kanamycin* Placebos*

Substance Determined	Drugs Causing Increased Values or False Positives	Drugs Causing Decreased Values or False Negatives

Bromsulphalein (B.S.P.) Retention (cont.)	Guanoxan
	Halogen compounds
	Heparin
	Hydroxyurea
	  suppresses renal tubular
	  function
	Indomethacin
	Kanamycin*
	Lipemia
	Mercaptopurine
	Meperidine (Demerol)
	Metaxalone
	  jaundice
	Methadone (Dolophine)
	Methotrexate
	Methyldopa (Aldomet)
	Mithramycin
	Monomine oxidase inhibitors
	  Isocarboxazid
	  Nialamide
	  Phenelzine sulfate
	  Trancylpromine sulfate
	Morphine
	Nicotinic acid (Niacin) (large doses)
	Novobiocin (Albamycin)
	Oxacillin
	Phenazopyridine (Pyridium)
	Phenolphthalein
	Phenolsulfonphthalein
	  (P.S.P.)
	Placebos*
	Probenecid (Benemid)
	Procainamide (Pronestyl)
	Progestational agents
	Progestin-estrogen combina-
	  tion (oral contraceptives)
	Pyridium
	Radiopaque contrast media
	  Bunamiodyl
	  Iopanoic acid (Telepaque)
	  Sodium ipodate
	Rifamycin
	Sulfonamides	

Calcium	Alkaline antacids Ammonium oxalate Anabolic/androgenic steroids Calcium salts Copper* Dihydrotachysterol Estrogens	Acetazolamide B.S.P.—interferes 24–48 hours after the test Citrate Corticosteroids Copper* Edathamil

Substance Determined	Drugs Causing Increased Values or False Positives	Drugs Causing Decreased Values or False Negatives
Calcium (cont.)	Iron* Parathyroid injection Potassium Progestins Sodium Thiazide diuretics (early in therapy) Vitamin D Zinc*	Fluorides Gentamicin Heparin Insulin Iron* Laxatives (excessive use) Lipomul (oil injection) Magnesium Methicillin Mithramycin Oxalate Phosphorus (large amounts) Sodium polystyrene sulfonate Sulfates Zinc*
Cephalin Floccula-tion	Ampicillin* Kanamycin* Oxacillin* Pargyline* Penicillamine* Placebo* Procainamide Thiabendazole Tolbutamide Troleandomycin (TAO) stop drug for 5 weeks Nicotinic acid (large doses)	
Chloride	Acetazolamide Ammonium chloride Boric acid Chlorides Ion exchange resins Oxyphenbutazone Phenylbutazone Protein Steroids Triamterene (prolonged use)	ACTH/corticosteroids Bicarbonate Bromides Ethacrynic acid Furosemide Mercurial diuretics Saline infusions Thiazide diuretics Triamterene Water, glucose infusions (prolonged)
Cholesterol	ACTH corticosteroids Aminopyrine Anabolic agents Androgens Bile salts Bilirubin Bromides Clofibrate Cortisone Epinephrine (indirect effect through ACTH stimulation)	ACTH/corticosteroids Aluminum nicotinate Aminopyrine bicamphorate Aminosalicylic acid (PAS) Androsterone Antidiabetic drugs Bile salts Chlortetracycline Cholestyramine resin Clofibrate Colchicine Cortisone

Substance Determined	Drugs Causing Increased Values or False Positives	Drugs Causing Decreased Values or False Negatives

Cholesterol (cont.)	Ether anesthesia
	Iodides
	Lipemia (Lipomul injection)
	Norepinephrine
	Paramethadione
	Penicillamine
	Phenothiazines
	  Chlorpromazine
	  Trifluoperazine
	Progestin-estrogen combination (oral contraceptives)
	Protein
	Salicylates
	Thiouracil
	Trimethadione
	Tryptophan
	Vitamin A
	Vitamin D
		Dextrothyroxine
		Diphenylhydantoin*
		EDTA
		Estrogens
		Glucagon
		Haloperidol
		Heparin
		Kanamycin
		Neomycin
		Nicotinic acid
		Nitrates
		Nitrites
		Paromomycin
		Pentylenetetrazol
		Phenformin
		Phenyramidol
		Salicylates

Creatine Phosphokinase (CPK)	Amphotericin B Ampicillin (I.M. administration) Carbenicillin (I.M. administration) Chlorpromazine (I.M. administration) Clofibrate	
Creatinine	p-Aminohippurate Amphotericin B Arginine Ascorbic acid Barbiturates B.S.P. Clofibrate Colistin Diacetic acid Gentamicin sulfate Glucose Hydroxyurea Kanamycin Levulose Lipomul (oil injection) Lithium carbonate Mannitol Methicillin Methyldopa Mithramycin Protein P.S.P. Pyruvate Streptokinase-streptodornase Triamterene	Marihuana Viomycin

Substance Determined	Drugs Causing Increased Values or False Positives	Drugs Causing Decreased Values or False Negatives
Glucose (Fasting)	ACTH Acetazolamide (prediabetics & diabetics) Aluminum nicotinate L-Arginine BAL (toxic levels) Caffeine Chlorthalidone Clopamide Corticosteroids Dextran Dextrothyroxine Diazoxide Diphenylhydantoin Epinephrine Estrogens Ethacrynic acid Ethionamide Ferrous ascorbinate Furosemide Imipramine Indomethacin (rare) Isoniazid (excessive doses) Lithium carbonate Morphine Nalidixic acid Nicotinic acid (large doses) Nicotinyl alcohol (large doses) Nitrofurantoin Paraldehyde (transient) Phenolpthalein Physostigmine Progestin-estrogen combination (oral contraceptives) Quinethazone Salicylates (toxic doses) Thiabendazole Thiazide diuretics Thyroid preparations/synthetic analogues Triamterene Trioxazine	Acetaminophen Acetohexamide (overdosage) Aminosalicylic acid (in diabetics) Anabolic steroids Ascorbic acid BAL (toxic levels) Carbutamide Chlorpropamide (overdosage) Clofibrate Cyproheptadine Dextropropoxyphene Ethacrynic acid (large doses) Ethanol Fructose Guanethidine Haloperidol Insulin (overdosage) Marihuana Metformin (overdosage) Monoamine oxidase inhibitors 　Nialamide 　Pargyline 　Phenelzine 　Tranylcypromine Phenformin Phosphorus Potassium chloride Potassium oxalate Potassium para-amino benzoate (prolonged use) Propranolol Propoxyphene Reserpine Salicylates (diabetics) (toxic doses) Sulfaphenazole Tolazamide Tolbutamide Tromethamine
Glucose Tolerance Curve	Corticosteroids* Estrogens (decrease tolerance) Ferrous ascorbinate Nicotinic acid and derivatives (resembles diabetic curve) Phenothiazines	Corticosteroids* Lithium carbonate Metyrapone

Substance Determined	Drugs Causing Increased Values or False Positives	Drugs Causing Decreased Values or False Negatives
Glucose Tolerance Curve (cont.)	Progestin-estrogen combination (oral contraceptives) increased peripheral resistance to hypoglycemic action of insulin Salicylates Thiazide diuretics	
17-Hydroxycorticosteroids (17-OHCS)	Acetazolamide (Diamox) Ascorbic acid (Vitamin C) Chloral hydrate (Noctec) Chloramphenicol (Chloromycetin) Chlordiazepoxide (Librium) Chlormerodrin Chlorthalidone (Hygroton) confirmation is needed Cloxacillin (Tegopen) more definitive information is needed Colchicine (modification of Reddy, Jenkins, Thorn) Erythromycin no supporting evidence Ethinamate (Valmid) Glutethimide (Doriden) interferes with absorbance Methenamine (Uritone, Mandelamine, Hipprex) Gonadotropins Hydroxyzine (Atarax, Vistaril) Hydralazine (Apresoline) Digitoxin Digoxin Cortisone Hydralazine (Apresoline) Digitoxin Digoxin	Aminoglutethimide Calcium gluconate Corticosteroids Diphenylhydantoin (Dilantin) Dexamethasone Mitotane Progestin-estrogen combination (oral contraceptives) Reserpine Phenothiazines (Chlorpromazine)
^{131}I Thyroid Uptake (24-hour)	Barbiturates Estrogens (not persistently) Lithium carbonate (3–4 months) Phenothiazine (1 week) Thyroid-stimulating hormone	ACTH Adrenocortical steroids Cortisone Corticosterone Desoxycorticosterone Prednisone Prednisolone (1 week or less) Aminosalicylic acid (prolonged use) (1 week) Amphenone (2–3 days)

Substance Determined	Drugs Causing Increased Values or False Positives	Drugs Causing Decreased Values or False Negatives

[131]I Thyroid Uptake (24-hour) (cont.)		Antihistamines
		  Chlortrimeton (1 week or less)
		Antithyroid drugs
		  Carbimazole
		  Iothiouracil
		  Mercazole
		  Methimazole
		  Methylthiouracil
		  Muracil
		  Propylthiouracil
		Chlordiazepoxide
		Cobalt (1 week or less)
		Coumarin anticoagulants
		Iodine-containing
		  compounds
		    general preparations
		    (1–3 weeks)
		    Antitussives
		    Diiodohydroxyquin
		    Enterosept
		    Indocyanine green
		    Iodochlorhydroxyquin
		    Iothiouracil
		    Lugol's solution
		    Neo-penil
		Isoniazid
		Meprobamate
		Mercurials (1 week)
		Nitrate
		Nitroprusside sodium
		Orinase
		Perchlorate (1 week)
		Phenothiazine (1 week)
		Phenylbutazone (1 week)
		Pentothal (1 week)
		Progesterone
		Radiopaque contrast media
		  Cholografin (3 months)
		  Diodrast (1–3 months)
		  Dionosil (2–4 months)
		  Hypaque (1–2 weeks)
		  Mediopaque (1–2 weeks)
		  Neo-iopax (1–2 weeks)
		  Oily solutions (up to 1 year
		    or more) (Ethiodol,
		    Iodochloral, Lipiodol,
		    Pantopaque, Visciodol)
		  Priodax (1–3 months)
		  Renographin (1–2 weeks)
		  Salpix (1 month)
		  Skiodan acacia

Substance Determined	Drugs Causing Increased Values or False Positives	Drugs Causing Decreased Values or False Negatives

[131]I Thyroid Uptake (24-hour) (cont.)		Resorcinol
		Salicylates
		Sulfonamides (1 week)
		Thiocyanates
		Thyroid medication (1–2 weeks)
		    Desiccated thyroid
		    Thyroglobuline
		    L-Thyroxine
		    Triiodothyronine

Iron and Iron Binding Capacity	Chloramphenicol Fluorides Iron dextran complex Oxalate Progestin-estrogen combination (oral contraceptives) Tungstate	Fluorides* Oxalate* Tungstate ACTH Hydroxyurea Steroids
Lactic Dehydrogenase	Codeine Clofibrate Meperidine Mithramycin Morphine Procainamide	Oxalate

Lipase	Cholinergics
	    Bentanechol
	    Methacholine
	Opiates and analogues
	    Codeine
	    Meperidine
	    Morphine	

Lipids (total)	Progestin-estrogen combination (oral contraceptives)	Cholestyramine resin Estrogens Fenfluramine (slight decrease)

Magnesium	Lithium carbonate
	Magnesium products
	    Magnesium antacids
	    Magnesium sulfate
	    Milk of magnesia
	Salicylates (prolonged use)
		Amphotericin B
		Aldosterone
		Calcium gluconate
		Ethacrynic acid
		Ethanol
		Insulin
		Mercurial diuretics
		    Mercaptomerin
		Neomycin

Nonprotein Nitrogen (N.P.N.)	Acetophenetidin (azotemia) Amphotericin B Capreomycin (reversible) Edathamil Gentamicin nephrotoxic	Nitrofurantoin*

Substance Determined	Drugs Causing Increased Values or False Positives	Drugs Causing Decreased Values or False Negatives
Nonprotein Nitrogen (N.P.N.) (cont.)	Lipomul (oil injection) Methicillin (azotemia) Kanamycin Neomycin Nitrofurantoin* Sulfonamides Tetracyclines Vitamin D	
pH	Potassium oxalate Sodium bicarbonate Sodium oxalate	Acetazolamide Ammonium chloride Ammonium oxalate Calcium chloride EDTA Methyl alcohol Paraldehyde Salicylates Sodium citrate
Phosphate (Inorganic Phosphorus)	Alkaline antacids Dilantin Heparin Lipomul (oil injection) Mannitol* Methicillin Pituitrin Vitamin D Tetracyclines	Aluminum hydroxide Epinephrine Insulin Mannitol* Mithramycin Parathyroid injection
Potassium	Aminocaproic acid Amiloride Boric acid Calcium Carbacrylamine resin Cephaloridine Copper Epinephrine Heparin Iron Isoniazid Lipomul (oil injection) Mannitol infusions Metformin Methicillin Penicillin G potassium Phenformin Protein Spironolactone Succinylcholine Triamterene Urea*	ACTH Acetazolamide Aminosalicylic acid (PAS) Ammonium chloride (rare) Amphotericin Amphotericin B Carbenoxolone Cathartics Chlorthalidone Corticosteroids Dextrose infusions Dichlorphenamide Diuretics (oral) Ethacrynic acid Furosemide Edathamil (EDTA) Epinephrine Glucagon Glucose Insulin Laxatives (excessive use) Licorice Lithium carbonate

Substance Determined	Drugs Causing Increased Values or False Positives	Drugs Causing Decreased Values or False Negatives
Potassium (cont.)		Methazolamide (prolonged use)
		Mithramycin
		Penicillin G sodium (massive I.V.)
		Phosphate
		Polymyxin B
		Salicylates
		Sodium glutamate
		Sodium phytate
		Sodium polystyrene sulfonate
		Sulfates
		Tetracyclines
		Thiazide diuretics
		Urea*
		Viomycin
Protein-Bound Iodine (P.B.I.)	ACTH	ACTH
	Barbiturates	Aminobenzoate
	Barium sulfate	Aminoglutethimide
	Bromide	Aminosalicylic acid
	B.S.P.	Anabolic agents
	Chlormadinone	Androgens
	Clofibrate*	Antithyroid drugs
	Cod liver oil	Methimazole
	Corticosteroids (large doses) (lasts 8 days)	Methylthiouracil
	Dextrothyroxine	Propylthiouracil
	Dimethisterone	B.S.P.
	Dithiazanine	Chlorate
	Erythrosine	Clofibrate*
	Estrogens	Cobalt
	Iodine-containing compounds	Corticosteroids (large doses) (lasts 8 days)
	Isopropamide	Diphenylhydantoin (1-week therapy) (lasts 7–10 days)
	Levodopa	Disulfiram
	Liothyronine	Ethionamide
	Meprobamate	Fluorides (massive dose)
	Metrecal (iodocasein in the preparation) (30 days)	Cold preparations
	Perphenazine (prolonged use)	Glucocorticoids
		Isoniazid
	Povidone iodine (even topically)	Lithium carbonate
	Progestin-estrogen combination (oral contraceptive)	Mercurial diuretics (effect lasts 2 days in vitro)
	Pyrazinamide	Mephenytoin
	Radiopaque contrast media (lasts from days to months to years)	Nitroprusside, sodium metabolite
		Phenothiazines (large doses)
		Phenylbutazone
		Resorcinol

Substance Determined	Drugs Causing Increased Values or False Positives	Drugs Causing Decreased Values or False Negatives

Protein-Bound Iodine (P.B.I.) (cont.)	Undeceylenium chloride-iodine (even topically)
	Thyroid therapy
	  L-thyroxine
	Vitamins A & D
		Salicylates (high dose)
		Sulfonamides
		Sulfonylurea (rare)
		Thiazide diuretics
		Thiocyanates
		Thyroid therapy
		  Triiodothyronine

Protein, Total	ACTH Anabolic steroids Androgenic steroids Bilirubin B.S.P. Clofibrate Corticosteroids Dextran Growth hormone Heparin Insulin Lipemia Mercuric chloride Penicillin (massive doses) Radiographic contrast media Thyroid preparations Tolbutamide	Ammonium ion Dextran Progestin-estrogen combination (oral contraceptives) Pyrazinamide Salicylates
Serum Glutamic Oxaloacetic Transaminase (S.G.O.T.)	Aluminum nicotinate Amantadine Aminosalicylic acid (PAS) Ampicillin Anabolic agents Androgens Carbenicillin (high dose) Cardiotonic glycoside Cephalothin Chlorquine Chloroquine Clindamycin Clofibrate Cloxacillin Colchicine Cortisone Cycloserine Desipramine Diphenylhydantoin Erythromycin Ethambutol Ethionamide Flurazepam Gentamicin Griseofulvin	Salicylates*

Substance Determined	Drugs Causing Increased Values or False Positives	Drugs Causing Decreased Values or False Negatives

Serum Glutamic Oxaloacetic Transaminase (S.G.O.T.) (cont.)	Guanethidine analogs
	Hydralazine
	N-hydroxyacetamide
	Ibufenac
	Indomethacin
	Isoniazid
	Lincomycin
	Lipemia (alcoholic patient)
	Methotrexate
	Methyldopa
	Mithramycin
	Nafcillin
	Nalidixic acid
	Nicotinic acid
	Nitrofurantoin
	Opiates
	  Codeine
	  Meperidine
	  Morphine
	Oxacillin
	Phenothiazines
	Placebo
	Polycillin
	Procainamide
	Progestin-estrogen combination (oral contraceptives)
	Propranolol
	Prostaphlin
	Pyrantel pamoate
	Rifampin
	Salicylates*
	Stibocaptate
	Sulfamethazole
	Tetracycline
	Theophylline
	Thiabendazole
	Thiothixene
	Troleandomycin (one week dose)
	Vitamin A	

Serum Glutamic Pyruvic Trans-aminase (S.G.P.T.)	Aluminum nicotinate Anabolic agents Androgens Carbenicillin (high doses) Cardiotonic glycosides Clofibrate Clindamycin Codeine Cycloserine Desipramine	Salicylates*

Substance Determined	Drugs Causing Increased Values or False Positives	Drugs Causing Decreased Values or False Negatives
Serum Glutamic Pyruvic Trans- aminase (S.G.P.T.) (cont.)	Erythromycin (lauryl salt) Ethionamide Flurazepam Gentamicin Guanethidine analogs N-hydroxyacetamide Ibufenac Indomethacin Isoniazid Lincomycin Lipemia Meperidine Methyldopa Mithramycin Morphine Phenothiazines Procainamide Progestin-estrogen combina- tions (oral contraceptives) Propranolol Pyrazinamide Rifampin Salicylates* Spectinomycin Stibocaptate Tetracycline Thiothixene Troleandomycin (effect lasts one week)	
Sodium	Anabolic agents Boric acid Calcium Copper Corticosteroids Glucose* Iron Marihuana Methyldopa Oxyphenbutazone Phenylbutazone Potassium Progestin-estrogen combina- tion (oral contraceptives) Protein Rauwolfia alkaloids Saline infusions Sulfate Urea*	Ammonium chloride Carbacrylamine resin Dichlorphenamide Diuretics (oral) Carbonic anhydrase inhibitors Ethacrynic acid Furosemide Glucose* Heparin Laxatives (excessive use) Mannitol Mercurial diuretics Phosphates Quinethazone Spironolactone Thiazide diuretics Triamterene Urea*

Substance Determined	Drugs Causing Increased Values or False Positives	Drugs Causing Decreased Values or False Negatives
Thymol Turbidity (Cephalin Flocculation)	Adrenocorticotropic hormones Aluminum nicotinate (large doses) (rare) Anabolic/androgenic steroids Bilirubin Cephalothin Chlorpropamide Clofibrate Erythromycin Florantyrone Growth hormone Heparin* Indomethacin Insulin Lincomycin Lipemia Nalidixic acid Penicillamine Thyroid preparation Tolbutamide Troleandomycin	Albumin (high) Heparin* Oxalated plasma
Thyroxine-Binding Globulin	Chlormadinone Progestin-estrogen combination (oral contraceptives)	Anabolic agents Androgens
Thyroxine T_4	Chloramidone Clofibrate Diethylstilbesterol Estradiol Estrogens Oral contraceptives Perphenazine Progestine	Aminosalicylic acid Cortisone Diphenylhydantoin Lithium Methylthiouracil Sulfonamides Chlorpromazine Reserpine Prednisone Testosterone Heparin Tolbutamide
Triiodothyronine (T_3) Uptake	ACTH (conflicting reports) Anabolic agents Androgens Anticoagulants, oral Corticosteroids (conflicting reports) Dextrothyroxine Diphenylhydantoin Heparin Iodate	ACTH (conflicting reports) Antithyroid drugs Methimazole Methylthiouracil Propylthiouracil BAL Chlordiazepoxide Corticosteroids (conflicting reports) Estrogens

Substance Determined	Drugs Causing Increased Values or False Positives	Drugs Causing Decreased Values or False Negatives

Triiodothyronine (T₃) Uptake (cont.)	Phenylbutazone
	Salicylates (high doses)
	Thyroid therapy
	   L-thyroxine
	   Triiodothyronine
		Ipodate
		Perphenazine
		Progestin-estrogen combination (oral contraceptives)
		Thiazide diuretics
		Sulfonylureas

Uric Acid	Acetazolamide
	Adrenocortical steroids
	Aluminum nicotinate
	Aminophylline
	Angiotensin
	Ascorbic acid
	Azathioprine
	Azathymine
	Bishydroxycoumarin
	Blood, whole
	Busulfan
	Coffee
	Corticosteroids
	Dextran
	Diazoxide
	Diuretics, oral
	Epinephrine
	Ethacrynic acid
	Ethambutol
	Ethanol
	Furosemide
	Fructose
	Gentamycin
	Glucose
	Griseofulvin
	Hydroxyurea
	Ibufenac
	Lead intoxication
	Levodopa
	Lipomul (oil injection)
	Mecamylamine
	Methicillin
	Methotrexate
	Methyldopa
	Norepinephrine
	Nicotinic acid
	Nitrogen mustards
	Phenothiazines
	Pyrazinamide
	Probenecid
	Purine analogue antimetabolites
	   Azathioprine
	   6-Mercaptopurine
	   6-Thioguanine
		ACTH
		Acetohexamide
		Adrenocortical steroids
		Allopurinol
		Anticoagulants
		Benziodarone
		Chlorine
		Chlorprothixene
		Chlorthalidone
		Cincophan
		Clofibrate
		Corticosteroids
		Coumarin
		Ethacrynic acid (I.V. administration)
		Furosemide
		Glucose
		Lithium carbonate (in manic depressives)
		Mannitol
		Marihuana
		Oxyphenbutazone
		Phenothiazines
		Phenylbutazone
		Piperazine
		Potassium oxalate
		Salicylates (large doses)
		Saline infusions
		Sodium oxalate
		Sulfinpyrazone
		Thiazide diuretics
		   Chlorothiazide (500 mg IV)
		Triamterene*

Substance Determined	Drugs Causing Increased Values or False Positives	Drugs Causing Decreased Values or False Negatives

Uric Acid (cont.)	Quinethazone
	Reducing substances
	Rifampin
	Salicylates (low doses)
	Spironolactone
	Thiazide diuretics
	  Chlorothiazide (1.5 g in
	  divided doses)
	Triamterene*
	Vincristine	

B □□ DRUGS AFFECTING RESULTS OF URINE STUDIES

*Substances with an asterisk in this table reportedly influence the laboratory test, but further study is needed to determine the exact effect and mechanism of action.

Substance Determined	Drugs Causing Increased Values or False Positives	Drugs Causing Decreased Values or False Negatives

Acetone	B.S.P.
	  color interference on nitro-
	  prusside test, Ketostix,
	  Labstix, Acetes,
	  Bili-Labstix
	Ether anesthesia
	Inositol and/or methionine
	Insulin (excessive doses)
	Isoniazid intoxication
	  produces acetonuria
	Isopropyl alcohol
	Levodopa (L-Dopa)
	  brown on Ketostix or
	  Labstix
	Metformin
	Paraldehyde
	  increased acetaldehyde;
	  nitroprusside reaction,
	  Acetest
	Phenazopyridine (Pyridium)
	  interfering colors on
	  Ketostix
	Phenformin
	P.S.P.
	  possible color interference
	  on nitroprusside test,
	  Ketostix, Labstix, Acetest,
	  Bili-Labstix	

Amino Acids	ACTH
	Ampicillin
	  false (+) spots on paper
	  chromatograms
	Cortisone
	Sulfonamide
	Tetracycline
		Epinephrine
		Insulin

Substance Determined	Drugs Causing Increased Values or False Positives	Drugs Causing Decreased Values or False Negatives
Benzidine	Bromides Copper Ferricyanide Formalin Iodides Permanganate	
Bile	Chlorzoxazone (Paraflex) Chlorprothixene Phenothiazines Thymol	
Bilirubin	Acetophenazine Chlorprothixine Ethoxazene (Serenium) reddish color (Bili-Labstix) Aspirin Flufenamic acid Mefenamic acid (Ponstel) Phenazopyridine (Pyridium) false (+)—"foam test"; atypical color reaction on talc-disk-Fouchet-spot test and Franklin's tablet- Fouchet test; red color– Ictotest, Bili-Labstix Phenothiazines Chlorpromazine (Bili-Labstix) Ictotest is unaffected Flufenazine Perphenazine	
Calcium	Cholestyramine Dihydrotachysterol Nandrolone (in some cancer patients) Parathyroid injection Vitamin D	Sodium phytate Thiazide diuretics Viomycin Alkaline urine
Catecholamines	Aminophylline Caffeine Carbon tetrachloride Chloral hydrate (Noctec) Epinephrine inhalation (Vaponephrine, Mehaler- Epinephrine, Dylephrin, Micronephrine) Erythromycin Ethanol Formaldehyde	Bethanedine Guanoxan Guanethidine (Ismelin) (elevated epinephrine, decreased norepinephrine) Reserpine

Substance Determined	Drugs Causing Increased Values or False Positives	Drugs Causing Decreased Values or False Negatives
Catecholamines (cont.)	Hydralazine (Apresoline) Guanethidine (Ismelin) (elevated epinephrine, decreased norepinephrine) Hypertensive agents Imipramine (Tofranil) Isoproterenol (Isuprel) Levodopa (L-Dopa) Methenamine (Hipprex) (Uritone) Methyldopa (Aldomet) Nitroglycerin Phenothiazines Quinidine Quinine Tetracyclines Chlortetracycline Oxytetracycline B complex vitamins Nicotinic acid, riboflavin Reserpine (large dose)	
Creatine and Creatinine	Androgens Corticosteroids Nitrofuran derivatives	Thiazide diuretics
Crystals	Acetazolamide Aminosalicylic acid Ampicillin Methenamine mandelate Sulfonamides (Sulfameter) renal damage Thiabendazole	
Diacetic Acid	Acetate* Antipyrine* Sodium bicarbonate* Cyanate* Coal tar drugs* Levodopa (L-Dopa) Phenazopyridine (Pyridium) Phenothiazines Salicylates	Acetate* Antipyrine* Sodium bicarbonate Cyanate*
Diagnex Blue	Aluminum salts Antacids Cremomycin Donnagel Kaolin Kaopectate Atabrine	Caffeine sodium benzoate Phenazopyridine

Substance Determined	Drugs Causing Increased Values or False Positives	Drugs Causing Decreased Values or False Negatives

Diagnex Blue (cont.)	Barium
	Potassium salts
	  large amounts
	Quinacrine (Mepacrine)
	Quinidine
	Quinine
	Sodium salts
	  large amounts
	B complex vitamins
	  Nicotinic acid
	  Riboflavin
	Calcium
	Iron
	Magnesium
	Methylene blue	

Estrogens	Phenothiazines*
	  Prochlorperazine
	    (Kober method)
	Tetracyclines*
	Vitamins
		Phenothiazines
		  Prochlorperazine
		Tetracyclines
		Vitamins*

Glucose	Ascorbic acid
	  large doses produce false
	  positive with Benedict's or
	  Clinitest
	Levodopa (L-Dopa)
	  Clinitest (+); glucose
	  oxidase (−)
	Cephaloridine (Loridin)
	Cephalothin (Keflin)
	  Clinitest—black brown,
	  interpreted as positive
	  glucose or interpreted as
	  false (−)
	Salicylates
	  (Clinitest) (+) (large doses)
	Phenazopyridine (Pyridium)
	  (glucose oxidase) (−);
	  (Tes-Tape) (+); copper
	  reduction test not affected
	Chlortetracycline
	Cinchophen
	Corticosteroids
	  Increased production of
	  glucose, lower renal
	  threshold
	Corticotropin
	Creatinine
	Dextrothyroxine (Choloxin)
	  pharmacologic effect
		Ascorbic acid
		Levodopa (L-Dopa)
		Cephaloridine (Loridin)
		Cephalothin (Keflin)
		Salicylates
		  (glucose oxidase) (−)
		Phenazopyridine (Pyridium)
		  (glucose oxidase) (−);
		  (Tes-Tape) (+); copper
		  reduction test not affected
		Meralluride sodium
		  (Mercuhydrin)
		  (glucose oxidase)

Substance Determined	Drugs Causing Increased Values or False Positives	Drugs Causing Decreased Values or False Negatives
Glucose (cont.)	Edathamil (EDTA)	
	Ephedrine (large doses)	
	Ethacrynic acid	
	Formaldehyde	
	Gluconates	
	Hippuric acid	
	Homogentisic acid	
	Hydrogen peroxide (Benedict's, glucose oxidase)	
	Hypochlorites (Benedict's, glucose oxidase)	
	Indomethacin	
	Isoniazid (INH) (Benedict's) Clinitest or glucose oxidase not affected; hyperglycemic and may produce true glucosuria	
	Phenothiazines	
	Probenecid reducing substance in the urine; (Benedict's, Clinitest) glucose oxidase not affected	
	Protein	
	Quinethazone glucosuria	
	Streptomycin (Benedict's, Clinitest) glucose oxidase not affected	
	Sulfonamides Sulfanilamide (Benedict's, Clinitest) large doses interfere with copper reducing method	
	Tetracycline large amounts of ascorbic acid in preparations of tetracycline (Benedict's, Clinitest) (+); (Clinistix, Tes-Tape) (−)	
	Thiazide diuretics	
	Trimethozine (Trioxazine) (Combistix, glucose oxidase)	
	Uric acid	
	Vaginal powders contain glucose	

Substance Determined	Drugs Causing Increased Values or False Positives	Drugs Causing Decreased Values or False Negatives

Glucose (cont.)	Acetanilid
	    (Benedict's)
	Amino acids
	Antipyrine
	Aminosalicylic acid (PAS)
	    reducing agent;
	    (Benedict's) glucose
	    oxidase not affected
	Aspidium oleoresin
	Bismuth
	Carbamazepine (Tegretol)
	Carinamide
	Chloral hydrate (Noctec)
	    (Benedict's) (large doses,
	    (+) Clinitest) glucose
	    oxidase not affected
	Chloramphenicol
	    (Chloromycetin)
	    Benedict's Clinitest
	Chloroform
	Lithium carbonate
	Metaproterenol
	Metaxalone (Skelexin)
	    reducing substance inter-
	    feres; (Benedict's, Clinitest)
	    glucose oxidase not
	    affected
	Methenamine products
	Methyldopa (Aldomet)*
	Morphine
	    (Benedict's)
	Nalidixic acid (NegGram)
	Nicotinic acid (large doses)
	Nitrofurans
	    Nitrofurantoin (Furadantin)
	    Furazolidine (Furoxone)
	        metabolite (Benedict's)
	Nucleoproteins
	Oxalic acid
	Penicillin
	    (Benedict's, Clinitest)
	Phenacetin
	Phenols	

Guaiac (Blood)	Bromides Copper Iodides Oxidizing agents (excreted in urine)	Ascorbic acid (high doses)

Substance Determined	Drugs Causing Increased Values or False Positives	Drugs Causing Decreased Values or False Negatives

17-Hydroxycorti- costeroids (17-OHCS)	Dextroamphetamine*
	 Iodides
	 Menadione
	 Meprobamate (Equanil)
	 Methyprylon (Noludar)
	 Metyrapone
	 Phenothiazines
	   (Chlorpromazine)
	 Potassium iodide
	 Spironolactone
	 Sulfamerazine
	 Thiazide diuretics
	   Chlorothiazide
	 Troleandomycin (TAO)
	 Quinidine
	 Quinine
	 Paraldehyde
	 Phenazopyridine (Pyridium)	

5-Hydroxyindole- acetic Acid (Serotonin)	Acetaminophen
	 Acetanilid
	 Caffeine
	 Fluorouracil (5-FU)
	 Glyceryl guaiacolate
	 Melphalan (Alkeran)
	 Mephenesin (Tolserol)
	 Methamphetamine
	   (Methedrine)
	 Methocarbamol (Robaxin)
	 Phenmetrazine (Preludin)
	 Phenacetin
	 Reserpine
	 Serotonin in food
	   (large amounts of serotonin
	   present in avocado,
	   bananas, plums, walnuts,
	   pineapples, and eggplants)
	 Methysergide maleate
	 Lugol's solution
		Corticotropin (ACTH)
		   pharmacologic effect
		 Chlorpromazine
		 Ethanol
		 Heparin
		 Imipramine (Tofranil)
		 Isoniazid (INH)
		 Methenamine mandelate
		   (Mandelamine)
		 Methyldopa
		 Monoamine oxidase
		   inhibitors
		 p-Chlorophenylalanine
		   (Fenclonine)
		 Phenothiazines
		   Chlorpromazine
		   Thorazine
		 Promethazine

17-Ketosteroids (17 KS)	Salicylates Secobarbital* Chlorothiazide* Nalidixic acid (NegGram) Methyprylon (Noludar) Metyrapone Penicillin G, large dose Phenaglycodol (Ultran) Phenazopyridine (Pyridium) Phenothiazines Spironolactone	Salicylates Secobarbital* Chlorothiazide* Estrogens Piperidine Progestin-estrogen combina- tion (oral contraceptives) Probenecid (Benemid) Pyrazinamide Quinidine Chlorpromazine

Substance Determined	Drugs Causing Increased Values or False Positives	Drugs Causing Decreased Values or False Negatives
	Testolactone	Meprobamate (Equanil, Miltown)
	Testosterone	Paraldehyde*
	Troleandomycin (TAO)	Quinine*
	Chlorpromazine	Aminoglutethimide
	Meprobamate (Equanil, Miltown)	Chlordiazepoxide (Librium)
	Paraldehyde*	Corticosteroids
	Quinine*	Cortisone derivatives of high potency
	Androgenic steroids	Betamethasone
	Chlorpromazine (Thorazine)*	Dexamethasone
	Cloxacillin (Tegopen)*	Diphenylhydantoin
	Corticotropin (ACTH)	Reserpine
	Cortisone	
	Dextroamphetamine*	
	Erythromycin*	
	Ethinamate (Valmid)	
	Gonadotropin	
Occult Urine Casts	Antimony compounds	
	Arsenicals	
	Bacitracin	
	renal tubular damage	
	Capreomycin	
	reversible renal toxicity	
	Chloroguanide	
	Colistimethate	
	Edathamil	
	Isoniazid	
	Kanamycin	
	nephrotoxic	
	Methicillin	
	Melarsopral	
	Neomycin	
	Paramethadione	
	Polymyxin B*	
	Rifampin	
	Trimethadione	
Phenolsulfonphthalein (P.S.P.)	Anthraquinone derivatives	Alkali (excess)
	B.S.P.	Carinamide
	Cascara	Diodrast
	urine discoloration	Diuretics
	Danthron	Iodopyracet
	Ethoxazene (Serenium)	Penicillin
	urine discoloration	Probenecid (Benemid)
	Formaldehyde-forming drugs	Salicylates
	Novobiocin	Thiazide diuretics
	Phenazopyridine (Pyridium)	Sulfonamides
	Phenolphthalein	
	Radiographic contrast media	

Substance Determined	Drugs Causing Increased Values or False Positives	Drugs Causing Decreased Values or False Negatives
Phenolsulfonphthal-ein (P.S.P.) (cont.)	Rhubarb extracts Sulfonamides Sulfinpyrazone	
Phenyl Ketone	Aminosalicylic acid Aspirin Bilirubin (high concentration) Chlorpromazine* Histidine metabolites Phenothiazines Salicylates*	Aminosalicylic acid Aspirin Bilirubin (high concentration) Chlorpromazine* Phenothiazines Salicylates*
Porphyrins	Acriflavine Alcohol Antipyretics Barbiturates Chloroquine Chlorpromazine Chlorpropamide Estrogens Ethoxazene Griseofulvin Oxytetracycline Phenazopyridine Phenothiazines Phenylhydrazine Penicillin Progestin-estrogen combina-tion (oral contraceptives) Procaine Sedatives and hypnotics Sulfonamides Sulphonal Tolbutamide	
Protein (as albumin)	Acetazolamide (Diamox) Aminosalicylic acid (PAS) Aminophylline Amphotericin B (Fungizone) Antimony compounds Arsenicals Bacitracin Bismuth triglycollamate Carbarsone Capreomycin Carbon tetrachloride Carbutamide Carinamide Cephaloridine (Loridine) Chlorpropamide Colistimethate Colymicin (Colistin)	

Substance Determined	Drugs Causing Increased Values or False Positives	Drugs Causing Decreased Values or False Negatives
Protein (as albumin) (cont.)	Corticosteroids	
	Dihydrotachysterol	
	Doxapram	
	Edathamil	
	Ethosuximide	
	Gentamicin	
	Gold salts	
	nephrotoxic	
	Griseofulvin	
	Iron sorbitex (Jectofer)	
	Isoniazid	
	Kanamycin	
	Lipomul (oil injection)	
	Lithium carbonate (Lithonate)	
	Mefenamic acid (Ponstel)	
	Mercuric chloride	
	Metahexamide	
	Metaxalone (Skelaxin)	
	Methenamine (large doses)	
	Methsuximide	
	Mithramycin	
	Mitotane	
	Neomycin	
	Paraldehyde	
	Paramethadione (Paradione)	
	Penicillamine (Cuprimine)	
	Penicillin (large doses)	
	Methicillin	
	Oxacillin	
	Phenacemide	
	Phenazopyridine	
	Phenindione (Hedulin)	
	Phenylbutazone (Butazolidin)	
	Phosphorus	
	Polymyxin B	
	Pyrazolone derivatives	
	Radiopaque contrast media	
	Sodium diatrizoate	
	(Hypaque)	
	Iopanoic acid (Telepaque)	
	Salicylates (overdosage)	
	Salyrgan-theophylline	
	Sulfonamides	
	Sulfameter	
	Sulfones	
	Suramin	
	Tetracyclines (degraded)	
	Theophylline sodium	
	glycinate (high doses)	
	Thiabendazole (Mintezol)	
	Thiosemicarbazones	

Substance Determined	Drugs Causing Increased Values or False Positives	Drugs Causing Decreased Values or False Negatives
Protein (as albumin) (cont.)	Thymol Tolbutamide (Orinase) Trimethadione (Tridione) Turpentine Viomycin Vitamin D Zoxazolamine (Flexin)	
R.B.C. or Hemoglobin	Phosphorus Phytonadione Polymyxin B Primaquine (high dosage) Probenecid Proguanil Pyrazoline derivatives Rifampin Sulfonamides Sulfones Suramin Thiabendazole (Mintezol) Thiazide diuretics Viomycin Aminosalicylic acid (large doses) Amphotericin B Bacitracin Chloroguanide Colistimethate (Colistin) Colchicine Corticosteroids	Ascorbic acid
R.B.C. or Hemoglobin (cont.)	Coumarin derivatives Cyclophosphamide Gold salts Indomethacin Kanamycin renal injury Lipomul (oil injection) Mandelic acid derivatives Mefenamic acid Mephenesin Mersalyl theophylline Methenamine Methicillin Mitotane Oxyphenbutazone Phenindione derivatives Phenylbutazone PhisoHex	
Specific Gravity	Dextran Radiopaque contrast media	

Substance Determined	Drugs Causing Increased Values or False Positives	Drugs Causing Decreased Values or False Negatives
Uric Acid	Bishydroxycoumarin Corticosteroids Mercaptopurine Methyldopa* Probenecid Salicylates Sulfinpyrazone Thiazide diuretics Thiothixene	Allopurinol Acetazolamide Ethacrynic acid Methyldopa* Triamterene Chronic alcohol consumption can interfere with test results
Urobilinogen	Acetazolamide (Diamox) Phenazopyridine Phenothiazines Formalin* Cascara Amidopyrine Aminosalicylic acid (PAS) Antipyrine Sulfonamides B.S.P. Hypaque Methenamine compounds (Hyprex, Mandelamine, Uritone) Novocaine Phenazopyridine Phenothiazines Procaine Pyradone Pyramidon Sodium bicarbonate Sulfonamides Chlorophyll Chlorpromazine (Thorazine) Diatrizoate Thoradex Drugs that cause hemolysis of R.B.C.'s	Formalin* Ammonium chloride Antibiotics Ascorbic acid Chloramphenicol (large doses) Tetracycline (possible)

Vanilmandelic Acid (VMA)	Aminosalicylic acid (PAS)
	Anileridine (Leritine)
	B.S.P.
	Cough medicines (some)
	Disulfiram (Antabuse)
	Epinephrine (Adrenaline)
	Foods and beverages
	  Bananas
	  Chocolate
	  Coffee
	  Tea
	  Vanilla extract
	Glyceryl guaiacolate (Robitussin)
		Chlorpromazine (Thorazine)
		Guanethidine (Ismelin)
		Imipramine (Tofranil)
		Monoamine oxidase inhibitors
		Morphine
		Pentobarbital (Nembutal)
		Reserpine

Substance Determined	Drugs Causing Increased Values or False Positives	Drugs Causing Decreased Values or False Negatives
Vanilmandelic Acid (VMA) (cont.)	Insulin (large doses) Levodopa (L-Dopa) Lithium carbonate Mandelamine Methocarbamol (Robaxin) Norepinephrine (Levophed) Nitroglycerin P.S.P. Salicylates Morphine Reserpine Mephenesin (Tolserol)	

Drugs Which May Affect Color of Urine

Color of Urine	Drug
Reddish-brown	Cascara and senna laxatives in acid urine
Orange	Amidopyrine Phenazopyridine
Orange to orange red	Ethoxazine Pyridium
Orange to purple red	Chorzoxozone
Orange yellow	Anisindione Phenedione Salicylazosulfopyridine in alkaline urine
Rust yellow to brownish	Nitrofurantoins Sulfonamides
Pink to red or red brown	Dilantin Doxidan Phenolphthalein (Ex-Lax) Phenothiazine
Magenta	Phenolphthalein (Ex-Lax)
Red	Aniline dyes, Amidopyrine, Desferal Pyridium, Prontosil, Neotropin, PSP and BSP dyes in alkaline urine Phenolphthalein and pyridium in acid urine,
Purple-red	Phenolphthalein (Ex-Lax) in alkaline urine

Color of Urine	Drug
Dark brown	Phenolic drugs Phenylhydrazine
Brown-black	Cascara Jecotofir, Amitriptyline Methylene blue Pyridium in alkaline urine Riboflavin
Pink to brown	Phenothiazine tranquilizers
Pale blue	Dyrenium (triamterene)
Dark colored	Iron salts
Urine that *darkens* on standing	Anti-Parkinsonian drugs Levodopa Sinemet
Blue or green	Methylene blue Amitriptylene
Bright yellow	Riboflavin Pyridium in alkaline urine

C □ DRUGS AFFECTING RESULTS OF FECAL STUDIES

Drugs Affecting Fecal Studies

Substance Determined	Drugs Causing Increased Values or False Positives	Drugs Causing Decreased Values or False Negatives
Stool Occult—for Blood—Benzidine or Guaiac Test	Boric acid (toxicity) Bromides Colchicine (toxicity) Iodine Iron, inorganic Oxidizing agents (excreted in urine)	Ascorbic acid (high doses)

Drugs that Affect Color of Feces

Color of Stool	Drug
Whitish discoloration or speckling	Antacids
Pink to red to black	Anticoagulants (excess dose), Salicylates, causing internal bleeding
Black	Bismuth salts, Iron salts, Charcoal
Brownish staining	Dihydroxyanthraquinones
Green to blue	Dithiazanine
Green	Mercurous chloride, Indomethacin, Calomel
Orange-red	Phenazopyridine,
Red	Phenolphthalein, pyruvium pamoate, Tetracyclines in syrup, Bromsulphalein
Yellow	Rhubarb, Santonin
Yellow to brown	Senna
Pink to red to black (resulting from internal bleeding)	Salicylates
Light	Sitosterols

D □□ DRUGS AFFECTING RESULTS OF HEMATOLOGIC AND SEROLOGIC STUDIES

Substance Determined	Drugs Causing Increased Values or False Positives	Drugs Causing Decreased Values or False Negatives
Bleeding Time	Dextran Mithramycin Pantothenyl alcohol and derivatives Streptokinase-streptodornase	
Coagulation Time	Mithramycin Tetracyclines Anticoagulants Azathioprine Carbenicillin (high doses in impaired renal function)	Corticosteroids Epinephrine

Coombs' Test	Cephalexin (Keflex)
	Cephaloglycin
	Cephaloridine (Loridine)
	Cephalothin (Keflin)
	Methyldopa
	  (effect lasts 6 months)
	Penicillin
	Rifampin
	Chlorpromazine
	Diphenylhydantoin
	Dipyrone
	Ethosuximide
	Hydralazine
	Isoniazide
	Levodopa
	Mefenamic acid
	Mephalan
	Oxyphenisatin
	Procainamide
	Quinidine
	Streptomycin
	Sulfonamides
	Tetracyclines
	All cause positive Coombs'
	  Test	

Substance Determined	Drugs Causing Increased Values or False Positives	Drugs Causing Decreased Values or False Negatives

Erythrocyte Count or Hemoglobin	Gentamicin
	Methyldopa (Aldomet)
		Acetaminophen
		Acetophenetidin
		Acetophenazine maleate
		Aminosalicylic acid
		Amphotericin B
		Antimony compounds
		Antineoplastic agents
		   Azathioprine
		   Florouracil
		   Floxuridine
		   Hydroxyurea
		   Mechlorethamine
		   Mithramycin
		   Triethylene Melamine
		   Urethan
		Arsenicals
		Carbamazepine
		Chloramphenicol
		Chloroquine
		Diiodohydroxyquin
		Doxapram
		Ethosuximide
		Furazolidone
		Glucosulfone
		Haloperidol
		Hydantoin derivatives
		Hydralazine
		Hydroxychloroquine sulfate
		Indomethacin
		Isoniazid (rare)
		MAO inhibitors
		Mefenamic acid
		Mepacrine (quinacrine)
		Mephenoxalone
		Mercurial diuretics
		   (prolonged use)
		Metaxalone
		Methaqualone
		Methsuximide
		Methyldopa (Aldomet)
		Nitrites
		Nitrofurantoin (rare)
		Novobiocin
		Oleandomycin
		Oxyphenbutazone
		Paramethadione,
		   trimethadione
		Penicillamine
		Penicillin
		Phenacemide
		Phenobarbital (rare)

Substance Determined	Drugs Causing Increased Values or False Positives	Drugs Causing Decreased Values or False Negatives
Erythrocyte Count or Hemoglobin (cont.)		Phenylbutazone Phytonadione (large doses in infants) Primidone Primaquine Pyrimethamine Pyrazolone derivatives Rifampin Radioactive agents (large doses) Spectinomycin Sulfonamides (rarely with sulfathiazole) Sulfameter Sulfones Sulfonylureas (oral hypoglycemic agents) Tetracycline Thiazide diuretics (rare) Thiocyanates Thiosemicarbazones Trimethadione Tripelennamine Troleandomycin Vitamin A (excess dose and use)

Leukocytes	Allopurinol (hypersensitivity)
	Aminosalicylic Acid
	Ampicillin
	Atropine (in children)
	Barbiturates (Vinbarbital, Talbutal)
	Capreomycin
	Cardiotonic glycosides
	Diethylcarbamacine
	Dipyrone
	Digitalis (rare)
	Epinephrine
	Erythromycin
	Florantyrone (in patients with pre-existing liver disease)
	Iron dextran injection (Imferon)
	Isoniazid
	Iodides
	Kanamycin
		Acetohexamide
		Acetaminophen
		Acetophenetidin
		Allopurinol (hypersensitivity)
		Aminoglutethimide
		Amodiaquine
		Aminopyrine
		Aminosalicylic acid
		Azathioprine
		Antineoplastic agents
		  Chlorambucil
		  Cyclophosphamide
		  Cytoxan
		  Florouracil
		  Floxuridine
		  Hydroxyurea
		  Mechlorethamine
		  Mithramycin
		  Triethylenemelamine
		Antipyrine
		Bismuth
		Chloramphenicol

Substance Determined	Drugs Causing Increased Values or False Positives	Drugs Causing Decreased Values or False Negatives

Leukocytes (cont.)	Lincomycin
	   one case reported
	Methicillin
	Nalidixic acid
	Potassium iodide
	Sulfonamides (long acting)
	Stibocaptate (antimony)
	Streptodornase-streptokinase
	Streptomycin
	Tetracyclines
	   (prolonged use)
	Triamterene
	Trifluperidol
	Vancomycin
	Viomycin
	Procainamide
	Procarbazine
	Cloxacillin
	Ristocetin
	Cephalothin
	Chlorpropamide
	Clindamycin (Cleocin)
	Desipramine, imipramine
	Diphenhydramine
	Gold compounds
	Hydantoin derivatives
	Primaquine
	Phenothiazines
	   (large dose)
	Novobiocin
	Methysergide
	Methyldopa
		Chlordiazepoxide
		Chloroquine
		Carbamazepine
		Carbimazole
		Chlorprothixene
		Chlorthalidone
		Clofibrate
		Colistin
		Corticosteroids
		   (reported for prednisolone)
		   Prednisone
		Diazepam
		Dichlorphenamide
		Diethazine
		Doxapram (Dopram)
		Diiodohydroxyquin
		Ethacrynic acid
		Ethoxzolamide
		Furosemide
		Glaucarubin
		Meprobamate
		Mercurial diuretics (rare)
		Metaxalone (Skelaxin)
		Methampyrone
		Methazolamide
		Methimazole
		Methocarbamol
		Methsuximide
		Methylthiouracil
		Methyprylon (metabolite)
		   Methicillin sodium
		   Oxacillin
		Metronidazole
		Nitrofurantoin (rare)
		Oleandomycin
		Oxandrolone
		Oxazepam
		Oxyphenbutazone
		Paraldehyde
		Penicillamine
		Penicillins
		Phenylbutazone
		Potassium perchlorate
		Primidone (rare)
		Propylthiouracil
		Protriptyline
		Pyrazolone derivatives
		Pyrimethamine (Daraprim)
		Pyrathiazine
		   (prolonged use)
		Quinine

Substance Determined	Drugs Causing Increased Values or False Positives	Drugs Causing Decreased Values or False Negatives
Leukocytes (cont.)		Radioactive agents
		Rifampin
		Sulfonylureas (oral hypoglycemic agents)
		Sulthiame
		Thiabendazole
		Thiazide diuretics (rare)
		Thiosemicarbazones
		Thiothixene
		Tripelennamine
		Vitamin A (prolonged use)
		Procainamide (both reported)
		Cephalothin
		Chlorpropamide
		Clindamycin (cleocin)
		Gold compounds
		Diphenhydramine
		Desipramine imipramine
		Glucosulfone
		Griseofulvin
		Haloperidol
		Hydralazine
		Hydroxychloroquine
		Idoxuridine (in high concentration)
		Indandione derivatives (oral anticoagulants)
		Indomethacin
		Iothiouracil
		Monoamine oxidase inhibitors
		Mefenamic acid
		Mepacrine (Quinacrine)
		Mepazine
		Mephenesin
		Novobiocin
		Phenothiazines (large doses)
		Primaquine
		Hydantoin derivatives
		Methysergide
		Methyldopa
		Cloxacillin
		Ristocetin
		Procarbazine
		Sulfonamides*

Substance Determined	Drugs Causing Increased Values or False Positives	Drugs Causing Decreased Values or False Negatives

Prothrombin Time	ACTH
	Alcohol
	  (large quantities)
	Aluminum nicotinate
	  (Nicalex) (50% decreased)
	Amidopyrine
	Aminosalicylic acid (PAS)
	Anabolic steroids
	Antibiotics
	Anticoagulants (oral)
	Benziodarones
	Carbenicillin
	  (high doses with renal
	  failure)
	Cathartics
	Chlorpromazine*
	Chloramphenicol
	  (Chloromycetin)
	Clofibrate (Atromid-S)*
	Diphenidol
	Diphenylhydantoin
	  (Dilantin)
	Edathamil
	Heparin
	Hydroxyzine
	Indomethacin (Indocin)
	Iothiouracil
	Kanamycin (Kantrex)
	Mefenamic Acid (Ponstel)
	Metandienone
	Methimazole
	Methyldopa (Aldomet)
	  (effect on liver)
	Methylthiouracil
	Mineral oil
	Mithramycin
	Monoamine oxidase
	  inhibitors
	Morphine
	Naloxone
	Neomycin
	Oxyphenbutazone
	  (Tandearil)
	Penicillin
	Phenylbutazone
	  (Butazolidin)
	Phenyramidol (Analexin)
	Phosphorus
	Propylthiouracil
	Pyrazinamide
	Reserpine
		Antihistamines
		  Diphenhydramine
		  (Benadryl)
		Barbiturates
		  enzyme induction
		Chloral hydrate
		Corticosteroids
		Digitalis
		  (in cardiac failure)
		Diuretics
		Griseolfulvin
		Glutethimide
		Progestin-estrogen combina-
		  tion (oral contraceptives)
		Rifampin
		Lipomul (oil injection)*
		Metaproterenol*
		Proteolytic enzymes*
		  (e.g., Papase, Ananase)
		Theophylline
		  xanthines may increase
		  plasma prothrombin and
		  factor V, but therapeutic
		  doses have small effect on
		  the response to oral anti-
		  coagulants
		Thiothixene
		Vitamin K

Substance Determined	Drugs Causing Increased Values or False Positives	Drugs Causing Decreased Values or False Negatives
Prothrombin Time (cont.)	Quinidine Quinine Salicylates Streptomycin Sulfonamides (Sulfameter) Tetracyclines Cholestyramine (Cuemid) Chlordiazepoxide (Librium)* Lipomul (oil injection)* Metaproterenol* Proteolytic enzymes* (e.g. Papase, Ananase) D-thyroxine (Choloxin) Thyroid hormones Vitamin A	
Sedimentation Rate Erythrocyte Sedimentation Rate (ESR)	Dextran Methysergide Methyldopa Penicillamine Procainamide Theophylline Trifluperidol Vitamin A Progestin-estrogen combination (oral contraceptives)	Ethambutol Quinine Salicylates Drugs that cause a high blood glucose level (cortisone and ACTH)

Thrombocytes (Platelets)	Aspirin	Acetazolamide
		Acetohexamide
		Aminosalicylic acid
		Amphotericin B
		Antazoline
		Antimony compounds
		Antineoplastic agents
		  Azathropine
		  Bulsulfan (Myleran) (large doses)
		  Chlorambucil
		  Cyclophosphamide (Cytoxan)
		  Florouracil
		  Floxuridine
		  Mechlorethamine
		  Mithramycin
		  Hydroxyurea
		Arsenicals
		Benzene
		Busulphan
		Bismuth
		Carbamazepine
		Cardiotonic glycosides

Substance Determined	Drugs Causing Increased Values or False Positives	Drugs Causing Decreased Values or False Negatives
Thrombocytes (Platelets) (cont.)		Chloramphenicol
		Chloroquine
		Chlorothiazide
		Chlorthalidone
		Chlorpropamide
		Colchicine
		DDT
		Dipyrone
		Diazoxide
		Ethacrynic acid
		Ethoxzolamide
		Diethylstilbestrol
		Diphenylhydantoin
		Gentamicin
		Gold salts
		Heparin
		Iothiouracil sodium
		Lincomycin
		Lipomul (oil injection)
		Mefenamic acid
		Mepazine
		Methimazole
		Mephenytoin
		Methimazole
		Methazolamide
		Methyldopa (Aldomet)
		Meprobamate
		Novobiocin (Albamycin)
		Methotrexate
		Oxyphenbutazone
		Penicillamine
		Penicillins
		Phenindione (indane derivative)
		Phenothiazines
		Phenylbutazone
		Potassium perchlorate
		Procainamide
		Prednisone
		Propranolol
		Propynyl-cyclohexanol carbamate
		Pyrazinamide
		Pyrimethamine
		Quinidine sulfate
		Quinine
		Rifampin
		Ristocetin A & B
		Salicylates
		Smallpox vaccine
		Sulphisoxazole

Substance Determined	Drugs Causing Increased Values or False Positives	Drugs Causing Decreased Values or False Negatives

Thrombocytes (Platelets) (cont.)		Sulfonamides
		  Sulfadimethoxine
		  Sulfameter
		Sulphamethoxypyridazine
		Sulfonyl ureas (oral hypo-
		  glycemic agents)
		Sulphamethoxazole
		Thiazide diuretics (rare)
		Thiourea
		Tolbutamide
		Toluene diisocyanate

E □□ DRUGS AFFECTING
CEREBROSPINAL FLUID STUDIES

Drugs Affecting Cerebrospinal Fluid Studies

Substance Determined	Drugs Causing Increased Values or False Positives	Drugs Causing Decreased Values or False Negatives
Proteins	Anesthetics (local) contaminant Chlorpromazine Salicylates Streptomycin Sulfanilamide Tryptophan	Albumin Acetophenetidin

A □ BLOOD CHEMISTRY AND
□ ELECTROLYTE ANALYSIS

Substance Determined	Normal Values	Clinical Implications	
		Increase	*Decrease*
Acid Phosphatase	1.0–4.0 King Armstrong μ/dl. 0.5–2.0 Bodansky or Gutman μ/dl. 0–1.1 Shinowara μ/ml. 0.1–0.73 Bessy Lowry μ/nk.	Significantly elevated nearly always indicative of metastatic cancer of prostate Moderately elevated values in: Paget's disease Gaucher's disease Hyperparathyroidism Multiple myeloma Any cancer that has metastasized to the bone Hepatitis Obstructive jaundice Acute renal impairment Sickle cell crisis Excessive destruction of platelets Cholecystitis Cholelithiosis Cancer metastatic to the liver Acute pancreatitis Cancer of the liver or bile duct Congestive heart failure Alcoholism Barbiturate use Lipoid nephrosis	
Alcohol	Negative	*Methyl Alcohol* 25 mg./dl. or greater: toxic 80 mg./dl. or greater: lethal	

| Substance | | Clinical Implications | |
Determined	Normal Values	Increase	Decrease
Alcohol (cont.)		*Ethyl Alcohol* 0.03–0.15 gm./dl.: "under the influence" or 30–150 mg./dl. Levels between 50–150 mg./dl. or .05–.015 gm./100 ml. exert unmistakable effects on behavior, especially driving.	
Alkaline Phosphatase	1.5–4.5 μ/dl. (Bodansky method) 4.3 μ/dl. (King-Armstrong method) 0.8–2.3 y./nk. (Bessey-Lowry method) 15.35 μ/ml. (Shinowar-Jones-Reinhart)	Liver Disease Bone Disease Hyperparathyroidism Infectious mono-nucleosis	Hypophosphatasia Malnutrition Hypothyroidism Pernicious anemia Scurvy Milk-alkali syndrome Placental insufficiency
Ammonia	40–110 mg./100	Liver disease Hepatic coma Severe heart failure Azotemia Cor pulmonale Erythroblastosis fetalis Pulmonary emphysema Acute bronchitis Pericarditis Myelocytic and lymphocytic leukemia	
Amylase	60–200 Somogyi units/100 ml.	Acute nonhemorrhagic pancreatitis Exacerbation of chronic pancreatitis Partial gastrestomy Obstruction of pancreatic duct Perforated peptic ulcer Alcohol poisoning Mumps Obstruction or inflammation of salivary duct or gland	Acute pancreatitis subsides Hepatitis Cirrhosis of liver Toxemia of pregnancy Severe burns Severe thyrotoxicosis

Substance Determined	Normal Values	Clinical Implications	
		Increase	Decrease
Amylase (cont.)		Acute choleytitis Intestinal obstruction with strangulation Ruptured tubal pregnancy Ruptured aortic aneurysm	
Barbiturate (Assay)	Negative	Toxic level of short-acting barbiturates— 3 mg./dl. Toxic level of long acting barbiturates such as phenobarbitol is 9 mg./dl.	

Bilirubin Icterus Index	Total: 0.3–1.3 mg./dl.
	Direct conjugated: 0.1–0.4 mg./dl.
	Free indirect unconjugated: 0.2–0.18 mg./dl.
	Newborn: 1–12 mg./dl.
	Icterus Index: 4–6 units
		Bilirubin elevations accompanied by jaundice due to hepatic, obstructive or hemolytic causes.
		Elevations of non-conjugated bilirubin levels occur in:
		Hemolytic anemias,
		   Trauma in the presence of a large hematoma,
		   Hemorrhagic pulmonary infarcts
		Elevated conjugated bilirubin in:
		Cancer of the head of pancreas
		Choledocholithiasis
		Crigler-Najjar syndrome
		Gilbert's disease
		Dubin-Johnson syndrome
		Elevation of both conjugated & non-conjugated in:
		Hepatic metastasis,
		Hepatitis,
		Lymphoma,
		Cholestasis secondary to drugs,
		Cirrhosis	

Substance Determined	Normal Values	Clinical Implications Increase	Decrease
Blood Urea Nitgrogen (BUN)	10–15 mg./100 ml.	Kidney disease or urinary obstruction from enlarged prostrate. Shock Dehydration GI hemorrhage Infection Diabetes Some malignancies Acute myocardial infarction Chronic gut Excessive protein uptake	Liver failure Negative nitrogen balance Impaired absorption Nephrotic syndrome Overhydration
Blood Volume Determination	Total blood volume 55–80 ml./kg. Red cell volume 20–35 ml./kg. (Greater in men than women) Plasma volume 30–45 ml./kg.	Increased total blood volume, plasma volume and red cell mass suggest polycythemia vera.	A normal total blood volume with a decreased red cell content would indicate the need for a transfusion of packed red cells. Normal or decreased total blood volume and plasma volume suggest secondary polycythemia.
Bromsulphalein (BSP)	5% BSP retention 45 minutes after injection of dye	Acute hepatitis Hepatic necrosis Chronic hepatitis Cirrhosis Cancer of liver Heart failure Shock Acute hemorrhage	
Calcium (Ca++)	Total 9.0–10.6 mg./dl. 4.5–5.3 mEq./l. Ionized 4.2–5.2 mg./dl. 2.1–2.6 mEq./l.	Cancer Hyperparathyroidism Addison's disease Hyperthyroidism Paget's disease of bone Prolonged immobilization Bone fractures combined with bedrest Excessive intake of Vitamin D Prolonged use of diuretics, thiazides Respiratory acidosis Milk-alkali syndrome	Pseudohypocalcemia Hypoparathyroidism Chronic renal failure Malabsorption Acute pancreatitis Alkalosis Osteomalacia Diarrhea Rickets

Substance Determined	Normal Values	Clinical Implications	
		Increase	Decrease
Carotene	50–300 μ/100 ml.	Myxedema Diabetes Mellitus Hypothyroidism Chronic nephritis Hyperlipidemia Excessive dietary intake	Fat malabsorption syndrome Steatorrhea Febrile illnesses Liver disease Poor dietary intake
Cephalin Floccula- tion Thymol Turbidity	Cephalin Floccu- lation—24 or less/negative Thymol Turbidity 0–4 units	Acute hepatitis Cirrhosis Multiple myeloma Sarcoidoses Hodgkin's disease Coccidiomycosis Subacute endocarditis Rheumatoid arthritis Lupus erythematosus Tuberculosis (hema- togenous) Histoplasmosis Malaria Lymphogranulo- vancrum	Liver abscess and neoplasms will give a negative result.
Chloride (Cl⁻)	95–105 mEq./l.	Dehydration Cushing's syndrome Hyperventilation Eclampsia Anemia Cardiac decompensa- tion Some kidney disorders	Severe vomiting Severe diarrhea Ulcerative colitis Pyloric obstruction Severe burns Heat Exhaustion Diabetic acidosis Addison's disease Fever Acute infections Drugs such as mercurial and chlorothiazide diuretics
Cholesterol	Total: 400–1000 mg./dl. Cholesterol 150– 250 mg./dl. Triglycerides 40–150 mg./dl. Phospholipids 150–380 mg./dl.	Cardiovascular disease Familial hypercholes- terolemia Obstructive jaundice Hypothyroidism Nephrosis Xanthomatosis Uncontrolled diabetes Markedly abnormal ratio of free to esteri- fied cholesterol in liver biliary tract, infectious diseases and extreme choles- terolemia	Associated with fat malabsorption syndrome Malabsorption Liver disease Hyperthyroidism Anemia Sepsis Stress Drug therapy Pernicious anemia Hemolytic jaundice Hyperthyroidism

Substance		Clinical Implications	
Determined	Normal Values	Increase	Decrease
Cholesterol (cont.)			Severe infections Terminal stages such as cancer Esterol fraction decreases in liver diseases, liver cell injury
Cortisone Glucose Tolerance	1 hour 160 mg./dl. 2 hours 140 mg./dl.	Pre-diabetic Carcinoma Hyperthyroidism Stress Obesity Cushing's syndrome	Liver disease Addison's disease Anterior pituitary hyposecretion Hypothyroidism
Creatine Phospho-kinase (CPK) Creatine Kinase (CK)	0–12 Sigma units/ml. Men: 5–35 ug./ml.; 20–140 I.U./l. Women: 5.25 ug./ml.; 10–100 I.U./l. MB isoenzyme: Less than 3 I.U./l.	Myocardial Infarction Progressive muscular dystrophy Dermatomyositis Delirium tremors Electric shock Myxedema Cardiac surgery Cardiac defibrillation Electromyography Convulsions Cerebral infarction Subarachnoid hemorrhage Hypokalemia Hypothyroidism Acute psychosis Central nervous system trauma Pulmonary infarction or edema	
Creatinine	0.2–0.5 mg./dl.	Impaired renal function Chronic nephritis Obstruction of the urinary tract Muscle disease Gigantism Acromegaly	Muscular dystrophy
Electrophoresis of LDH (LD)	LDH 1/5 29% LDH 2/4 38% LDH 3 19% LDH 4/2 8% LDH 5/1 5%	Increased LD_1 and LD_2, indicates myocardial infarction Increased LDH_3 indicates pulmonary infarction	

Substance Determined	Normal Values	Clinical Implications	
		Increase	Decrease
Electrophoresis of LDH (LD) (cont.)		Increased LDH_4 and LDH_5 indicates liver disease	
Folic Acid (Folate)	5.9–21.0 ng./ml.		Drugs which are folic acid antagonists Megaloblastic anemia Hemolytic anemia Liver disease Sprue Celiac disease Idiopathic steatorrhea Malignancies Malnutrition Elderly persons with inadequate diets Hyperthyroidism Vitamin C deficiency Febrile states Chronic dialyses
Gastrin	92–275 pg./ml.	Stomach cancer Gastric and duodenal ulcers Zollinger-Ellison syndrome Pernicious anemia End-stage renal disease In elderly patients	
Glucose Fasting Blood Sugar (FBS)	70–110 mg./dl. (serum) 60–100 mg./dl. (whole blood)	Diabetes Cushing's disease Acute stress Pheochromocytoma Pituitary adenoma Hyperthyroidism Adenoma of pancreas Pancreatitis Brain trauma Chronic liver disease	Overdose of insulin Addison's disease Bacterial sepsis Islet cell carcinoma of pancreas Hepatic necrosis Hypothyroidism Glycogen storage disease Psychogenic causes
Glucose Tolerance	FBS (Fasting Blood Sugar below 100 mg./100 ml. ½ hr. 155 mg./ 100 ml. 1 hour 165 mg./ 100 ml.	Maturity onset diabetes Overt diabetes	Hypoglycemia

Substance Determined	Normal Values	Clinical Implications Increase	Decrease
Glucose Tolerance (cont.)	2 hours 140 mg./ 100 ml. 3 hours 80 mg./ 100 ml. All urines are negative for glucose		
Lactic Acid Dehydrogenase (LD, LDH)	80–120 Wacker Units 120–340 I.U./l. 150–450 Wroblewski Units	Myocardial Infarction Pulmonary Infarction Acute leukemia Hemolytic anemias Malignant neoplasms Acute renal infarctions and chronic renal disease Hepatic disease Skeletal muscle necrosis Sprue Shock with necrosis Myxedema Extensive cancer	
Lipase	0–1 unit/ml.	Pancreatitis Obstruction of the pancreatic duct Pancreatic carcinoma Acute cholecystitis Cirrhosis Severe renal disease	
Magnesium (Mg^{++})	1.8–3.0 mg./dl. 1.5–2.5 mEq./l.	Renal failure Diabetic coma Hypothyroidism Addison's disease Adrenalectomy Controlled diabetes in older people Use of antacids containing magnesium Dehydration Use of thiazides Use of ethracynic acid	Chronic diarrhea After hemodialysis Chronic renal disease Hepatic cirrhosis Chronic pancreatitis Use of diuretics Aldosteronism Ulcerative colitis Hyperaldosteronism Toxemia of pregnancy Hyperparathyroidism Hypoparathyroidism Excessive lactation Cirrhosis of liver
Mucoproteins (Seromucoid)	83–203 mg./l.	Cancer Rheumatoid arthritis Infections Ankylosing spondylitis	Infectious hepatitis Infectious cirrhosis

Substance Determined	Normal Values	Clinical Implications	
		Increase	Decrease
Oleic Acid Test (^{131}I Absorption test)	8–12% in blood in 3–4 hours.		Malabsorption
Phosphate/ Inorganic Phosphorus (P) (PO$_4$)	Adult: 2.5–4.8 mg./dl. Child: 3.5–5.8 mg./dl.	Renal insufficiency Severe nephritis Hypoparathyroidism Hypocalcemia Excessive intake of alkali Excessive intake of vitamin D Fractures in the healing stage Bone tumors Addison's disease Acromegaly	Hyperparathyroidism Rickets Diabetic coma Insulin administration Continuous intravenous glucose in a nondiabetic patient.
Plasma Lipids (Total) Cholesterol, Triglycerides, Phospholipids	Total: 400–1000 mg./dl. Cholesterol 150–250 mg./dl. Triglycerides 40–150 mg./dl. Phospholipids 150–380 mg./dl.	Hyperlipidemia	Associated with fat malabsorption syndrome
Potassium (K$^+$)	3.5–5.0 mEq./l.	Burns Addison's disease Acute renal failure Selective hypoaldosteronism Internal hemorrhage Uncontrolled diabetes Acidosis	Diarrhea Pyloric obstruction Starvation Malabsorption Severe vomiting Severe burns Primary aldosteronism Excessive ingestion of licorice Renal tubular acidosis Diuretic administration Steroids Estrogen Familial periodic paralysis Liver disease with ascites Chronic stress, Crash dieting without K$^+$ Chronic fever

Substance		Clinical Implications	
Determined	Normal Values	Increase	Decrease
Protein- Bound Iodine (PBI) Butanol- Extractable Iodine (BEI)	4.0–8.0 μg./dl. PBI 3.5–6.5 g./dl. BEI	Hyperthyroidism Acute thyroiditis	Hypothyroidism Chronic thyroiditis Myxedema Nephrosis
Proteins, Al- bumin and Globulin; A/G Ratio	Total: 6–8 gm./dl. Albumin 4–4.5 gm.% Globulin 1.5–3 gm.% A/G ratio 1.5:1– 2.5:1	*Increased albumin levels* generally not observed *Increase in Total Protein* Hemoconcentration as a result of dehydra- tion from loss of body fluid Lupus erythematosus Rheumatoid arthritis Collagen diseases Chronic infections Acute liver disease Multiple myeloma	*Decreased albumin* Edema Hypocalcemia Inadequate iron intake Severe liver diseases Malabsorption Diarrhea Eclampsia Nephrosis Exfoliative dermatitis Third degree burns Starvation Excessive IV glucose in water *Decrease in Total Protein* Increased loss of albumin in urine Decreased formation in liver Insufficient protein intake Severe hemorrhage Malabsorption Diarrhea Exfoliative dermatitis Severe burns Excessive IV admin- istration of glucose in water
Radioactive Iodine (RAI) Uptake Test	1–13% absorbed after 2 hrs. 2–25% absorbed after 6 hrs. 15–45% ab- sorbed after 24 hrs.	Hyperthyroidism	Hypothyroidism

| Substance | | Clinical Implications | |
Determined	Normal Values	Increase	Decrease
Radioactive Triolein Uptake (Triolein ^{131}I Absorption Test)	8–12% tagged triolein in blood in 3–4 hrs. Less than 2% tagged triolein in feces in 48 hrs.		Pancreatic insufficiency Chronic pancreatitis Malabsorption syndrome
Red Blood Cell Survival Time Test	25–35 days	Abnormality of red cell production Prior Splenectomy	Blood loss Hemolysis Removal of red blood cells by the spleen
Salicylate	Negative	Therapeutic level is 20–25 mg./dl. Toxic level is more than 30 mg./dl. A lethal level is more than 60 mg./dl.	
Schilling Test	Excretion of 8% or more of test dose of Cobalt-tagged Vitamin B_{12} in urine.	Absence of intrinsic factor Defective absorption in the ileum of radioactive vitamin B_{13}	
Serum Glutamic Oxaloacetic Transaminase (SGOT) Aspartate Transaminase	5–40 Sigma Frankel μ/ml. 0–36 I.U./l., lower in women	Myocardial Infarction Liver Disease Acute pancreatitis Trauma and irradiation of skeletal muscle Acute hemolytic anemia Acute renal disease Severe burns Cardiac catheterization Recent brain trauma Crushing injuries Progressive muscular dystrophy	Beriberi Uncontrolled diabetes mellitus with acidosis Liver disease on occasion may cause a decrease instead of the expected increase
Serum Glutamic Pyruvic Transaminase (SGPT) Alanine Transaminase (ALT)	0–48 I.U./l. 5–35 Sigma Frankel μ/ml.	Hepatocellular disease Active cirrhosis Metastatic liver tumor Obstruction jaundice/biliary obstruction Infection or toxic hepatitis Liver congestion Pancreatitis Hepatic injury in myocardial infarction complicated by shock	

Substance Determined	Normal Values	Clinical Implications Increase	Decrease
Sodium (Na^+)	136–142 mEq./l. in adults under 65 years of age 132–140 mEq./l. in adults older than 65 years	Dehydration and insufficient water intake Primary aldosteronism Coma Cushing's disease Diabetes insipidus Tracheo-bronchitis	Severe burns Severe diarrhea Vomiting Excessive IV's of non-electrolyte fluids Addison's disease Severe nephritis Pyloric obstruction Malabsorption syndrome Diabetic acidosis Drugs Edema Excessive sweating accompanied by large amounts of water by mouth Stomach suction accompanied by water or ice chips by mouth
T_3 and T_4 Uptake Test and Thyroid Binding Globulin (TBG) Test	T_3 25–35% T_4 3.8–11.4% TBI 0.9–1.1	T_3 increased in hyperthyroidism T_4 increased in hyperthyroidism TBI increased in hypothyroidism	T_3 decreased in hypothyroidism T_4 decreased in myxedema TBI decreased in hyperthyroidism
Testosterone	406–954 mg./dl. Men 40–120 mg./dl. Women	Adrenogenital syndrome in women Stein-Leventhal syndrome in women when virilization is present Adrenal neoplasms Ovarium tumors	Male hypogonadism Klinefelter's syndrome
Theophylline	None should be present	20 mg./l. is a toxic level Therapeutic level is 5–20 μ/l., depending on time and dosage	
Thyroid Stimulation Test TSH (Thyroid Stimulating Hormone) Test	RAI and T_4 uptake is increased within 8–10 hours after TSH is given TSH—less than 5μ U/ml.	Primary untreated hypothyroidism Hashimoto's thyroiditis	Normal in: Secondary hypothyroidism Hypothalamic hypothyroidism Pituitary hypothyroidism TSH cannot be detected in thyrotoxicosis

Substance Determined	Normal Values	Clinical Implications Increase	Decrease
Thyroid Stimulation Test (cont.)			No response to TSH administration in cases of diminished thyroid reserve
Triglyceride	40–150 mg./100 ml.	Familial hyperlipidemia Liver disease Nephrotic syndrome Hypothyroidism Poorly controlled diabetes Pancreatitis Glycogen storage Myocardial infarction	Malnutrition Congenital a-beta lipoproteinemia
Two Hour Post Prandial Blood Sugar (2 hr. P.P.B.S.)	Less than 145 mg./dl.	Malnutrition Advanced cirrhosis of liver Cushing's syndrome Acromegaly Hyperthyroidism Pheochromocytoma Lipoproteinemias Myocardial or cerebral infarction Some malignancies Pregnancy Anxiety states	Anterior pituitary insufficiency Islet cell adenoma Steatorrhea Addison's disease
Uric Acid	Women: 3.0–7.5 mg./100 ml. Men: 7–8.5 mg./100 ml.	Decreased kidney function Gout Leukemia Acute stages of infectious diseases Lymphomas Metastatic cancer Severe eclampsia Starvation Shock Alcoholism Chemotherapy for cancer Excessive X rays Multiple myeloma Metabolic acidosis Diabetic ketosis Lead poisoning	Patients who are treated with uricosuric drugs

B □ SEROLOGIC STUDIES

Substance		Clinical Implications	
Determined	Normal Values	Increase	Decrease
AGM Test for Immuno-globulins IgG, IgA, and IgM	IgG—700–1350 mg./dl. IgA—75–370 mg./dl. IgM—35–200 mg./dl. IgD—very small amount IdE—small amount	**IgG** Chronic granulomatous infections Infections of all types Hyperimmunization Liver disease Malnutrition (severe) Dysproteinemia Disease associated with hypersensitivity gran-ulomas, dematologic disorders, and IgG myeloma **IgD** Chronic infections IgD myelomas **IgE** Atopic skin diseases such as eczema Hay fever Asthma Anaphylactic shock E-myeloma **IgA** Wiskott-Aldrich syn-drome Cirrhosis of the liver Collagen and other autoimmune dis-orders Chronic infections not based on immuno-logic deficiencies IgA myeloma **IgM** Waldenstrom's macro-globulinemia Trypanosomiasis Actinomycosis Carrion's disease	**IgE** Congenital agam-maglobulinemia Hypogammaglobu-linemia **IgA** Hereditary ataxia telangiectasia Immunologic defi-ciency states Malabsorption syndromes **IgM** Agammaglobu-linemia Lymphoproliferative Lymphoid aplasia IgG and IgA myeloma

Substance Determined	Normal Values	Clinical Implications	
		Increase	Decrease
AGM Test for Immuno-globulins IgG, IgA, and IgM (cont.)		IgM (cont.) Malaria Infectious mononu-cleosis Dysgammaglobulin-emia	IgM (cont.) Dysgammaglobu-linemia
Alpha₁-anti-trypsin Test	159–400 mg./dl.	Acute and chronic in-flammatory illnesses After infections of typhoid vaccine Cancer Thyroid infections Use of oral contracep-tives Stress syndrome Hematologic abnor-malities	Early-onset chronic pulmonary em-physema in adults Liver cirrhosis in children Pulmonary disease Severe hepatic damage Nephrotic syndrome Malnutrition
Antinuclear Antibody (ANA, ANF) Anti-DNA Antibody Tests	Negative	Positive Test: a titer of 1:10 or 1:20 Positive tests are asso-ciated with: Systemic lupus erythematosus Rheumatoid arthritis Chronic hepatitis Perarteritis nodosa Dermatomyositis Scleroderma Atypical pneumonia Tuberculosis Anaplastic car-cinomas or lymphomas Raynaud's disease Sjogren's syndrome	
Anti-Strepto-lysin O (ASO), Strepto-zyme, Strepto-nase-B, ASLO Test	200 I.U. or less than 160 Todd units Levels are age-dependent Preschool 1:60 School age 1:70 Adult 1:85	Focus of streptococcal infection Rheumatic fever Glomerulonephritis	
Blood Groups	O, A, B, AB		
Carcinoem-bryonic Antigen (CEA)	2.5–3.0 ng./ml.	Carcinoma of the liver Carcinoma of the pan-creas Inflammatory bowel disease	After treatment

Substance Determined	Normal Values	Clinical Implications	
		Increase	Decrease
Carcinoem-bryonic Antigen (CEA) (cont.)		Cirrhosis Chronic cigarette smoking Other cancers Without evident cause (at times)	
Cold Agglu-tinins	0–8	Above 16 is significant Atypical pneumonia Congenital syphilis Severe hemolytic anemia Cirrhosis Lymphatic leukemia Malaria Peripheral vascular disease	
Coombs' Antiglo-bulin Test	Direct Coombs' Test—negative on RBC Indirect Coombs' Test—negative on serum	Direct Coombs' Test Positive tests in: Erythroblastosis fetalis Autoimmune hemolytic anemia Transfusion reaction Cephalothin therapy and some penicillin Drugs like alpha methyl dopa—aldomet	Negative test in: Nonautoimmune hemolytic anemias
C-Reactive Protein (CRP)	Trace amounts	Any titer is significant Rheumatoid arthritis Lupus erythematosus Myocardial infarction Active, widespread malignancy Pneumonia Bacterial and viral infections (acute)	
Crossmatch (Compati-bility Test)	Absence of clumping or hemolysis when serum and cells are appropriately mixed and in-cubated in the laboratory.	Transfusion reaction when incompatible blood is transfused. Red cell destruction	

Substance Determined	Normal Values	Clinical Implications Increase	Decrease
Entamoeba Histolytica (Amebiasis) Detection and HK9 Antigens	Negative	May reflect only past not current infections Positive in: Amebic liver abscess Amebic dysentery	
Febrile Agglu- tinating Antigen Test	Negative	Typhoid and salmonella fever Typhus Brucellosis Tularemia A titer of 1:60 or 1:80 is considered signifi- cant	
Fungal Anti- body Tests (HP and CM) (for detection) of coccidio- idomycosis blastomy- cosis, and histoplas- mosis	Negative	Antibodies to coccidio- mycosis, and blasto- mycosis, and histoplasmosis appear early in dis- ease (from the first to the fourth week)	
Hemagglu- tination In- hibition (HI or HAI) Test (for deter- mination of immun- ity to rubella)	1:10 susceptible to rubella in- fection 1:20 previous rubella infec- tion and there- fore protection from rubella		
Hepatitis- Associated Antigen (HAA) Tests	Negative	Chronic active hepatitis whether or not prior acute hepatitis has occurred Patients receiving renal dialysis Institutionalized patients with Down syndrome Patients receiving immunosuppressive medication (certain cases)	

| Substance | | Clinical Implications | |
Determined	Normal Values	Increase	Decrease
Human Trans- ferrin Test (Total Iron- Binding Capacity (TIBC)	250–450 mg./dl.	Inadequate dietary iron Iron-deficiency anemia due to hemorrhage Acute hepatitis Polycythemia Oral contraceptives	Pernicious anemia Thalassemia Sickle cell anemia Chronic infection Cancer Hepatic disease Uremia Rheumatoid arthritis
L.E. Test	Negative	Positive in: Lupus erythematosus Rheumatoid arthritis Scleroderma Blood-sensitivity reac- tions Hepatitis (certain types)	

Rh Antibody
Titer Test
	Negative—no
	antibody
		If the Rh antibody titer
		   in the pregnant
		   woman is <1:64, an
		   exchange transfusion
		   is considered	

Rheumatoid
Factor (RA
Factor)
Rheumaton
	Negative (<1:20)	Tentative diagnosis of
		   early rheumatoid
		   arthritis
		Inactive rheumatoid
		   arthritis
		Lupus erythematosus
		Endocarditis
		Tuberculosis
		Syphilis
		Sarcoid
		Cancer
		Viral infections
		Diseases affecting the
		   liver, lung or kidney	

Rh Factor; RH
Typing
	Whites: 85% Rh-
	positive 15%
	Rh-negative
	Blacks: 90%
	Rh-positive
	10% Rh-nega-
	tive
		Significance of Rh
		   factors is based on
		   their capacity to im-
		   munize in trans-
		   fusions or pregnancies	

Syphilis De- tection Tests	Nonreactive: negative	Positive for syphilis	

Substance Determined	Normal Values	Clinical Implications	
		Increase	*Decrease*
Tests for Infectious Mononucleosis Monospot and Heterophile Antibody Titer Test Monoscreening-Mono-Diff	Negative	Titer of 1:56 is suspicious A titer of 1:2224 or > is diagnostic of infectious mononucleosis	
Thyroid Hemagglutination Test	Negative or 1:20	Hashimoto's thyroiditis Graves' disease Pernicious anemia Lupus erythematosus Rheumatoid arthritis Connective tissue diseases	
TPM Test (for detection of toxoplasmosis)	Negative or <1:64 titer	Positive for toxoplasmosis Titer is 1:256 or higher	

C □□ HEMATOLOGIC STUDIES

Substance Determined	Normal Values	Clinical Implications	
		Increase	*Decrease*
Autohemolysis Erythrocyte Fragility	0.4–4.5 0–0.7 glucose added 0–15 ATP added		Hereditary spherosis
Basophils	0.5–1.0% total WBC 25–100/cu. mm.	Most commonly with: Granulocytic & basophilic leukemia & myeloid metaphasia Less commonly with: Chronic inflammation Polycythemia vera Chronic hemolytic anemia Following splenectomy The healing phase of inflammation Following radiation	Acute allergic reactions Hyperthyroidism Stress reactions Hypersensitivity reactions Following prolonged steroid therapy
Bleeding Time (Duke and Ivy Methods)	3–10 minutes in most laboratories Duke Method <8 minutes-usually 1–6 minutes Ivy Method 2–9.5 minutes	Thrombocytopenia Platelet dysfunction syndromes Vascular defects Severe liver disease Leukemia Aplastic anemia DIC disease	
Buffy Coat Smear	Atypical Mononuclear cells, Megakaryocytes, Metamyelocytes, Normal cell components: The buffy coat of of the blood of healthy people contains these cells.	Abnormal cells are an indication of: Leukemia Cancer metastatic to the bone Lupus erythematosus	

Substance Determined	Normal Values	Clinical Implications	
		Increase	Decrease
Clot Retraction	Nearly complete in 4 hours and definitely completed in 24 hrs.	Severe anemia and hypofibrinogenia	Thrombocytopenia von Willebrand's disease Disorders due to increase in red cell mass
Coagulation Time (CT) Whole Blood Clotting Time; Lee-White Clotting Time	5 to 10 minutes	Afibrinogenemia and marked hyper-heparinemia	
Eosinophils	1–4 of total WBC 50–250 cu. mm.	Allergies Parasitic diseases Addison's disease Lung and bone cancer Chronic skin infections Myelogenous leukemia Hodgkin's disease Polycythemia Subacute infections Familial eosinophilia Polyarteritis nodosa Many tumors	Infectious mono-nucleosis Hypersplenism Congestive heart failure Cushing's syndrome Aplastic and perni-cious anemia Certain drugs Infections with neutrophilia
Erythrocyte Sedimentation Rate (ESR)	Method Westegren Men: 0–15 mm./hr. Women: 0–20 mm./hr. Children: 0–10 mm./hr. Cutler Men: 0–8 mm./hr. Women: 0–10 mm./hr. Children: 4–13 mm./hr. Landon Adams Men: 0–6 mm./hr. Women: 0–9 mm./hr.	Collagen diseases Infections Inflammatory diseases Carcinoma Acute heavy metallic poisoning Cell or tissue destruc-tion Toxemia Syphilis Nephritis Pneumonia Severe anemia Rheumatoid arthritis	Polycythemia vera Sickle cell anemia Congestive heart failure Hypofibrinogemia Acute phase of rheu-matic fever

Substance		Clinical Implications	
Determined	Normal Values	Increase	Decrease

Erythrocyte Sedimentation Rate (ESR) (cont.)	Landon Adams (cont.) Children: 0–20 age 4-11–12 mm./hr. age 12-15– 7.5 mm./hr. Wintrobe Men: 9mm./hr. Women: 0–15 mm./hr. Children: 0–13 mm./hr. Smith Adults: 0–10 mm./hr.		
Fetal Hemoglobin (Hemoglobin F) (Alkali Resistant Hemoglobin)	Adults: 0–2% Newborns: 60– 90% Before age 2: 0–4%	Thalassemia Hereditary familial fetal hemoglobinemia Spherocytic anemia Sickle cell anemia Hemoglobin H disease Anemia Leakage of fetal blood into the maternal bloodstream	
Heinz-Ehrlich Body Stain (Beutler's Method) Negative	Negative	G6PD deficiency Splenectomized patients Acute hemolytic crisis Drugs related to hemolytic anemias	
Hematocrit (HCT) Microhematocrit	Men: 40–54/100 ml Women: 37–47/ 100 ml. Men: 45–47 Women: 42–44 Infant: 44–62	Erythrocytosis Polycythemia Severe dehydration Shock	Anemia Leukemia Hyperthyroidism Cirrhosis Hemolytic reaction
Hemoglobin (Hgb)	Women: 12–15 gm./100 ml. Men: 14–16.5 gm./100 ml. Newborn: 14–20 Gm./100 ml.	Hemoconcentration of the blood Chronic obstructive pulmonary disease Congestive heart failure	Anemia states Hyperthyroidism Cirrhosis of the liver Severe hemorrhage Hemolytic reactions
Hemoglobin S (Sickle Cell Test)	Normal Adult: 0		Positive Test in sickle cell disease and trait

Substance Determined	Normal Values	Clinical Implications	
		Increase	*Decrease*
Histiocyte Smear	None in circulatory blood	Subacute bacterial endocarditis Typhoid fever Hemolytic anemia Hodgkin's disease Reticulum cell sarcoma Severe diarrhea in children Tuberculosis Leprosy Fat storage disease Lymphoma Some parasitic diseases Histiocytic leukemia	
Leukocyte Alkaline Phosphatase Stain (LAP) Alkaline Phosphatase Stain	30–130	Neutrophilic leukemoid reactions, Polyerythemia vera Thrombocytopenia infection, Myelofibroses	Acute and chronic granulocytic leukemia Paroxysmal nocturnal hemoglobinuria Aplastic anemia Infectious mononucleosis Hereditary hypophosphatasia Many infections
Lymphocytes (Monomorphonuclear lymphocytes)	20–40% total WBC or 1000–4000/cu. mm.	Most viral upper respiratory infections Other viral diseases Bacterial infections Hormonal disorders Lymphocytic leukemia Diarrhea	Hodgkin's disease Lupus erythematosus Administration of ACTH and cortisone After burns or trauma Chronic uremia Cushing's syndrome Early acute radiation syndrome
Mean Cell Hemoglobin (MCH)	27–32 picograms (pg.)	Macrocytic anemia	Iron-deficiency anemia
Mean Corpuscular Hemoglobin Concentration (MCHC)	32–36 gm./100 ml.	Spherocytosis	Iron-deficiency anemia Macrocytic anemias Hypochromic anemia Pyridoxine responsive anemia Thalassemia

Substance Determined	Normal Values	Clinical Implications Increase	Decrease
Mean Corpuscular Volume (MCV)	87–103 cubic microns (μ^3)	Liver diseases Alcoholism Sprue Anti-metabolite therapy Deficiency of folate or Vitamin B_{12}	Iron-deficiency anemia Pernicious anemia Thalassemia Anemia of chronic blood loss Chlorasis
Methemoglobin (Hgb M) Sulfhemoglobin Carboxyhemoglobin	2% of total hemoglobin or 0.5% gm./dl. 0 in normal persons 0–2.3% of total hemoglobin	Hereditary methemoglobinemia Acquired Methemoglobinemia Oxidant drugs and excessive intake of Bromo-Seltzer Smokers and carbon monoxide poisoning	
Monocytes	2–6% of total WBC or 100–60 cu. mm.	Viral infections Bacterial and parasitic infections Collagen diseases	Not usually identified with specific diseases
Osmotic Erythrocyte Fragility	Hemolysis begins at 0.45–0.39% end at 0.33–0.30%	Hereditary spherocytosis Hemolytic jaundice Auto immune anemia Chemical poisons Burns	Obstructive jaundice Thalassemia Sickle cell anemia Iron-deficiency anemia Polycythemia vera Liver disease Following splenectomy 46-C disease
Partial Thromboplastin Time (PTT) Activated Partial Thromboplastin Time (APTT)	PTT 30–45 sec. APTT 16–25 sec.	PTT: Coagulation defects of Stage II von Willebrand's disease APPT: Hemophilia Vitamin K deficiency Liver disease Presence of circulating anticoagulants DIC disease	APTT: Extensive cancer Acute hemorrhage
Periodic Acid Schiff Stain (PAS)	Granulocytes stain PAS positive. Agranulocytes stain PAS negative.	Positive in: Acute lymphocytic leukemia Erythroleukemia Severe iron-deficiency anemia Thalassemia Amyloidosis Malignant lymphoma	

Substance Determined	Normal Values	Clinical Implications	
		Increase	*Decrease*
Platelet Count	15,000–350,000/ cu. mm.	Cancer Chronic myelogenous and granulocytic leukemia Polycythemia vera Splenectomy Trauma Asphyxiation Rheumatoid arthritis Iron-deficiency and posthemorrhagic anemia Acute infections Heart disease Cirrhosis Chronic pancreatitis Tuberculosis	Idiopathic thrombocytopenic purpura Pernicious, aplastic, and hemolytic anemias After massive blood transfusion Pneumonia Allergic conditions Exposure to DDT and other chemicals During cancer chemotherapy Infection Lesions involving the bone marrow Toxic effects of many drugs
Prothrombin Consumption Test (PCT) Serum Prothrombin Time	15 seconds or more measured 1 hour after coagulation. 80% consumed in one hour		Circulating anticoagulants Hemophilias Hypoprothrombinemia Thrombocytopenia Thrombocytopathies DIC disease
Prothrombin Time (PRO TIME PT)	11–16 seconds or 100%	Prothrombin deficiency Vitamin K deficiency Hemorrhagic disease of the newborn Liver disease Anticoagulant therapy Biliary obstruction Salicylate intoxication Hypervitaminosis A DIC disease	
Red Blood Cell Count (RBC) (Erythrocyte Count)	Men: 4.2–5.4 million/cu. mm. Women: 3.6–5.0 million/cu. mm.	Polycythemia vera Secondary polycythemia Severe diarrhea Dehydration Acute poisoning Pulmonary fibrosis During and immediately following hemorrhage	Diseases of bone marrow function Lupus erythematosus Addison's disease Rheumatic fever Subacute endocarditis Anemias
Reticulocyte Count	Adults: 0.5–1.5% of total erythrocytes	Hemolytic anemias Sickle cell disease Metastatic carcinoma	Iron-deficiency anemia Untreated pernicious anemia

Substance Determined	Normal Values	Clinical Implications	
		Increase	Decrease
Reticulocyte Count (cont.)	Children: 0.5–4.0% of total erythrocytes Infants: 2–5% of total erythrocytes Reticulocyte index = one	Leukemia Following hemorrhage Hereditary spherocytosis After splenectomy	Chronic infection Radiation therapy
Rosette Test For T and B Lymphocytes	B-cells 10–30% of total lymphocytes T-cells 70–90% of total lymphocytes	T-cells: Grave's disease	T-cells: DeGeorge syndrome Hodgkin's disease Chronic lymphocytic leukemia Long-term immunosuppressive drug therapy
		B-cells: Active erythematosus	B-cells: X-linked agammaglobulinemia Myeloma Chronic lymphocytic leukemia
Screening Acid Serum Test for PNF Presumptive Acid Serum Test & Ham Test-Acidified Serum Test for PNF	Negative	Positive in PNF, Paroxysmal nocturnal hemoglobinuria	
Segmented Neutrophils PMN "Segs" "Polys"	50–60% of WBC 3000–7000 per cu. mm.	Bacterial and parasitic infections Metabolic disturbances Blood disorders Hemolysis Drugs Tissue breakdown Allergies	Acute viral infections Blood diseases Toxic agents Hormonal diseases Massive infections in debilitated patients
Sudan Black B Stain (SBB) for phospholipids	Lymphocytes will not stain with this method. Granulocytes cells will stain with this method.	SBB positive in acute granulocytic leukemia	SBB negative in acute lymphocytic leukemia

Substance Determined	Normal Values	Clinical Implications	
		Increase	*Decrease*
Thrombin Time: Thrombin clotting time	15 seconds	Hypofibrinogenemia Anticoagulant therapy Dysproteinemias such as multiple myeloma	
Tourniquet Test: Rumpel-Leede-Positive Pressure Test; Negative Pressure Test; Capillary Fragility Test	Occasional petechiae or none	Most commonly in thrombocytopenia Less commonly in thrombasthenia, vascular purpura, scurvy	
White Blood Cell Count (WBC) (Leukocyte count)	5000–10,000 cu. mm.	Acute infection Hemorrhage Trauma Malignant disease Toxins Drugs Serum sickness Circulatory disease Tissue necrosis Leukemia	Viral infections Hypersplenism Bone marrow depression due to drugs Cancer chemotherapy Heavy metals Radiation Agranulocytosis Pernicious and aplastic anemia Multiple myeloma Alcoholism Diabetes

D ☐ ☐ URINE STUDIES

Substance Determined	Normal Values	Clinical Implications	
		Increase	*Decrease*
Addis Count	Adults: WBC and epithelial cells up to 1,000,000/12 hrs. RBC up to 500,000/12 hrs. Casts up to 0–5,000/12 hrs. Children: WBC up to 2,000,000/12 hrs. RBC up to 600,000/12 hrs. Casts up to 10,000/12 hrs.	Bacterial infection Infection of urinary tract or in an area having access to the tract Kidney disease	
Amino Acid	50–200 mg./24 hrs.	Aminoacidurea Fanconi syndrome Cystinosis Wilson's disease Cystinuria Muscular dystrophies Leukemia Maple syrup urine disease Hartnup disease Phenylketenuria Glycinuria Liver disease Megaloblastic anemias Lead poisoning Oxalosis Tyrosinosis Pyridoxine deficiency Folic acid deficiency	
Amylase Excretion	35–260 Somogyi u./hr.	Acute pancreatitis Choledocholethiasis	

Substance Determined	Normal Values	Clinical Implications	
		Increase	*Decrease*
Bilirubin	Negative—0.02 mg./dl.	Liver disease due to infections or toxic agents Obstructive biliary disease	
Blood or Hemoglobin (HEME)	Negative	Renal disease Extensive burns and crushing injuries Transfusion reactions Febrile intoxication Chemical agents and alkaloids Malaria Irrigation of operated prostatic bed with water Hemolytic anemias Paroxysmal hemoglobinuria Drugs that are toxic to the kidneys Drugs that cause actual bleeding Drugs that cause hemolysis of RBC's	
Calcium	100–250 mg./24 hr. average diet 150 mg./24 hr. low calcium diet	Hyperparathyroidism Sarcoidosis Primary cancers of breast and lung Metastatic malignancies Myeloma with bone metastasis Wilson's disease Renal tubular acidosis Glucocorticoid excess	Hypoparathyroidism Vitamin D deficiency Malabsorption syndrome
Chlorides Cl (24 hours)	110–250 mEq./24 hrs. 10–20 gm. NaCl/24 hrs. 9 gm./l. (0.9 gm./100 ml.	Addison's disease Dehydration Starvation Salicylate toxicity Mercurial and chlorothiazide diuretics	Malabsorption syndrome Pyloric obstruction Prolonged gastric suction Diarrhea Diaphoresis Congestive heart failure Emphysema
Color	Yellow, straw, amber	Many disease states	Many disease states

Substance Determined	Normal Values	Clinical Implications	
		Increase	Decrease
Concentration	Fishberg test— 1:024 or higher Vohhard—1.025 or higher Mosenthal— 1.020		Renal disease Potassium deficiency Hypercalcemia due to sarcoidosis Bone disease Hyperparathyroidism
Creatinine Clearance	115 to 120 ml./ min. or 0.7 to 1.5 mg./ml.		Impaired kidney function
Crystals	Acid urine-urates, uric acid, calcium oxalate Alkaline urine Amorphous and calcium phosphates Ammonium biurate	Cystine Leucine or tyrosine, Cholestin, drug crystals are abnormal	
D-Xylose Absorption	Urine—more than 1.2 gm. Blood—25–40 mg./100 ml. in 2 hrs.		Enterogenous steatorrhea Malabsorption
Epithelial Cells and Epithelial Casts	Occasional	Nephrosis Eclampsia Amyloidosis Poisoning from heavy metals and other toxins	
Follicle Stimulating Hormone (FSH) and Luteinizing Hormone (LH)		Turner's syndrome (ovarian dysgenesis) Hypogonadism	Ovarian tumors
Granular Casts	Occasional	Acute tubular necrosis Advanced glomerulonephritis Pyelonephritis Malignant nephrosclerosis Chronic lead poisoning	
Hyaline Casts	Occasional	Possible damage to the glomerular capillary membrane	

Substance Determined	Normal Values	Clinical Implications	
		Increase	*Decrease*
Hyaline Casts (cont.)		Fever Nephrotic syndrome	
5-Hydroxy-indoleace-tic Acid (5-HIAA)	Negative 2–10 mg./24 hr. 60–100 mEq./24 hr.	Large carcinoid tumor Hemorrhage Thrombosis Nontropical sprue Severe pain of sciatica or skeletal and smooth muscle spasm	
Ketone Bodies (Acetone)	Negative	Ketoacidosis and possible diabetic coma Fever Anorexia Gastrointestinal disturbances Fasting Starvation Prolonged vomiting Following anesthesia	
17-Ketoste-roids (17 KS)	*17 Ketosteroids (17 KS)* Men: 8–18 mg./24 hrs. Women: 5–15 mg./24 hrs. *17-Hydroxycorti-costeroids (17 OHCS)* 10 mg./24 hrs. *17 Ketogenic steroids (17 KGS)* Men: 5.5–23 mg./24 hrs. Women: 3–15 mg./24 hrs.	Precocious puberty Surgery Burns Infection KGS 17 OHCS Hyperplasia of adrenal cortex, tumor, cancer, variation of the adrenogenital syndrome Steroid level in Cushing's syndrome, eclampsia, acute pancreatitis, and ACTH therapy	
Morphine (Assay)	Negative	Positive for heroin or morphine Codeine Poppy seeds	
Odor	Aromatic	Acetone in diabetic ketosis Heavily infected urine Unpleasant odor Maple sugar urine disease	

Substance Determined	Normal Values	Clinical Implications	
		Increase	Decrease
Osmolality	Dilute urine— less than 200 mM. Concentrated urine—more than 850 mM.	Post surgery Hepatic cirrhosis Congestive heart failure Addison's disease IV sodium High protein diets Inappropriate ADH secretion	Aldosteronism Diabetes insipidus Hypokalemia Hypercalcemia Compulsive water drinking IV 5% dextrose and water
pH	4.6–8	Urinary tract infections Pyloric obstruction Salicylate intoxications Renal tubular acidosis Chronic renal failure Severe alkalosis	Acidosis Uncontrolled diabetes Pulmonary emphysema Diarrhea Starvation Dehydration Respiratory diseases
Phenosulfonphthalein (PSP) Excretion	15 min.—30–35% 30 min.—20–25%—more than 15 min. spec. 60 min.—10–15%—more than 30 min. spec.		Renal tubular disease or diminished renal plasma
Phenylketonuria (PKU)	Urine—Negative	Positive test for PKU Urine positive in PKU	
Porphyrins and Porphobilinogens	Porphobilinogens 2 mg./24 hrs. Porphyrins 50–300 mg./24 hrs. DLA or ALA 1.0–710 mg./24 hrs.	Porphyrias Porphyrins ALA and DLA excretion in acute intermittent porphyria Lead poisoning Cirrhosis Infectious hepatitis Hodgkin's disease Some cancers Central nervous system disorders Heavy metal poisoning Carbon tetrachloride or benzine toxicity	

| Substance | | Clinical Implications | |
Determined	Normal Values	Increase	Decrease
Potassium	40–80 mEq./24 hrs.	Chronic renal failure Diabetic and renal tubular acidosis Dehydration Starvation Primary aldosteronism Cushing's disease Salicylate toxicity Mercurial chlorothiazide	Malabsorption syndrome Diarrhea Acute renal failure Adrenal cortical insufficiency Excessive mineralcorticoid activity Potassium deficiency
Pregnancy Tests	Negative, blood and urine	Positive Pregnancy Choriocarcinoma Hydatidiform mole Testicular tumors Chorioepithelioma Chorioadenoma destruens Conditions with a high ESR such as acute salpingitis	
Pregnanediol	Women: Proliferative phase—0.5–1.5 mg./24 hrs. Luteal phase—2–7 mg./24 hrs. Postmenopausal —0.2–1.0 mg./24 hrs. Men: 1.5 mg./24 hrs.	Luteal cysts of ovary Arrhenoblastoma of the ovary Hyperadrenocorticism	Amenorrhea Sometimes in threatened abortion Fetal death Toxemia
Pregnanetriol	4 mg./24 hrs.	Congenital adrenocortical hyperplasia Stein-Leventhal syndrome	
Protein (Albumin)	Negative or 2–8 mg./dl. 10–100 mg./24 hrs.	Nephritis Nephrosis Polycystic kidney Tuberculosis and cancer of the kidney Ascites Fever Trauma Severe anemias and leukemia Abdominal tumors Convulsive disorders	

| Substance | | Clinical Implications | |
Determined	Normal Values	Increase	Decrease
Protein (Albumin) (cont.)		Hyperthyroidism Intestinal obstruction Cardiac disease Poisoning	
Red Cells and Red Cell Casts	1 or 2	Pyelonephritis Lupus Renal stones Cystitis Prostatitis Tuberculosis and malignancies of the genitourinary tract Hemophilia Acute glomerulo-nephritis Renal infarction Collagen disease Kidney involvement in subacute bacterial endocarditis	
Sodium (Na), Quantitative	130–200 mEq./ 24 hrs.	Dehydration Starvation Salicylate toxicity Adrenal cortical insufficiency Mercurial and chloro-thiazide diuretics Chronic renal failure Diabetic acidosis	Malabsorption syndrome Congestive heart Pyloric obstruction Diarrhea Diaphoresis Acute renal failure Pulmonary emphysema Aldosteronism Cushing's disease
Specific Gravity	1.003–1.035 1.025–1.030 (concentrated urine) 1.001–1.010 (dilute urine)	Diabetes mellitus or nephrosis Excessive water loss	Diabetes insipidus Absence of anti-diuretic hormone (ADH) Glomerulonephritis Pyelonephritis Severe renal damage
Sugar (Glucose)	Negative 100 mg./24 hr.	Diabetes mellitus Brain injury Myocardial infarction	
Tubular Reabsorption Phosphate (TRP)	>78% on normal diet >85% on a low phosphate diet	Hyperparathyroidism	Hypoparathyroidism
Turbidity	Clear	Urinary tract infections	

Substance Determined	Normal Values	Clinical Implications	
		Increase	*Decrease*
Uric Acid, Quantitative	0.4–1.0 gm./24 hrs. on normal diet 0.2–0.5 gm./24 hrs. on a purine free diet 2.0 gm./24 hrs. on a high-purine diet	Gout Chronic myelogenous leukemia Polycythemia vera Liver disease Febrile illnesses Toxemias of pregnancy Fanconi Syndrome Cytoxic drugs	Kidney disease
Urobilinogen (Quantitative Urobilin and Estimate)	Random: 0.3–3.5 mg./100 ml. 2 hour: 0.3–1.0 Ehrlich units/ 2 hrs. 24 hour: 1–4 mg./ 24 hrs.	Hemolytic anemias Pernicious anemias Malaria Infectious and toxic hepatitis Pulmonary infarct Biliary disease Cholangitis Hemolytic jaundice and anemia Chemical injury to liver Cirrhosis Congestive heart failure Infectious mononucleosis	Cholelithiasis Severe inflammatory disease Cancer of the head of pancreas Antibiotic therapy Severe diarrhea Renal insufficiency
Vanillylmendelic Acid (VMA)	VMA up to 9 mg./ 24 hrs. Epinephrine 100–230 mg./ 24 hrs. Norepinephrine 100–230 mg./ 24 hrs. Metanephrine 24–96 mg./24 hrs. Normetanephrine 12–288 mg./ 24 hrs.	*VMA levels:* In pheochromocytoma Neuroblastomas Ganglioneuromas Ganglioblastomas *Catecholamines* In pheochromocytoma Neuroblastomas Ganglioneuromas Ganglioblastomas Progressive muscular dystrophy Myasthenia gravis	
Waxy Casts	Negative	Chronic renal disease Tubular inflammation and degeneration	
White Cells and white cell casts	3 or 4 WBC casts	White cells usually indicate bacterial infection in the urinary tract White cell casts indicate renal parenchymal infection	

E □□ FECAL STUDIES

Substance Determined	Normal Values	Clinical Implications Increase	Decrease
Blood	Negative	Chronic nonspecific ulcerative or colitis, carcinoma of the colon. Diaphragmatic hernia Diverticulitis, gastric carcinoma, and gastritis	
Color	Brown	Color changes in: Severe diarrhea Bleeding into the upper gastrointestinal tract Blockage of the common bile duct and pancreatic insufficiency Bleeding from the lower gastrointestinal tract	
Consistency, shape	Plastic, soft, formed Shape	Diarrhea mixed with mucus and blood in: Typhus Typhoid Cholera Amebiasis Large bowel cancer Diarrhea mixed with mucus and pus in: Ulcerative colitis Regional enteritis Shigellosis Salmonellosis Hard stools due to increased absorption of fluid because of delayed transit time	"Pasty" consistency with a high fat content A narrow, ribbonlike stool suggests spastic bowel or rectal narrowing or stricture, decreased elasticity; a partial obstruction

Substance Determined	Normal Values	Clinical Implications	
		Increase	*Decrease*
Fat	18% colorless fatty acid crystals and soaps	Enteritis and pancreatic diseases Surgical removal of a section of the intestine Malabsorption syndromes	
Mucus		Spastic constipation Mucous colitis Emotionally disturbed patients Excessive straining at stool Ulcerative colitis Bacillary dysentery Ulcerating cancer of colon Acute diverticulitis Intestinal tuberculosis	
Odor and pH	Characteristic odor varies with the pH of stool Normal pH— neutral or weakly alkaline	Carbohydrate fermentation changes the pH to acid	Protein breakdown changes the pH to alkaline
Parasites	Negative	Parasitic diseases	
Pus	Negative	Chronic ulcerative colitis Chronic bacillary dysentery Localized abscesses Fistulas to sigmoid rectum or anus	
Undigested food, meat fibers, starch trypson	Negative	Intestinal motility	

F □□ CEREBROSPINAL FLUID STUDIES

Substance Determined	Normal Values	Clinical Implications Increase	Decrease
A/G ratio (albumin to globulin)	8:1		
Bilirubin	Negative		
Calcium	2.1–2.7 mEq./l.	Tuberculous meningitis	
Chloride	118–132 mEq./l.		Tuberculous meningitis Bacterial meningitis
Cholesterol	0.2–0.6 mg./dl.		
Color	Crystal clear, colorless	Abnormal in: Subarachnoid Cerebral hemorrhage Bilirubinemia Subarachnoid block Acute meningitis Cloudiness Cryptococcal infection	
Creatinine	0.5–1.2 mg./dl.		
Glucose	45–85 mg./dl. (20 mg./dl. less than blood level)	Mump encephalitis Cerebral trauma Brain tumors accompanied by increased intracranial pressure Hypothalamic lesions	Pyrogenic, tuberculous and fungal meningitis Toxoplasmosis Sarcoidosis Subarachnoid hemorrhage Primary brain tumors Lymphomas Leukemia Melanoma Viral meningoencephalitis

Substance Determined	Normal Values	Clinical Implications	
		Increase	Decrease
Pressure	75–150 mm. H_2O	Intracranial tumors Purulent or tuberculous meningitis Low grade inflammatory processes Encephalitis Neurosyphilis	Hydrocephalus when there is a small pressure drop that is indicative of a large CSF pool.
Protein	15–45 mg./dl. (lumbar) 15–25 mg./dl. (cisternal) 5–15 mg./dl. (ventricular)	Purulent meningitis Guillain-Barre syndrome Froin's syndrome Tuberculous meningitis Aseptic meningitis Syphilis Brain tumors and abscesses Subarachnoid hemorrhage Congenital toxoplasmosis	
Total Cell Count and Differential Cell Count of CSF	0–8 cu. mm.	Purulent infection Viral infections Syphilis of CNS Tuberculous meningitis Multiple sclerosis Tumor or abscess Subarachnoid hemorrhage	Abnormal cells in: Brain tumors Inflammatory processes Multiple sclerosis Leukoencephalitis Delayed hypersensitivity responses Subacute viral encephalitis Meningitis (tuberculous or fugae) Cranial infarcts Surgical procedures or trauma to the Central Nervous System
Urea	7–15 mg./dl.	Uremia	
Urea nitrogen	6–16 mg./dl.		
Uric acid	0.5–4.5 mg./dl.		

G □ PULMONARY FUNCTION STUDIES

Substance Determined	Normal Values	Clinical Implications	
		Increase	Decrease
Body Plethysmography	Men: 0.081 (H)– 2.94 Women: 0.135 (H)–0.008 (W)–4.74 TGV = approx. 2400 ml. (Thoracic Gas Volume) C = 0.2 L/cm. H_2O RAW = 0.6 to 2.4 cm./H_2O/l/sec.	C—Obstructive diseases TGV—Obstructive pulmonary disease RAW—asthma, emphysema, bronchitis and other forms of obstruction	C—Fibrotic diseases, restrictive diseases, pneumonia, congestion, atelectasis
Carbon Dioxide CO_2 Response	3-fold increase		Unresponsiveness suggests a disturbance in the normal physiological pathway of ventilatory changes and hypercapnia.
Carbon Monoxide Diffusing Capacity of the Lung (DLCO)	Approximately 25 ml./min./ torr		Multiple pulmonary emboli Emphysema Anemia Lung restriction Pulmonary fibroses Sarcoidosis Scleroderma Systemic lupus erythematosus Asbestosis
Closing Volume (CV)	About 10% of vital capacity	In diseases in which the airway is decreased, in pulmonary edema, in chronic smokers, and in old patients	

Substance Determined	Normal Values	Clinical Implications	
		Increase	Decrease
Expiratory Reserve Volume (ERV)	Approximately 1200–1500 ml.		Chest wall restriction due to nonpulmonary causes Elevated diaphragms as seen in massive obesity, ascites, or pregnancy Massive enlargement of the heart, pleural effusion, kyphoscoliosis, and thoracoplasty
Flow Volume Loops	Normal loops are characteristic of absence of lung disease.		Abnormal flow volume loops are indicative of: Obstructive lung disease; Small airway obstructive disease as in emphysema and asthma. Large airway obstructive disease such as tumors of trachea and bronchioles Restrictive diseases when the disease is far advanced
Forced Vital Capacity (FVC) or Forced Expiratory Volume (FEV)	Approximately 4800 ml.	Restrictive lung disease can be normal or elevated	Obstructive lung disease such as emphysema, pulmonary fibrosis and asthma
Functional Residual Capacity (FRC)	Approximately 2400–3000 ml.	Obstructive airway disease represents hyperinflation from emphysematous changes, asthmatic or fibrotic obstruction of the bronchioles, compensation for surgical removal of lung tissue, or a thoracic deformity.	Restrictive disease

Substance Determined	Normal Values	Clinical Implications	
		Increase	*Decrease*
Inspiratory Capacity (IC)	Approximately 2500–3600 ml.	Changes usually parallel increases or decreases in the vital capacity	
Maximum Voluntary Ventilation (MVV)	Approximately 170 l./min.		Obstructive defects, chronic pulmonary disease (COPD), abnormal neuromuscular control, and poor patient effort.
Methacholine Challenge	Negative response	Asthma	
Peak Expiratory Flow Rate (PEFR)	An average 300 l./min.		Obstructive disease such as emphysema. Usually normal in restrictive lung disease, except in severe restriction, when it is reduced.
Peak Inspiratory Flow Rate (PIFR)	An average of at least 300 l./min.		Neuromuscular disorders, weakness, poor effort and extrathoracic airway obstruction. Substernal thyroid, tracheal stenosis and laryngeal paralysis
Residual Volume (RV)	1200–1500 ml.	Young asthmatics Emphysema Chronic air trapping Chronic bronchial obstruction	Sometimes in diseases that occlude many alveoli
Total Lung Capacity (TLC)	Approximately 5500 ml.	Obstructive defect Normal or increased in broncheolar obstruction with hyperinflation and in emphysema	Edema Atelectasis Neoplasms Pulmonary congestion Pneumothorax or thoracic restriction
Vital Capacity (VC)	4000–4800 ml.		Depression of the respiratory center in the brain, neuro-

Substance Determined	Normal Values	Clinical Implications	
		Increase	*Decrease*
			muscular diseases, pleural effusion, ascites, pneumothorax, pregnancy, limitations of thoracic movement due to pain
Volume of Isoflow (V_{Iso})	Values cover a wide range based on age and sex.	Mild airway obstruction Small airways disease	

H □□ BLOOD GAS STUDIES

Substance Determined	Normal Values	Clinical Implications Increase	Decrease
Alveolar to Oxygen Gradient (A-a DO$_2$ RATIO)	9 torr or less in a patient breathing room air.	Mucus plugs Bronchospasm Airway collapse in: Asthma Bronchitis Emphysema Hypoxemia caused by: Pneumothorax Atelectasis Emboli Edema	
Base Excess/ Deficit	(Plus or minus 3 mEq./l.)	Nonvolatile acid deficit	Nonrespiratory or metabolic disturbance nonvolatile acid accumulation due to a dietary intake, lactic acid, ketoacidosis
Blood pH	Arterial blood— 7.35–7.45 Venous blood— 7.34–7.41	Alkalemia Loss of gastric juice Vomiting Potassium or chloride depletion Excessive bicarbonate or lactate administration Hyperventilation Hysteria Lack of oxygen Toxic stimulation of the respiratory centers: High fever Cerebral hemorrhage Excessive artificial respiration Salicylates	Acidemia Renal failure Diabetic ketoacidosis Lactic acidosis Anaerobic metabolism Hypoxia Diarrhea Depression of respiratory Centers: Drug overdose Barbiturate toxicity Anesthetics Interference with mechanized function of thoracic cage Deformity of thoracic cage Kyphoscoliosis

Substance Determined	Normal Values	Clinical Implications Increase	Clinical Implications Decrease
Blood pH (cont.)			Airway obstruction: Extra thoracic tumors Asthma Bronchitis Emphysema Circulatory disorders: Congestive heart failure Shock
Carbon Dioxide (CO_2) Total Carbon Dioxide (CO_2)	24–30 mEq/l.	Severe vomiting Emphysema Aldosteronism Mercurial diuretics	Severe diarrhea Starvation Acute renal failure Salicylate toxicity Diabetic acidosis Chlorothiazide Diuretics
Oxygen (O_2) Content	Arterial blood— 15–22 Vol % Venous blood— 11–16 Vol %		Chronic obstructive lung disease Respiratory complications postoperatively Flail chest Kyphoscoliosis Neuromuscular impairment Obesity hypoventilation
Oxygen Saturation (SO_2)	(SaO_2) 95% or higher (S_vO_2) = 75%		
Partial Pressure of Carbon Dioxide (PCO_2)	$PaCO_2$ 35–45 torr P_vCO_2 41–51 torr	Hypoventilation Obstructive lung disease Chronic bronchitis Emphysema Reduced function of respiratory center Over reaction Head trauma Anesthesia Pickwickian syndrome	Hyperventilation Hypoxia Nervousness Anxiety Pulmonary emboli Pregnancy
Partial Pressure of Oxygen (PO_2)	PaO_2 80 torr or greater PvO_2 30–40 torr	Polycythemia Hyperventilation Increased frequency of breathing	Anemias Cardiac decompensation Insufficient atmospheric oxygen

Substance Determined	Normal Values	Clinical Implications	
		Increase	Decrease
Partial Pressure of Oxygen (PO_2) (cont.)			Intracardiac shunts Chronic obstructive or Restrictive pulmonary disease Hypoventilation due to neuromuscular disease Decreased arterial PO_2 With normal or decreased Arterial blood PCO_2 Tension in: Diffuse interstitial Pulmonary infiltration Pulmonary edema Pulmonary embolism Postoperative extracorporeal circulation

□ APPENDIX THREE □
Abbreviations of Basic Quantities, Equivalents, and Units of Measurements in Normal Values

Symbol	Definition
mol.	mole
m.	meter
kg.	kilogram
m.^{2}	square meter
mm.^{2}	square millimeter
m.^{3}	cubic meter
l.	liter
cm.^{3}	cubic centimeter
c	centi-
cu	cubic
cu. mm.	cubic millimeter
d	deci-
dl.	deciliter
m	milli-
μ	micron
μ^3	cubic micron
n	nano
p	pico
sec.	second
mg./l.	milligram per liter
g./l.	gram per liter
k	kilo
kg./l.	kilogram per liter
mol./l.	mole per liter
mOsm./l.	milliosmole per liter
l./sec.	liter per second
SI units	International system of units
<	less than
>	greater than
g. or gm.	gram
I.U.	International Unit
mEq.	milliequivalent
mg.	milligram
ml.	milliliter
mM.	millimole
torr	millimeters of mercury
mm. H_2O	millimeters of water

Symbol	*Definition*
ml.U.	milliInternational Unit
mμ	millimicron
ng.	nanogram
pg.	picogram
μEq.	microequivalent
μg.	microgram
μl.U.	microInternational Unit
μl.	microliter
μU.	microunit

INDEX

Numerals in *italics* indicate a figure; *t* following a page number indicates a table.